HANDBOOK OF

Veterinary
Pain Management

NOTICE

Veterinary medicine is an ever-changing field. Standard safety precautions must be followed, but as new research and clinical experience broaden our knowledge, changes in treatment and drug therapy may become necessary or appropriate. Readers are advised to check the most current product information provided by the manufacturer of each drug to be administered to verify the recommended dose, the method and duration of administration, and contraindications. It is the responsibility of the licensed veterinarian, relying on experience and knowledge of the patient, to determine dosages and the best treatment for each individual patient. Neither the publisher nor the editor assumes any liability for any injury and/or damage to persons or property arising from this publication.

HANDBOOK OF

Veterinary
Pain Management

JAMES S. GAYNOR
DVM, MS, DIPL ACVA

Associate Professor and Section Chief, Anesthesiology
Department of Clinical Sciences
College of Veterinary Medicine and Biomedical Sciences
Colorado State University, Fort Collins, Colorado

WILLIAM W. MUIR III
DVM, PHD, DIPL ACVA, ACVECC

Head Section of Anesthesia and Pain Management
Professor of Veterinary Clinical Sciences
College of Veterinary Medicine Veterinary Teaching Hospital
The Ohio State University, Columbus, Ohio

with 70 illustrations

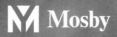

An Affiliate of Elsevier

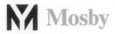

An Affiliate of Elsevier
11830 Westline Industrial Drive
St. Louis, Missouri 63146
HANDBOOK OF VETERINARY PAIN MANAGEMENT

Library of Congress Cataloging-in-Publication Data

Gaynor, James S.
    Handbook of veterinary pain management / James S. Gaynor,
William W. Muir.
        p.   cm.
    Includes bibliographical references and index.
    ISBN-13: 978-0-323-01328-4   ISBN-10: 0-323-01328-7
    1. Pain in animals—Treatment—Handbooks, manuals, etc.
I. Muir, William, 1946-   II. Title

    SF910.P34 G38 2002
    636.089'60472—dc21

                                                    2002067781

ISBN-13: 978-0-323-01328-4
ISBN-10: 0-323-01328-7

Acquisitions Editor: Elizabeth M. Fathman
Developmental Editor: Teri Merchant
Publishing Services Manager: Pat Joiner
Design Coordinator: Mark A. Oberkrom
Designer: Renée Duenow
Cover Design: Studio Montage

TG/RRD
Printed in the United States of America

Last digit is the print number: 9   8   7   6   5   4

Contributors

Steven Budsberg, DVM, Dipl ACVS
Small Animal Medicine
College of Veterinary Medicine
University of Georgia, Athens, Georgia

James S. Gaynor, DVM, MS, Dipl ACVA
Associate Professor and Section Chief, Anesthesiology
Department of Clinical Sciences
College of Veterinary Medicine and Biomedical Sciences
Colorado State University, Fort Collins, Colorado

Peter W. Hellyer, DVM, MS, Dipl ACVA
Associate Professor of Anesthesiology
Department of Clinical Sciences
College of Veterinary Medicine and Biomedical Sciences
Colorado State University, Fort Collins, Colorado

Leigh Lamont, DVM
Resident in Anesthesiology
Department of Veterinary Clinical Medicine
University of Illinois, Urbana, Illinois

Khursheed R. Mama, DVM, Dipl ACVA
Assistant Professor
Department of Clinical Sciences
College of Veterinary Medicine and Biomedical Sciences
Colorado State University, Fort Collins, Colorado

William W. Muir III, DVM, PhD, Dipl ACVA, ACVECC
Head Section of Anesthesia and Pain Management
Professor of Veterinary Clinical Sciences
College of Veterinary Medicine Veterinary Teaching Hospital
The Ohio State University, Columbus, Ohio

Bernard E. Rollin, PhD
Professor of Veterinary Clinical Sciences
University Distinguished Professor of Philosophy
Professor of Biomedical Sciences
Professor of Animal Sciences
Colorado State University, Fort Collins, Colorado

Richard A. Sams, PhD
Professor of Veterinary Clinical Sciences
College of Veterinary Medicine
The Ohio State University, Columbus, Ohio

Roman T. Skarda, DMV, PhD, Dipl ACVA, ECVA, CVA
Associate Professor, Anesthesiology
Department of Veterinary Clinical Sciences
College of Veterinary Medicine
The Ohio State University, Columbus, Ohio

Mary O. Smith, BVM & S, PhD, Dipl ACVIM (Neurology)
Affiliated Veterinary Specialists, Maitland, Florida

William Tranquilli, DVM, MS, Dipl ACVA
Professor of Veterinary Clinical Medicine
Director of the Pain Management Program
Veterinary Teaching Hospital
College of Veterinary Medicine
University of Illinois, Urbana, Illinois

Ann E. Wagner, DVM, MS, Dipl ACVA, ACVP
Associate Professor of Anesthesiology
Department of Clinical Sciences
College of Veterinary Medicine and Biomedical Sciences
Colorado State University, Fort Collins, Colorado

*This textbook is dedicated to
all those animals that needlessly suffer from pain
and the countless individuals who have devoted
their efforts and careers to its alleviation.*

A Companion's Pain

*Labored into the world
Vibrant life ripped from flesh
Flung towards days of wagging ease.
Comfort razed in an instant
A shrouded attack within
Writhe, recoil
Stifled whimper
Not too close! Trust growls distant
Flee, retreat, curl up close
Wrapped tight while hope tremors.
Pleading glance; lights wane and ebb
The tearless eye reveals nature's sting
On stoic souls;
Bearing it wisely
Grasping on instinct
Eased by the graciousness of man
On Mercy*

Kristine J. McComis

Preface

The science of pain and its therapy has garnered everyone's attention and interest during the past several decades due in no small part to the literal exponential growth of scientific information and the ever increasing number of therapeutic modalities. Although all veterinarians take an oath to use their scientific knowledge and skills for "the relief of animal suffering," the treatment and prevention of pain has only recently become a singular objective. Excellent textbooks describing the neuroanatomy, neurophysiology, pathophysiology, and treatment of pain have been published only since the early 1980s. These textbooks, particularly *The Textbook of Pain,* edited by Patrick D. Wall and Ronald Melzack, serve as the foundation of current understanding and practice. The goal of this *Handbook* is not to replace these textbooks but to supplement them by providing a rapid, clinically applicable resource for use by all who witness and treat animal pain. The *Handbook* serves as a quick reference for pertinent physiologic and pharmacologic information, including drugs and alternative therapeutic modalities used to treat pain. Uniquely, this *Handbook* also provides an extensive array of acute and chronic case examples that should help practicing veterinarians, professional students, interns, residents, and veterinary technical support staff understand, evaluate, and treat pain. The contributors have attempted to provide current information that has been generated from animals, particularly dogs, cats, and horses. Significantly and somewhat unfortunately, some information has been extrapolated from the human experience. Ideally, future basic and clinical investigations conducted in animals will remedy this shortcoming, since most if not all therapies are tested in animals before they are applied to humans.

We would like to thank all of the contributors for the time and effort they have dedicated to making this *Handbook* a reality. We also greatly appreciate the talented efforts of Tim Vojt and Dr. Michelle Murray, whose artwork has made written concepts visually under- standable. Finally, we would like to thank our families, who have given us the time and emotional support to bring this *Handbook* to completion.

James S. Gaynor
William W. Muir III

Veterinarian's Oath

Being admitted to the profession of veterinary medicine,

I solemnly swear to use my scientific knowledge and skills for the benefit of society through the protection of animal health, the relief of animal suffering, the conservation of livestock resources, the promotion of public health, and the advancement of medical knowledge.

I will practice my profession conscientiously, with dignity, and in keeping with the principles of veterinary medical ethics.

I accept as a lifelong obligation the continual improvement of my professional knowledge and competence.

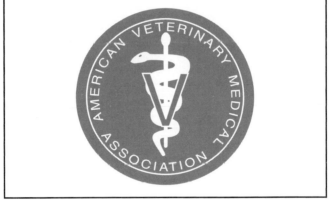

Adopted by the American Veterinary Medical Association (AVMA) House of Delegates, July, 1969.

Contents

PART THREE
Therapy for the Alleviation of Pain

PART FOUR
Acute and Chronic Pain Management

PART ONE

Principles of
Pain Management

1

The Ethics of Pain Management

BERNARD E. ROLLIN

HISTORY OF ETHICS OF ANIMAL TREATMENT

For most of human history, civilized society has expressed a social ethic consensus regarding animal treatment, albeit a minimalistic one. This ethic, found even in the Bible, forbids cruelty toward animals, where *cruelty* is defined as deliberate, purposeless, willful, sadistic, deviant, unnecessary infliction of pain and suffering, such as muzzling an ox when it is being used to thresh grain. Historically the concept of cruelty has been used in part to protect the animals but in equal measure to identify sadists and psychopaths who, both common sense and recent science tell us, begin by torturing animals and graduate to harming people. In this spirit, "accepted," "necessary," and "nondeviant" infliction of pain and suffering have been invisible to the anticruelty laws and ethic they instantiate. Thus practices such as steel-jawed trapping, hot iron branding, castration without anesthesia, training of animals with severe negative reinforcement, poisoning, fracturing, or invasive use of animals in research—in short, as one law put it, "anything done to minister to the necessities of man," do not fall under the purview of cruelty.

During the past 30 years, however, society has considerably expanded the old ethic. For a variety of reasons, the public, at least in North America, Western Europe, and Australia and New Zealand, has grown increasingly concerned about a wide array of animal suffering, well beyond what arises out of cruelty. Most evident, perhaps, are the laws and policies that have been adopted to protect the interests of research animals in Great Britain, the United States, the Netherlands, Sweden, Australia, New Zealand, Switzerland, and Germany, all aimed at minimizing the pain and suffering of animals used in science. Laws and bills relevant to control of animal pain and suffering in all areas of human use have proliferated all over the world, ranging from the abolition or severe curtailment of confinement agriculture to protection of dolphins from tuna nets.

All of this marks a major departure from traditional social concern with cruelty alone. For example, in the 1890s, a judge refused to stop a service club–sponsored tame pigeon shooting competition under the anticruelty laws on the grounds that the people participating were upstanding citizens, working for charity, who were no threat to the community. In today's world, in most urban and suburban jurisdictions, such an activity, if not stopped by the judge, would be eliminated by public pressure or a city council mandate, merely because of the unnecessary suffering and pain incurred by the animals.

Today's social ethic is thus concerned first of all with eliminating unnecessary pain and suffering in a much broader sense than the traditional anticruelty ethic. As society has become more urbanized, more sensitive, and less tolerant of animal suffering, the bar for what counts as cruelty has naturally been lowered. Since 1986, 32 states have elevated animal cruelty from a misdemeanor to a felony offense, and what counts as cruelty has been significantly expanded. Consider one example. In 1997, during the United States Department of Agriculture's (USDA) attempt to bolster dairy prices by buying a large number of dairy cows, the agency did not trust the farmers not to rebuy the cattle and return them to their herds. In an attempt to forestall such undercutting of the program, the USDA mandated face branding of all purchased milk cows with a USDA identification mark. Dairy farmers (who generally do not brand any part of the cow) and Humane Society members were appalled by this barbaric decree and brought the USDA to court in New York State on charges of cruelty. The judge ruled that the agency was in fact guilty of cruelty, for it had failed to examine or use alternative, less invasive methods of identification. In earlier eras, although society always defined cruelty as inflicting "unnecessary" suffering, it defined *necessary* as that which was inconvenient, too expensive, or not customary to alleviate. Today that definition has changed radically, and increasingly, when someone says that "unnecessary suffering" is unacceptable, he or she means suffering that is possible, if inconvenient, to alleviate. Necessary suffering, then, is suffering that is impossible to alleviate. In another era, it might have been

considered acceptable to train a horse by using considerable negative reinforcement. Today, because our sensitivities and expertise in
training have increased, we are aware that positive reinforcement
can accomplish more than negative reinforcement. Thus someone
who beats a horse severely in the process of training is likely to be
seen as cruel by society in general, even if some of his or her peers
endorse such training methods.

Today society is far less willing to tolerate animal pain and suffering in any area of animal use, regardless of whether such use is
seen as frivolous (and hence possible to eliminate) or as essential to
human well-being, as in the case of research and agriculture (and
hence not seen as possible to eliminate), but traditionally exempt
from the purview of anticruelty laws. These latter uses have elicited
new ethical principles in the form of legislation (ethics "written
large," as Plato said), aimed at minimizing animal pain and suffering attendant on these activities.

For example, consider the 1985 federal laboratory animal laws.
On one hand, society realizes that researchers are not cruel and yet
also sees that some pain, suffering, and death must inevitably and
necessarily accompany the study of disease, toxicity, new surgical
procedures, stress, and so on. Society was unwilling to forsake the
benefits of biomedicine, despite the inevitability of some animal suffering and thus would not forbid animal experimentation. Society
also did not believe that researchers were doing the best they could
for animals used in research, however. This belief was evident when
it was discovered that analgesics were rarely used, social animals
such as chimpanzees were housed in tiny individual cages, atroci-
ties were documented, and so on. Society acted to "write large" in
law its moral commitment to the best possible treatment of animals
consonant with biomedical use by mandating pain control, eliminating multiple use, preventing the administration of paralytic agents
without anesthetics, and providing enriched environments.

The key moral concept encoded both in the 1985 amendments to
the Animal Welfare Act and in the National Institutes of Health
(NIH) Reauthorization Act, the latter putting the NIH Guidelines
for Laboratory Animal Care and Use into law, is in fact the need to
control laboratory animal pain not directly required by the nature
of the research (for example, pain research). In some countries, such
as Great Britain, the research must be terminated if the animal
experiences intractable pain. In the United States, such a move

depends on the discretion of the Institutional Animal Care and Use Committee, which may move to stop research under conditions of uncontrollable pain but need not do so. However the laws are written, it is manifest that society wants to see virtually all pain managed. Because this moral mandate is encoded in federal law, the highest law of the land, it therefore becomes the standard of practice for veterinary medicine. The ethic embodied in the laboratory animal laws has or will have ramifications for all veterinary practice.

The same point about minimizing pain and suffering holds true for animal agriculture in Europe. People do wish to consume animal products, but as the 1965 British Brambell Commission stated, they also wish to see animals live decent lives, such as those provided by husbandry agriculture. Industrialized agriculture grew without people explicitly realizing what it entailed. As soon as they did (e.g., in Great Britain and Sweden), laws were passed that underscored public commitment to decent lives for animals, abolished sow stalls, veal crates, and battery cages, and also required pain control for management procedures.

Research is seen by society as essential to human life, and animal agriculture is seen as essential to the food supply (most people are not prepared to be vegetarians). Thus society deploys the new ethic to shape these activities. Horse tripping, tame pigeon shoots, and dog fighting are not seen as essential or desirable by most citizens but are seen to cause animal suffering; therefore society moves to abolish them.

VETERINARY MEDICINE'S ROLE IN PAIN CONTROL

This ethic suggests that a fundamental role for veterinary medicine in society is finding modalities to control pain and suffering in our use of animals because such control seems to be the main point of the new ethic and the laws it has engendered. The track record of veterinary medicine in this area is not good, however. The reasons for this neglect are worth detailing because relatively few veterinarians have actively thought them through.

First, in the twentieth century, both human and veterinary medicine became increasingly science-based, essentially perceived as applied biologic science, with physics and chemistry serving as the exemplar of ideal science. In this light, emphasis on both the individual and idiosyncratic aspects of a disease (what comprised the "art of medicine") became subordinate to the universal captured in medical science. Second, in keeping with an ideological emphasis on science dealing only with what is testable and observable, talk of subjective states, such as pain and suffering, tended to disappear as unscientific. Even psychology became the science of observable behavior. Third, physicians and veterinarians measured success by prolonging life or function, focusing on quantity of life rather than quality of life, and emphasizing cure rather than care because quality is difficult to measure and impossible to quantify. Pain became more of a concern to the patient than to the clinician. Several articles by Frank McMillan have eloquently documented the untoward effects of this attitude in veterinary medicine. Thus in essence, control of pain became increasingly irrelevant in scientific medicine, a tendency that unfortunately continues to this day.

The most dramatic and egregious example of the supposed irrelevance of pain in the history of human medicine is the failure to control pain in 80% of human patients with cancer, even though 90% of such pain is controllable. Equally horrifying is the fact that until the late 1980s, neonatal surgeons regularly performed open heart surgery on newborns after administration of paralytic drugs and still perform a variety of procedures from colonoscopy and setting broken limbs to bone marrow aspiration with the use of nonanesthetic, nonanalgesic amnesiacs such as short-acting benzodiazepines (diazepam [Valium], midazolam [Versed, Dormicum]).

If human medicine was cavalier in dealing with pain and suffering in its patients during most of the twentieth century (the term *suffering* does not even appear in medical dictionaries), this is even more true of veterinary medicine because for most of the twentieth century, society placed little moral value on control of animal pain.

Until the late 1960s, veterinary medicine was overwhelmingly ancillary to agriculture, and the veterinarian's task was strictly dictated by the economic value of the animal; the control of pain was not of concern to producers and thus not expected of veterinary medicine. This attitude is epitomized in Merillat's 1905 veterinary surgery textbook in which he laments the almost total disregard of anesthesia in veterinary practice, with the episodic exception of the canine practitioner, whose clients presumably valued their animals enough in noneconomic terms to demand anesthesia.

These practical considerations were further compounded by the persistence of the Cartesian belief that possession of language is a precondition for the ability to feel pain, a notion that until recently (2001) existed in the International Pain Society's definition of pain.

The denial of the experience of pain by animals in veterinary medicine was so powerful that when the first textbook of veterinary anesthesia (by Lumb and Jones) was published in the United States in 1972, it did not list the control of felt pain as a reason for using anesthesia.

Many veterinarians who are more than 40 or 50 years of age still use the phrase *chemical restraint* as synonymous with *anesthesia;* some were trained in the 1960s to castrate horses using curariform (paralytic) drugs such as succinylcholine, which not only do not mask or diminish pain but probably intensify it by the fear they create. Others erroneously speak of anesthesia as *sedation,* although most sedatives neither mask nor diminish pain.

Of equal concern are the ideologic rationalizations still invoked by some (particularly older) veterinarians to justify withholding postsurgical or posttraumatic analgesia from animals. These rationalizations include the belief that anesthesia is more stressful than the surgical procedure performed without anesthesia. Also, postsurgical analgesics are not needed because animals supposedly will eat immediately after surgery. Analgesics are not to be used because without the pain, the animal will inexorably reinjure the damaged body part. Postsurgical howling and whining are not signs of pain; they are aftereffects of anesthesia. Anatomic differences, such as the presence of an anatomic mesenteric sling, vitiate the need for pain control after abdominal surgery in the dog. Animals do not need postsurgical analgesia because we can watch them behave normally after surgery. Young animals feel less pain than older ones and thus do not need surgical anesthesia for procedures such as tail docking or castration, which are performed with "bruticaine." Analgesia deadens the coping ability of predators and thus is more discomfiting to an animal than the pain is. Liver biopsies do not hurt, and so on.

Although adequate, even definitive, responses to this spurious reasoning exist, they persist as barriers to pain management. One drug company executive has even told me that, by the company's reckoning, approximately one third of veterinarians do not use analgesia. This is buttressed by a statement made by the executive director of one large state veterinary association who expressed amazement that so many veterinarians fail to supply pain control, even though it is easy to achieve, lucrative, and causes remarkable changes in the animal's demeanor.

Finally, many veterinarians do not know a great deal about pain management. In a 1996 study, Dohoo and Dohoo showed that veterinarians' knowledge is quite limited and that what practitioners do know is typically not acquired in veterinary school, although I suspect that this is rapidly changing as society increases its demand for pain control in animals. In fact, a variety of factors provide strong arguments in favor of the idea that pain control is one of the chief issues facing veterinary medicine.

The Changing Social Ethics

As previously discussed, society has become increasingly concerned about animal welfare. Central to the new ethic is the realization that uncontrolled pain and suffering probably represent the greatest harm we can visit upon animals, and thus control of pain and suffering in all areas of animal use is a major moral imperative.

New Philosophical Reflections on Animal Experience

Better philosophy than we have had in the past strongly argues in favor of the view that animals have thoughts, mental states, and feelings. The fact that some such mental states are in many ways probably not like ours, since animal thoughts and feelings are not mediated by language, does not obviate the need for serious concern about their pain, fear, and distress. It is possible that animal pain is worse than human pain because, lacking language and sophisticated reasoning skills and temporal concepts, animals cannot understand the reasons for and causes of pain, and thus lack the ability to hope for and anticipate its cessation.

Laws

New laws articulating the new ethic have specifically flagged pain control as the major moral concern about animal treatment. The essence of the 1985 U.S. laboratory animal laws, originally the first laws in America articulating the new ethic for animals, embody the control of pain and distress as their major edict. Unfortunately, before the advent of these laws, virtually no literature on animal pain control existed. Thus this goal of pain control needs to be sought not only for research animals but for animals in all other areas of human use, including farm and companion animals. Countries such as Sweden have articulated the need for pain control in farm animals. Treatment of companion animals may be the only area in which concern for pain in animals is not trumped, diluted, or submerged by economic considerations and can be wholly realized.

Prevention of Suffering

If we keep these animals to give and receive love, as members of our families, we have an insurmountable obligation to not let them suffer. Equally important, it is now definitively known that uncontrolled pain is not only morally problematic when allowed to persist in humans or animals, it is biologically deleterious. Unmitigated pain is a major biologic stressor and affects numerous aspects of physical health, from wound healing to resistance to infectious disease. One remarkable study showed that when pain in rats with cancer was controlled with analgesia versus not controlled, the rats given analgesia had 80% fewer metastatic lesions. The conclusion is inescapable: uncontrolled pain damages health and well-being and can even, if pain is severe enough, engender death. Ironically, the new edition of Lumb and Jones's veterinary textbook stresses this dimension of pain management, a major salubrious change since the publication of the 1970s edition.

Preserving the Role of Veterinarians as the Recognized Health Care Providers for Animals

One of the unexpected consequences of ignoring pain and suffering in human and animal medicine in the twentieth century has been the fueling of the development of alternative, nonevidence-based, nonscientific "therapies." To put it crudely, patients and animal owners have reasoned that if doctors do not worry about human or animal suffering, they will find others who will. Also, many alternative practitioners do approach human and animal patients with empathy and understanding of the full significance of pain and suffering. Unfortunately, however, compassion is not cure and is only part of care. Recognition that a being is suffering is not alleviation of that suffering, although it is surely a necessary condition for such alleviation. If veterinary clients are drawn to alternative unproven therapies that may be fueled by compassion but do not work to control pain, the animal may be cheated of a proven modality for pain control, creating an intolerable moral situation for the animal owner and a loss of credibility for veterinarians because clients may not be able to judge when pain is (or is not) alleviated. If veterinarians will not manage pain, they also risk a grave loss of credibility among the public, who may then seek to remove the special status of scientifically based veterinary medicine and open animal medicine to the forces of the free market, at an incalculable cost in animal suffering.

Meeting One's Professional Obligations

It does not appear that animals fear death, lacking after all the concepts to understand, in Heidegger's masterful phrase, "the possibility of the impossibility of their being." Yet they clearly fear pain. We urge death in veterinary medicine as a merciful tool for escape from pain. (There is reason to believe that humans also fear pain more than death, and it is often suggested that if we truly attacked pain in terminally ill patients with all of our medical armamentarium and with no absurd fears that they will become addicted, people would not seek euthanasia as much as they do and would die with far more dignity, as the hospice movement has shown.) It is thus reasonable to say of animals that letting them live in unalleviated pain is the worst thing we can do to them. If the veterinarian's raison d'etre is, as is so often remarked, the health and well-being of the animals in his or her care, then the assiduous pursuit of eliminating or at least managing pain should be his or her top priority. The fact that it has not been so in the past only makes it all the more imperative to make it so in the future.

Sources of Information Regarding Regulations Governing Animal Welfare

- Animal Welfare Act and Regulations
  Animal Welfare Information Center
  United States Department of Agriculture
  Agricultural Research Service
  National Agricultural Library
  http://www.nal.usda.gov/awic/legislat/usdaleg1.htm

- 2000 Report of the AVMA Panel on Euthanasia (American Veterinary Medical Association, 2000)
  http://www.nal.usda.gov/awic/pubs/noawicpubs/avmaeuth.htm

- USDA Animal and Plant Health Inspection Animal Care Policy Manual
  http://www.aphis.usda.gov/ac/polman.html

- Office of Laboratory Animal Welfare
  http://grants.nih.gov/grants/olaw/olaw.htm

SUGGESTED READINGS

Dohoo SE, Dohoo IR: Factors influencing the postoperative use of analgesics in dogs and cats by Canadian veterinarians, *Can Vet J* 37(9):552-556, 1996.

Dohoo SE, Dohoo IR: Postoperative use of analgesics in dogs and cats by Canadian veterinarians, *Can Vet J* 37(9):546-551, 1996.

Ferrel BR, Rhiner M: High-tech comfort: ethical issues in cancer pain management for the 1990s, *J Clin Ethics* 2:108-115, 1991.

Humane Society of Rochester v. Ling, 633f. Supp. 480, U.S. District Court, WDNY, NY 1986.

Kitchell R, Guinan M: The nature of pain in animals. In Rollin B, Kesel M, editors: *The experimental animal in biomedical research,* vol 1, Boca Raton, Fla, 1989, CRC Press.

McMillan F: Comfort as the primary goal in veterinary medical practice, *J Am Vet Assoc* 212(9):1370-1374, 1998.

McMillan F: Effects of human contact on animal well-being, *J Am Vet Assoc* 215(11):1592-1598, 1999.

McMillan F: Influence of mental states on somatic health in animals, *J Am Vet Assoc* 214(8):1221-1225, 1999.

McMillan F: Quality of life in animals, *J Am Vet Assoc* 216(12):1904-1910, 2000.

Merillat LA: *Principles of veterinary surgery,* Chicago, 1906, Alexander Eger.

Page GG, Ben-Eliyahu J, Yirmiyah R, et al: Morphine attenuates surgery-induced enhancement of metastatic colonization in rats, *Pain* 54:21-28, 1993.

Rollin BE: *Animal rights and human morality,* ed 2, Buffalo, 1992, Prometheus Books.

Rollin BE: Pain and ideology in human and veterinary medicine, *Semin Vet Med Surg (Small Animal)* 12(2):56-60, 1997.

Rollin BE: *The unheeded cry: animal consciousness, animal pain, and science,* ed 2, Ames, 1998, Iowa State University Press.

Rollin BE: Some conceptual and ethical concerns about current views of pain, *Pain Forum* 8(2):78-83, 1999.

Rollin BE: *Veterinary medical ethics: theory and cases,* Ames, 1999, Iowa State University Press.

Rollin BE: Equine welfare and emerging social ethics, *J Am Vet Assoc* 216(8):1234-1237, 2000.

Rollin BE: The ethics of pain control in companion animals. In Hellebrekers L, editor: *Animal pain: a practice-oriented approach to an effective pain control in animals,* Utrecht, Netherlands, 2000, Van Der Wels.

2

Physiology and Pathophysiology of Pain

WILLIAM W. MUIR III

Pain is a sensory experience that is frequently but not always associated with nerve or tissue damage. The study of pain encompasses all the individual biologic basic sciences, especially anatomy, physiology, pharmacology, and pathology. A functional appreciation of each of these areas as they pertain to the generation, transmission, and recognition of painful stimuli is fundamental to understanding pain and pain processes. The following discussion is meant to provide an overview of the important aspects of the nervous system and the sensory processing of nonpainful and painful stimuli. As in all areas of biologic science, jargon will be used, such as *afferent* (toward the central nervous system [CNS]) and *efferent* (away from the CNS), and all terms will be defined when first mentioned. Pain itself is usually described as a noxious stimulus, meaning a damaging or potentially tissue-damaging stimulus. One term frequently encountered in descriptions of the effects of pain is *neuroplasticity.* This term implies that the nervous system can be changed (shaped or molded), depending on the environment (outside) and biologic processes (inside) that are responsible for painful sensations. The neuroplasticity of the nervous system should be kept in mind during attempts to assess the severity of pain, especially chronic pain, and in the design of treatment protocols. Another term that arises during discussions of pain management in animals is *anthropomorphize,* which means to attribute a human form or personality to an animal. It is human nature to project our own experiences and feelings onto our animal patients because they cannot verbally describe to us how they feel;

13

however, it is inappropriate to attribute human feelings to something not human. Alternatively, it is morally and ethically appropriate to adopt an anthropocentric viewpoint (i.e., humanity or the human mind is the center or ultimate, such as when the instincts of animals are interpreted as analogous to human instincts) when assessing and treating pain in animals.

PART 1: NEUROPHYSIOLOGY OF SENSATION

Peripheral nerves can be thought of as the tentacles of the CNS, consisting of sensory, motor, and autonomic nerve fibers. The terminal ends of sensory nerve fibers recognize and transform (transduction) various environmental stimuli into electrical signals (action potentials) that are carried (transmission) to the dorsal horn of the CNS, where they are immediately changed (modulation) and relayed (projection) to the brainstem and brain where the signal is integrated, recognized, and identified (perception) and transformed (secondary modulation) into appropriate self-preserving experiences and motor responses that are remembered (Fig. 2-1).

Transduction

The detection of innocuous and noxious information is accomplished by specialized encapsulated and bare (free) nerve endings that transform or transduce environmental stimuli into electrical signals called *action potentials* (Table 2-1). These receptors vary in their sensitivity to mechanical, thermal, and chemical stimuli (low- and high-threshold), providing a seamless transition from innocuous to noxious sensations.

Threshold

The minimum stimulus required to elicit a transmittable electrical signal (action potential) from a peripheral receptor is considered to be its *threshold.* The peripheral receptors of A-beta (Aβ), A-delta (Aδ), and C fibers demonstrate a large degree of overlap, providing for a continuum of sensations. Once the threshold for the receptor is reached, the greater the strength of the stimulus, the more electrical signals (action potentials) are produced; the longer the duration of the stimulus, the longer is the train of electrical signals produced (Fig. 2-2).

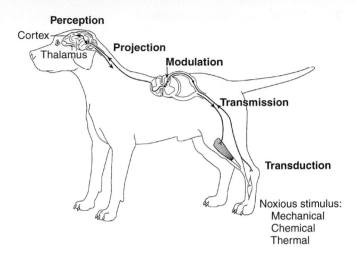

Fig. 2-1 Pathways involved in producing painful sensations. Noxious stimuli (mechanical, chemical, thermal, electrical) are transduced (transduction) into electrical signals that are transmitted (transmission) to the spinal cord, where they are modulated (modulation) before being relayed (projection) to the brain for final processing and awareness (perception). Descending pathways from the brain modulate sensory input, and outputs from the spinal cord regulate skeletal muscle contraction.

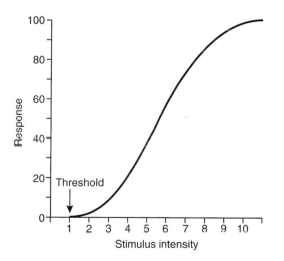

Fig. 2-2 The pain threshold is the point at which stimulus intensity is just strong enough to be perceived as painful. Stronger stimuli elicit greater and greater responses until the maximum response possible is produced.

TABLE 2-1

Important Receptors in Somatic Sensation

Receptor	Modality	Nerve Fiber Type
Cutaneous and Subcutaneous	**Touch**	
Pacinian's	Vibration	Aα,β
Ruffini's	Skin stretch	Aα,β
Merkel's	Pressure	Aα,β
Meissner's	Stroking	Aα,β
Muscle and Skeletal Mechanoreceptors	**Limb Proprioception**	
Muscle spindles	Muscle length and stretch	Aα,β
Golgi tendon	Muscle contraction	Aα
Joint capsule	Joint angle	Aβ
Stretch	Excess stretch	Aδ
Thermal	**Temperature**	
Heat nociceptors	Hot temperature	Aδ
Cold nociceptors	Cold temperature	C
Nociceptors	**Pain**	
Mechanical	Sharp, pricking	Aδ
Thermal-mechanical	Burning, freezing	Aδ, C
Polymodal	Slow burning	C

Specialized Nerve Endings

Specialized low-threshold nerve endings or receptors (e.g., Meissner's, Merkel's, Pacinian's, Ruffini's) in the skin, muscles, and joints respond to innocuous mechanical stimulation. These receptors are primarily concerned with touch, vibration pressure, movement, and proprioception. The information transduced by these nerve endings is conveyed to the CNS by Aβ nerve fibers. The nerve terminals of Aβ fibers are responsible for transducing innocuous sensory information but may become involved in chronic pain states.

Free Nerve Endings

Aδ and C nerve fibers terminate as free nerve endings in the skin, subcutaneous tissue, periosteum, joints, muscles, and viscera.

Free nerve endings respond to both low-intensity (nonpainful) and high-intensity (painful) mechanical, thermal, and chemical stimuli. The terminals of Aδ and C nerve fibers are essential for the detection of acute pain, and with few exceptions, are responsible for conducting all pain sensations. Approximately 75% of the Aδ-fiber and 10% to 15% of the C-fiber free nerve endings respond to low-threshold stimuli. The remainder respond only to high-threshold tissue-threatening or tissue-damaging (nociceptive) events and are referred to as *nociceptors* (pain receptors). Some nociceptors respond only to intense mechanical stimulation and are referred to as *high-threshold mechanical nociceptors,* whereas others respond to noxious mechanothermal stimulation, and still others respond to noxious mechanical, thermal, and chemical stimuli (polymodal nociceptors).

Aδ Nociceptors. Aδ nerve terminals can be nociceptive or nonnociceptive and are composed of both low- (<75%) and high-threshold (>25%) mechanoreceptors and mechanothermal receptors. The latter are referred to as *Aδ heat nociceptors.* High-threshold Aδ nociceptors respond only to tissue-threatening or tissue-damaging stimulation. Many of the Aδ nociceptors respond only to specific stimuli, whereas others are polymodal and respond to mechanical, chemical, and thermal stimulation. Aδ-fiber nociceptors respond with higher discharge rates than C-fiber nociceptors, providing more discriminative information to the CNS, and are responsible for the pricking and sharp qualities associated with the initiation of pain ("first pain"). Activation of both Aδ-fiber and C-fiber nociceptors is necessary for perception of acute pain.

C-Fiber Nociceptors. Almost all C-fiber nociceptors are high-threshold and polymodal. C-fiber nociceptors are found in large numbers in the skin and in skeletal muscle and joints. Although they are abundant, fewer C fiber nociceptors are found in visceral tissues. C-fiber activation is responsible for the second (slow) pain that occurs after the initial insult and is characterized by a burning, aching quality, which signals damaged or inflamed tissue. The pain produced by tissue damage and inflammation promotes avoidance reactions, guarding (protective) behaviors, and rest. Tissue damage and inflammation also intensify the sensation of pain (activate silent receptors), producing hyperalgesia.

Silent or Sleeping Nociceptors. Aδ-fiber and C-fiber nociceptors that are not activated by tissue-damaging events are referred to as "silent" or "sleeping" nociceptors. These receptors are activated by tissue inflammation and are particularly sensitive to mechanical stimulation. They are believed to be important in the development of hyperalgesia and guarding behaviors.

Transmission

Sensory and motor nerve impulses (action potentials) are transmitted by peripheral nerves. Peripheral nerves contain both afferent (sensory) and efferent (motor) nerve fibers. The peripheral processes of sensory nerves diverge to form multiple branches, ending in specialized (low-threshold) or free (high-threshold) nerve endings (see "Free Nerve Endings"). Near the spinal cord, the afferent (sensory) fibers of peripheral nerves separate to form the afferent (sensory) dorsal root. The efferent (motor) fiber from the spinal cord forms the ventral root (Fig. 2-3). The area of the skin innervated by the dorsal root is called a *dermatome*. Adjacent dermatomes overlap, minimizing sensory deficits that may occur as a result of dorsal root injuries.

Once a peripheral afferent nerve is activated and the stimulus is transduced into an electrical signal (action potential), it is transmitted to the dorsal horn of the spinal cord. Peripheral nerves are categorized according to their anatomy, size, and mean conduction velocity (Table 2-2). Under normal circumstances, nonnoxious sensory information is transmitted by myelinated Aβ nerve fibers, whereas nonnoxious and some noxious information is transmitted by minimally myelinated Aδ nerve fibers. Noxious information is transmitted by unmyelinated C fibers. The central process of a primary afferent nerve constitutes the dorsal root, which divides into multiple nerve rootlets that connect with the spinal cord (see Fig. 2-3).

Receptive Fields

The receptive field defines the area innervated by a sensory nerve fiber and increases with animal size. The receptive fields of high-threshold nociceptors consist of collections of 2 to 20 spots, each with an area of less than 1 mm^2. Receptive fields are small on the face and head (1 to 2 mm^2), are larger on the body surface, and provide discriminatory capability. The receptive fields of C-fiber nociceptors are generally much smaller than those of Aδ-fiber nociceptors, and considerable overlap exists between Aδ-fiber and C-fiber nociceptive fields. Nociceptive afferent nerve fibers from the thoracic and abdominal viscera are few compared with cutaneous fibers and constitute less than 10% of the nervous input to the

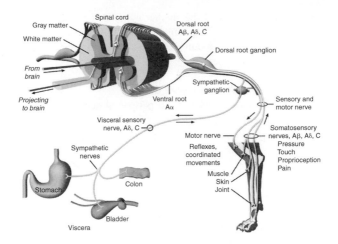

Fig. 2-3 A simplified illustration of sensory (visceral and somatic) nerve fibers (Aβ, Aδ, C) as they travel to the dorsal root ganglia and then via the dorsal root nerves to the gray matter of the spinal cord. Many of the Aδ and C sensory nerve fibers innervating the viscera travel with the sympathetic nerves, passing through the sympathetic ganglia before reaching the dorsal root ganglia.

TABLE 2-2

Classification of Nerve Fibers

Group	Innervation	Myelination	Velocity (m/sec)
Aα	Motor to skeletal muscle	Myelinated	70-120
Aβ	Sensory: touch, vibration, pressure, proprioception	Myelinated	30-70
Aγ	Motor to muscle spindles	Myelinated	15-30
Aδ	Mechanoreceptors, thermo-receptors, nociceptors	Thinly myelinated	12-30
B	Sympathetic Preganglionic	Unmyelinated	3-15
C	Mechanoreceptors, thermoreceptors Sympathetic postganglionic Nociceptors	Unmyelinated	0.5-3

spinal cord. Furthermore, the smaller number of visceral afferent fibers innervates a much larger area and demonstrates almost 100% overlap, which helps explain the diffuse nature of many visceral pain sensations.

Dorsal Root and Cranial Nerve Ganglia

The cell bodies of sensory afferent peripheral nerve fibers are located in the dorsal root ganglia of the spinal nerves and sensory ganglia of the cranial nerves (V, VII, IX, and X). The nerve branches divide as they leave the cell body, with one branch traveling centrally to the spinal cord and the other branch traveling through the formed peripheral nerve and its divisions to reach the sensory organs in the skin, subcutaneous tissues, muscles, bones, and joints. These branches are called *somatic sensory fibers.* Some of the sensory processes of sensory afferent nerves accompany the sympathetic and parasympathetic nerves to innervate the viscera and are called *visceral sensory nerve fibers* (see Fig. 2-3). The cell bodies of the dorsal root ganglion (DRG) produce a variety of enzymes and neurotransmitters that are important in signal transmission and transformation and nerve cell viability. Among the more prevalent are substance P, calcitonin gene-related peptide (CGRP), cholecystokinin (CCK), somatostatin (SOM), vasoactive intestinal peptide (VIP), bombesin (BOM), galanin (GAL), dynorphin (DYN), endorphin (END), enkephalin (ENK), and corticotropin-releasing factor (CRF).

Modulation

Peripheral sensory nerve impulses are modulated (amplified or suppressed) in the spinal cord. The spinal cord is divided into white matter (axons of nerve fibers) and gray matter (nerve cells). The gray matter is divided into three distinct regions: the dorsal horn, the intermediate zone, and the ventral horn. The gray matter of the dorsal horn contains interneurons (interconnecting nerves) and ascending neurons that receive, transmit, and project sensory information to the brain. The ventral horn contains interneurons and motor neurons that control skeletal muscle function, and the gray matter of the intermediate zone contains autonomic preganglionic neurons that mediate visceral control and transmit information to higher centers. Primary sensory afferent nerve fibers enter the spinal cord through the dorsal nerve root and synapse with neurons in the dorsal horn of the gray matter. Many of the sensory afferent nerve fibers bifurcate, sending branches that ascend and descend several spinal cord segments (Lissauer's tract) before entering and synapsing in the dorsal horn. Sensory nerve fibers can synapse directly with projection neurons in the gray matter, which relay incoming sensory information to the brain, or indirectly with local excitatory and inhibitory interneurons that regulate and modify sensory information before it is relayed to projection neurons and higher centers.

Gray Matter

The gray matter of the spinal cord has been subdivided into 10 laminae (Rexed's laminae) based on the presence of neuronal cells with similar function. Gray matter sensory neurons are basically of two types: (1) those that process high-threshold, nociceptive-specific information and have small receptive fields that are organized somatotopically and (2) those that process low- and high-threshold information *(wide-dynamic-range neurons),* are nociceptive-nonspecific, and have large receptive fields. Information from the various peripheral sensory nerve fiber types (Aβ, Aδ, C) is transmitted to the various laminae where amino acids (glutamate) and peptides (substance P) activate a variety of postsynaptic receptors.

- The gray matter of the dorsal horn contains projection neurons, propriospinal neurons, and interneurons that relay sensory information to the brain and activate descending control systems, which control the sensitivity of dorsal horn neurons to excitatory and inhibitory impulses. Propriospinal neurons transfer sensory information from one segment of the spinal cord to the next and ultimately to the brain, and local interneurons modulate (excite and inhibit) and transmit sensory information for a short distance within the spinal cord.
- The gray matter of the ventral horn contains interneurons and motor neurons that control skeletal muscle activity.
- The gray matter of the intermediate zone contains preganglionic neurons of the autonomic nervous system that control visceral functions and transmit afferent information to the brain.

White Matter

The white matter contains the axons of the spinal cord and has been anatomically divided into three bilaterally paired spinal columns that relay information to and from the brain.

- Dorsal columns: The dorsal columns are medial to the dorsal horn and relay somatic sensory information to the medulla.
- Lateral columns: The lateral columns are lateral to the gray matter, relay somatic sensory information to the brain, and contain nerve fibers from sensory, motor, and autonomic control centers in the brain.
- Ventral columns: The ventral columns are medial to the ventral horns and are primarily composed of neurons descending from the brain that control skeletal muscle.

Spinal Cord Laminae *(Fig. 2-4)*

Laminae I to VI comprise the dorsal horn, lamina VII comprises the intermediate zone, and laminae VIII to IX comprise the ventral horn. These laminae extend the entire length of the spinal cord and fuse cranially in the medulla. Lamina X surrounds the central canal of the spinal cord. The laminar anatomy refers to the location of specific cell bodies.

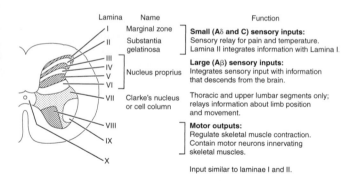

Fig. 2-4 The gray matter of the spinal cord is divided into functionally distinct nerve cells (Rexed's laminae). The dorsal horn of the gray matter receives sensory input from Aβ, Aδ, and C nerve fibers. The ventral horn of the spinal cord contains motor nerves that innervate and regulate skeletal muscle contraction. The white matter that surrounds the gray matter is divided into columns of myelinated nerves. The dorsal column relays somatic sensory information to the brain. The intermediate column contains sensory motor and autonomic nerve fibers descending from the brain and sensory pathways ascending to the brain. The ventral column contains nerve fibers descending from the brain that control skeletal muscle contraction.

- Lamina I: The most superficial lamina, or marginal layer, of the dorsal horn serves as an important sensory relay junction for pain and temperature. Lamina I contains nociceptive-specific neurons, wide-dynamic-range neurons, and projection neurons. This lamina receives the majority of its input from sympathetic Aδ and C fibers originating in the skin, skeletal muscle, joints, viscera, and trigeminal structures.
- Lamina II: Known as the *substantia gelatinosa,* lamina II is divided into outer (IIo) and inner (IIi) layers, which receive afferent sensory information, predominantly from small nonmyelinated C fibers and thinly myelinated Aδ fibers that project to lamina I. Lamina II contains a large number of second-order multireceptive or wide-dynamic-range neurons, almost all of which are interneurons; this suggests the importance of lamina II as a site for the modulation of synaptic transmission. Few visceral afferent nerves terminate in lamina II.
- Laminae III to VI: Known as *the nucleus proprius,* lamina III integrates sensory input with information descending from the brain and contains neurons that project sensory information to the brain. Lamina IV receives sensory information from large-diameter Aβ fibers from the skin, which synapse with low-threshold mechanoreceptors responding to innocuous tactile and thermal stimuli. It also receives some input from small-diameter Aδ and C fibers in the skin, muscle, and viscera. Lamina V predominantly contains wide-dynamic-range neurons, which receive sensory information from Aβ fibers and sympathetic Aδ and C fibers, which synapse with neurons that project to the brain.
- Laminae VII to IX: Laminae VII, VIII, and IX contain interneurons that are important in regulating skeletal muscle contraction and limb movement.
- Laminae X: Lamina X surrounds the central canal and receives sensory information similar to that received by laminae I and II.

Spinal Cord Neurotransmitters and Receptors
As stated previously, the dorsal horn of the spinal cord receives and processes sensory information and relays this information to the brain. A multitude of neurotransmitters—including peptides (substance P, CGRP, SOM, neuropeptide Y, GAL), excitatory (aspartate, glutamate) and inhibitory (gamma-aminobutyric acid [GABA], glycine) amino acids, nitric oxide (NO), prostaglandins, adenosine

triphosphate (ATP), endogenous opioids, and monoamines (sero-tonin, norepinephrine)—are responsible for transmitting peripheral information to spinal cord neurons. These neurotransmitters act on excitatory (α-amino-3-hydroxy-5-methyl-4-isoxazole propionic acid [AMPA], kainate [KAI], N-methyl-D-aspartate [NMDA]) and in-hibitory (GABA, glycine) receptors on neurons that relay sensory information to the brain.

- AMPA, KAI, and neurokinin receptors: Most transmission be-tween the periphery and dorsal horn of the spinal cord occurs as a result of glutamate acting on postsynaptically located AMPA and KAI ionotropic receptors. Activation of AMPA and KAI re-ceptors is responsible for tactile sensations, and with neurokinin (NK) receptors, the acute response to brief and tonic noxious sensations. The activation of AMPA and NK receptors is be-lieved to be responsible for signaling the location, intensity, and duration of peripheral stimuli.

- NMDA receptors: The activation of ionotropic glutamate NMDA receptors, caused by prolonged afferent input from Aδ and C fibers, is responsible for the development of slower-onset and longer-lasting or chronic pain states. NMDA receptors are involved in long-term potentiation and central sensitization and are facilitated by the simultaneous activation of substance P–sensitive AMPA and NK receptors, which remove the normally present physiologic magnesium (Mg^{2+})–dependent block of NMDA receptors.

- Metabotropic receptors: Activation of metabotropic glutamate receptors (mGluR) stimulates the production of intracellular sec-ond messengers (inositol-1,4,5-triphosphate [IP_3], DAG, NO), which increase intracellular calcium levels, leading to increases in cellular metabolism, potentiation in synaptic transmission, and alterations in gene expression (central neuroplasticity). Activa-tion of NMDA and mGluR is believed to be responsible for in-tegrating spatial and temporal pain-related events.

- GABA and glycine receptors: Activation of GABA and glycine receptors modulates and reduces (inhibits) the effects of excita-tory sensory input to the spinal cord.

Spinal Cord Modulation of Sensory Input

The complexity of neural inputs (peripheral, local, ascending, de-scending) and networks (parallel, converging, diverging) within the spinal cord suggests that sensory homeostasis is maintained by a balance of activity between peripheral nerve inputs and descending excitatory and inhibitory influences from the brain. Although this description may seem overly simplistic, the selective stimulation of peripheral afferent nerve input, the release of local endogenous modulators of synaptic transmission, and the activation of descending inhibitory pathways modify sensory input and the response to a painful stimulus (Table 2-3).

- Gate control theory (Fig. 2-5): This theory, first proposed by Melzack and Wall, suggests that low-threshold Aβ fibers and high-threshold C fibers modulate the activity of inhibitory interneurons located in the spine. Inhibitory interneurons normally reduce the output of spontaneously active projection

---

TABLE 2-3
Modulators of Excitatory and Inhibitory Synaptic Transmission

Modulator	Effect
Excitatory	
GABA	Inhibition
Opioid	Inhibition
Serotonin:	
5-HT$_1$	Inhibition
5-HT$_2$	Facilitation
Norepinephrine	Inhibition
ATP	Facilitation
Tachykinin:	
Substance P	Facilitation
Neurokinin A	Facilitation
Prostanoids	Facilitation
BDNF	Facilitation
Kainate	Inhibition
Inhibitory	
Serotonin	Facilitation
Norepinephrine	Facilitation
Acetylcholine	Facilitation
Adenosine	Inhibition

BDNF, Brain-derived neurotrophic factor; *5-HT,* 5-hydroxytryptamine (serotonin).

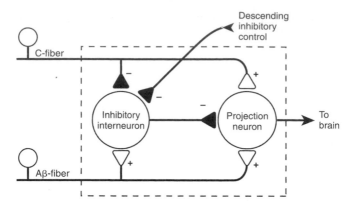

Fig. 2-5 The gate control theory is a simplified view of pain modulation in the CNS. Inputs from large myelinated Aβ sensory nerve fibers, which normally transmit innocuous sensory information (touch), activate (+) inhibitory interneurons in the spinal cord, inhibiting projection neurons to the brain. Note that the activation of Aδ and C sensory nerve fibers, which carry noxious inputs, inhibits (−) the inhibitory interneurons.

neurons, which relay sensory information to the brain. Activation of the low-threshold Aβ fibers, which normally transmit nonpainful stimuli, increases inhibitory interneuron effects on projection neurons, thereby reducing the transmission of painful stimuli to the brain.

- Endogenous opioids: Painful stimuli can initiate the release of endogenous opioids (e.g., ENK, END, DYN). These chemicals act at a variety of opioid receptors (μ, δ, κ) to suppress nociceptive responses in the periphery, spinal cord, and brain. One of the effects of these chemicals is to inhibit the release of local excitatory neurotransmitters, including glutamate and substance P.

- Modulators of excitatory and inhibitory spinal cord transmission: Both excitatory and inhibitory synaptic transmission are modulated in the spinal cord by various neuromodulators. GABA, opioids, serotonin, and norepinephrine inhibit excitatory synaptic transmission, whereas ATP, substance P, and prostanoids are facilitatory. Conversely, serotonin, norepinephrine, and acetylcholine facilitate inhibitory synaptic transmission, and ATP is inhibitory (see Table 2-3).

Supraspinal Modulation of Sensory Input

Descending axons of serotoninergic and noradrenergic neurons from the brain synapse with opioid containing inhibitory interneurons. Once activated by a stressful event (e.g., pain, fear, hypoxia), opioid-like analgesic effects are produced. Activation of these pathways is thought to be responsible for "stress-induced analgesia." Interestingly and somewhat paradoxically, activation of these same pathways suppresses the release of the inhibitory neurotransmitter GABA from inhibitory interneurons, leading to local disinhibitory effects and a potential increase in pain perception. This latter effect is believed to be more important in chronic, rather than acute, pain states.

Projection

Nociceptive information is conveyed to the brain by bundles of neurons (nerve tracts) that originate in the laminae of the dorsal horn. Some controversy exists regarding the relative importance of the various nerve tracts in nociceptive processing, so only the pathways of primary importance are mentioned.

- Spinothalamic tract: The spinothalamic tract is the most prominent ascending nociceptive pathway and originates from laminae I and IV to VII of the spinal cord. It contains axons of nociceptive-specific and wide-dynamic-range neurons, which terminate in the thalamus.
- Spinoreticular tract: Spinoreticular tract axons originate at locations similar to those of the spinothalamic tract neurons but terminate in the reticular formation and the thalamus.
- Spinomesencephalic tract: Axons of the spinomesencephalic tract originate in laminae I and V and terminate in the midbrain (periaqueductal gray region, limbic system, hypothalamus).
- Spinohypothalamic tract: Axons originating from neurons in laminae III and IV project information to the hypothalamus and ventral forebrain.

Perception

The integration, processing, and recognition of sensory information (perception) occurs in multiple specific areas of the brain, which communicate via interneurons to produce an integrated response that reflects the coordinated contributions of arousal, somatosensory input, and autonomic and motor output (Fig. 2-6). Somatosensory modalities take specific routes to the brain: the dorsal column–medial lemniscal system and the anterolateral system. The use of several neural pathways (redundancy) to convey information from a specific body part is called *parallel processing* and helps to ensure adequate input to the CNS. Neurons in the dorsal column–medial lemniscal system originate from laminae III, IV, and V; ascend to synapse with neurons in the caudal medulla (brainstem); and relay information concerning tactile sensation, including touch, vibration, and limb proprioception.

- The reticular activating system (RAS), located in the brainstem, is a critical center for the integration of these sensory experiences and the subsequent affective and motivational aspects of pain through projections to the medial thalamus and limbic system. The RAS also mediates motor, autonomic, and endocrine responses. The anterolateral system originates from neurons in

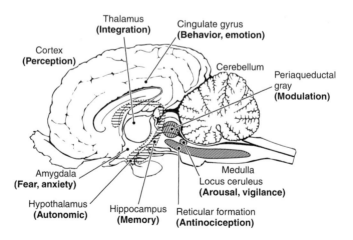

Fig. 2-6 Regions of the brain that are linked to various functions and responses. The thalamus serves as the central integrating and transmission point for pain perception and subsequent responses.

laminae I and V, which synapse in the reticular formation of the pons and medulla, the midbrain (periaqueductal gray matter [PAG]), and the thalamus. Both the PAG and thalamus serve as relay points for sensory information transfer: the former transfers information to the thalamus and hypothalamus, and the latter transfers information to the cerebral cortex. The three major pathways of the anterolateral system are the spinothalamic, spinoreticular, and spinomesencephalic tracts (see "Projection" section), which are primarily involved in relaying painful and temperature-related sensations.

- The thalamus relays information to the somatosensory cortex, which in turn projects the information to adjacent cortical association areas, including but not limited to the limbic system. The limbic system includes the cingulate gyrus (behavior, emotion), amygdala (conditioned fear, anxiety), hippocampus (memory), hypothalamus (sympathetic autonomic activity), and locus ceruleus (arousal, vigilance, behavior) (see Fig. 2-6). The caudal extension of the limbic system, the PAG, receives descending information from the cortex, amygdala, and hypothalamus and ascending projections from the medulla, reticular formation (including the locus ceruleus), and spinal cord.

- The PAG is considered to be an important relay for descending facilitatory and inhibitory (endogenous opioid) modulation of nociceptive input. The PAG connects with the rostral ventromedial medulla (RVM) and medullary reticular formation (RF), from which adrenergic and serotoninergic fibers descend to the dorsal horn of the spinal cord, inducing inhibitory or analgesic effects. Descending facilitation from the RVM is thought to be a critical component of many chronic pain states.

- Collectively these centers process sensory information that elicit fear, anxiety, and aggression and activate efferent pathways, which mediate autonomic, neuroendocrine, and motor (skeletal and visceral) responses. Furthermore, all of these areas can be conditioned by visual, olfactory, auditory, and somatic or visceral stimuli that prepare the CNS for fearful or stressful (painful) events. The physiologic, biochemical, cellular, and molecular changes that occur in response to stressful or noxious events emphasize the tremendous plasticity of the CNS and highlight the importance of chronic stress in the development of pathologic pain.

Memory

The memory of pain is shaped by several factors, including the animal's behavior pattern, the environment, the expectation of pain, and the intensity of pain. The peak intensity of pain is the single most important factor in determining the memory of pain. *Neuroplasticity* refers to the ability of the nervous system to change its biochemical and physiologic functions in response to internal and external stimuli: the implication is that multiple minor sensory events or a single major sensory event can change the stimulus-response characteristics of the nervous system. Patients who have an inherent memory of pain or of a significant painful event are harder to treat, and those patients in whom pain has been allowed to persist for periods of more than 12 to 24 hours often respond poorly to analgesic therapy.

PART 2: PAIN

Pain has been and remains difficult to define, both in scope and consequence (see Chapter 4). The complexity of its ubiquity is highlighted by the myriad of neurochemical, peripheral, and central neuroanatomic and biochemical events involved in pain production. Pain is not nociception (the detection of tissue damage by specialized receptors [nociceptors]) but is the conscious experience of nociception, which is only partly determined by the stimulus-induced (mechanical, thermal, chemical, electrical) activation of afferent neural pathways. Pain encompasses nociception, the perception of pain, suffering, and pain-related behaviors, and is defined by the International Association for the Study of Pain as "an unpleasant sensory and emotional experience associated with actual or potential tissue damage, or described in terms of such damage." The inability to communicate (verbally or because of altered consciousness) in no way negates the fact that pain may exist. Pain can occur in the absence of input from peripheral nociceptors (e.g., phantom limb pain, CNS-induced pain) and depends on but is not limited to somatic and visceral sensory input, conditioned environmental cues, memory, and activity. In other words, pain is not homogenous but represents a continuum of varied physiologic and behavioral responses that are unique to each animal.

Taxonomy

Pain has been categorized on the basis of disease (arthritis, pancreatitis, cancer), anatomy (bladder, pancreatic, back, orthopedic), general location (superficial, visceral, deep), duration (transient, acute, chronic), intensity (mild, moderate, severe), and response to manipulation (palpation, response to commands, algesiometers). Each category attempts to suggest potential causes for pain, its severity, and by association, the most appropriate therapy. Although they are descriptive, none of these methods identify the mechanism(s) responsible for pain and therefore provide minimal therapeutic insight. Ultimately, pain should be categorized on the basis of the mechanism(s) responsible for its production. Current conceptual mechanisms include alterations in nociceptive transduction, peripheral sensitization, altered excitability, central sensitization, phenotypic modulation, synaptic reorganization, and disinhibition. As these mechanisms are studied and become better understood, rational pain therapy will follow. Until that time, the best approach to categorizing pain is to understand its evolution from purely physiologic and protective to pathologic and harmful.

- Physiologic pain is frequently referred to as *nociceptive pain* because it is dependent on the activation of high-threshold peripheral pain receptors (nociceptors) by excessive pressure, heat, cold, chemical, or electrical irritants. This is the type of pain an animal feels when it is pinched, poked, or aggressively palpated or when it briefly comes in contact with a potentially harmful entity. Physiologic or nociceptive pain is highly localized, often transient, serving to warn the body of potential danger or tissue damage, which is why its intensity is highly correlated to reflex withdrawal responses. All other types of pain can be considered pathologic or clinical, arising for the most part from tissue (inflammatory) or nerve (neuropathic) damage.

- Pathologic pain can occur in the absence of a stimulus or in response to innocuous stimuli (allodynia), often producing an exaggerated (hyperalgesia) and prolonged (hyperpathia) response. The acute form of pathologic pain, like physiologic pain, serves a protective function leading to disuse, rest and recuperation, guarding, and avoidance, thereby minimizing further injury and promoting repair processes (Fig. 2-7). Exaggerated (extensive trauma) or prolonged (chronic) pain, however, far exceeds any protective role and disrupts homeostasis, initiating considerable suffering and producing abnormal and unexpected behaviors that may contribute to the clinical decision to euthanize an animal. In fact, abnormal or unexpected behaviors (aggression) are

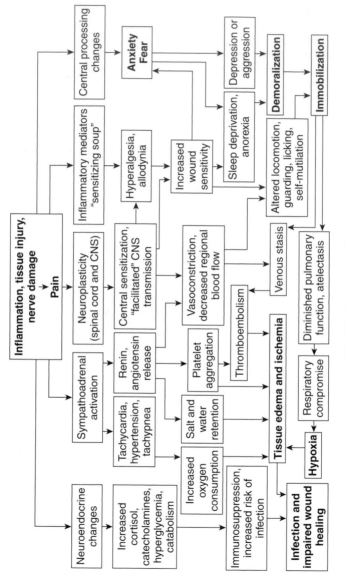

Fig. 2-7 Consequences of pain.

relatively common in small animal veterinary practice in spite of or because of the administration of analgesic drugs, emphasizing the need for careful evaluation before selection of the appropriate analgesic therapy.

- Aggression is recognized as one of the most common abnormal behaviors in dogs and cats and can be induced by pain and many drugs used to produce analgesia and sedation (release of suppressed behavior). Aggression is particularly common in dogs and cats when they are frightened, experiencing pain, during the postoperative period when they are recovering from anesthesia, are semiconscious, and are under the influence of anesthetic drugs. It is during this time that the clinician or veterinary technician must be particularly astute in identifying abnormal behavior and determining whether it is pain-related, thereby facilitating appropriate therapy and avoiding unnecessary drug administration.

- The inability to adequately treat pathologic pain and control suffering is a potential cause for euthanasia (relinquishment) in animals.

Painful Sensations

Although truly rational therapeutic approaches cannot be developed until most, if not all, of the specific mechanisms responsible for physiologic and pathologic pain are known, the use of simple yet detailed pain scoring systems can help categorize the intensity, duration, and topography of pain, thereby suggesting potential treatments or the benefits of treatment (see Chapter 6). Pain scoring systems, however, are of little value in suggesting therapy until the evaluator has a general understanding of the physiologic and pathophysiologic processes involved in the production of pain. An understanding of these processes implies an understanding of the reasons for tissue hypersensitivity, peripheral sensitization, primary and secondary hyperalgesia, central sensitization, allodynia, spontaneous and referred pain, and the differences between somatic and visceral pain. All of these changes modify the gain of the system and can lead to CNS modification and phenotypic (physical characteristics) changes. To rephrase an often-quoted saying, "No gain, no pain."

- Pain is produced by activation of functionally specialized $A\delta$ and C nerve terminal nociceptors, which transduce noxious stimuli dependent on distinct thermal, mechanical, chemical, and electrical thresholds. The free nerve endings of these afferent pain processing fibers encode noxious stimuli, depending on the modality, intensity, duration, and location of the stimulus.

- The intensity of the stimulus that produces pain is considerably greater than that required to elicit innocuous sensations and is the most important factor in determining the severity of pain. It can be quantitatively defined by a stimulus intensity–response relationship similar to that of other somatosensatons (see Fig. 2-2).

- In the absence of tissue damage, nociceptor-mediated pain is considered to be physiologic, warning the animal of potentially harmful stimuli (Fig. 2-8). Most pathologic pain occurs after tissue or nerve damage, and as stated previously, has been clinically categorized as inflammatory or neuropathic.

- Unlike physiologic pain, pathologic pain can be produced by stimulation of large myelinated Aβ nerve fibers, which normally do not transmit painful sensations. The temporal aspects of pathologic pain continuously change (dynamic plasticity) and are characterized by a reduction in the intensity of the stimulus required to initiate pain (hypersensitivity) and a leftward shift in the stimulus-response curve (Fig. 2-9). The development of tissue hypersensitivity (nociceptive sensitization) is responsible for allodynia, hyperalgesia, and hyperpathia.

Peripheral Sensitization

Peripheral sensitization is produced by neurochemical alterations caused by tissue damage and inflammation at the site of injury and in the immediately surrounding tissues, resulting in hyperalgesia at the site of injury (primary hyperalgesia). The release and activation of intracellular components from damaged cells, inflammatory cells

---

Fig. 2-8 Physiologic pain: Non–tissue-damaging stimuli activate peripheral pain receptors (nociceptors; R), which produce electrical signals that are transmitted by Aδ and C sensory nerve fibers to the spinal cord and brain. Glutamate is the primary neurotransmitter released at the nerve terminal in the spinal cord (central terminals). Glutamate primarily activates AMPA/KAI, producing transient or temporary ("ouch") pain.

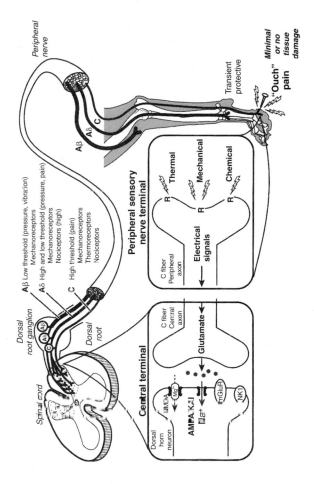

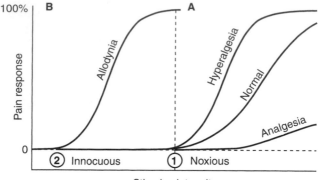

Fig. 2-9 The normal stimulus intensity-pain response curve is shown (**A**). Increased responsiveness to a given stimulus that shifts the curve to the left is termed *hyperalgesia*. A decrease in the response to a given stimulus that shifts the curve to the right or flattens the curve is termed *analgesia* or *anesthesia*. A large left shift in the curve such that innocuous stimuli begin to elicit a painful response (**B**) is termed *allodynia*.

(lymphocytes, neutrophils, mast cells, macrophages), postganglionic sympathetic efferent nerve terminals, and the primary nerve fiber itself both excite and increase the sensitivity of peripheral nociceptors (Table 2-4). Direct tissue damage results in the local release and spread of ATP, ions (H^+, K^+), prostaglandins, bradykinin, and nerve growth factors (NGFs). Lymphocytes, neutrophils, and macrophages release cytokines (interleukin 1 [IL-1], IL-6, and tumor necrosis factor alpha [TNF-α]). Mast cell degranulation increases the local concentration of 5-hydroxytryptamine (5-HT; serotonin) and histamine. Sympathetic nerve fibers release substances (catecholamines, neuropeptide Y) that potentiate inflammatory mediators that amplify the local inflammatory response. Primary afferent sensory nerve fibers release neuropeptides (substance P, CGRP), which cause degranulation of mast cells, local vasodilation, and plasma extravasation, resulting in a further amplification of the inflammatory response and a spread of hypersensitivity to surrounding tissues (secondary hyperalgesia). Together these substances produce a "sensitizing soup,"

TABLE 2-4

**Activation and Sensitization of Nociceptors
("Sensitizing Soup")**

Substance	Origin	Effect
Hydrogen ion	Damaged cells	Activation
Potassium ion	Damaged cells	Activation
Prostaglandins (PGE_2)	Damaged cells	Sensitization
Leukotrienes	Damaged cells	Sensitization
Bradykinin	Plasma	Activation
Serotonin	Platelets, mast cells	Activation
Histamine	Mast cells	Activation
Substance P	Sensory nerve endings	Sensitization
Nerve growth factor	Sensory nerve endings	Sensitization

---

which changes high-threshold nociceptors to low-threshold nociceptors and activates the so-called silent nociceptors (10% to 40% of the total nociceptor population) found in joints and visceral and cutaneous tissues, amplifying the pain response (Fig. 2-10).

Central Sensitization

Central sensitization is produced by a change in the excitability of neurons in the spinal cord and/or activation of spinal cord glial cells and therefore contributes to primary hyperalgesia, but more importantly, it is responsible for pain hypersensitivity outside the area of primary hyperalgesia (secondary hyperalgesia, extraterritorial pain). Mild, infrequent, noxious stimuli generate fast excitatory potentials within the CNS (spinal cord, brainstem, and brain) that indicate the onset, duration, intensity, and location of the painful stimulus (Box 2-1). This fast excitatory transmission is transmitted by Aδ and C fibers and is mediated by glutamate acting on AMPA and KAI ligand–gated ion channels within the dorsal horn of the spinal cord. The sensory input is focused by descending activation of inhibitory neurons that co-release glycine and GABA, two CNS inhibitory neurotransmitters. Frequent (chronic) or severe peripheral nociceptor input initiated by inflammation or tissue damage, by contrast, results in the central release of neuromodulators (substance P,

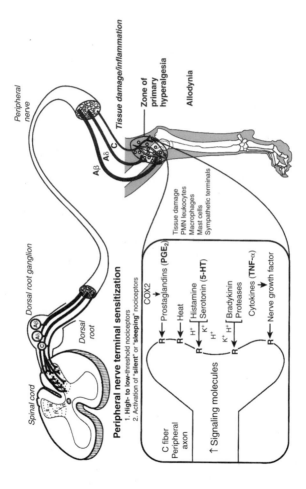

Fig. 2-10 Inflammation and tissue damage produce a variety of nociceptor-sensitizing substances, including prostaglandins, histamine, serotonin, bradykinin, proteases, cytokines (TNF-α), and nerve growth factor. This "sensitizing soup" lowers the nociceptor threshold to painful stimuli and activates "silent" or "sleeping" nociceptors, resulting in hyperalgesia and allodynia.

BOX 2-1

Mechanisms Responsible for Prolonged and Exaggerated Pain

- Peripheral sensitization (inflammatory soup)
- "Wind-up" (temporal summation of sensory inputs)
- Central sensitization
- Increased sympathetic innervation and excitation of dorsal root ganglion (DRG)
- Disinhibition of inhibitory modulation of sensory inputs
- Redistribution of Aβ inputs from laminae III/IV to lamina II
- Abnormal patterns of spinal cord interneuronal communication
- Altered phenotype of damaged sensory nerve fibers
- Abnormal patterns of peripheral nerve regeneration after trauma

---

neurokinin A, CGRP) including glutamate, which activates NMDA (removes the Mg^{2+} block), neurokinin, and mGluR, providing for temporal and spatial summation ("wind-up") of noxious stimuli and a prolonged increase in sensitization (long-term potentiation [LTP]) of neurons in the dorsal horn of the spinal cord. Sensitization of dorsal horn neurons can last for hours and is believed to be responsible for increases in the receptive field properties (spatial, threshold, temporal, modality), secondary hyperalgesia, and allodynia (Fig. 2-11). Decreases in phasic and tonic inhibition from higher CNS centers and a loss of segmental inhibitory interneurons in the dorsal horn can also contribute to dorsal horn hyperexcitability, resulting in the perception of pain from otherwise innocuous stimuli carried by Aβ nerve fibers (receptive field plasticity). Nerve injury can stimulate

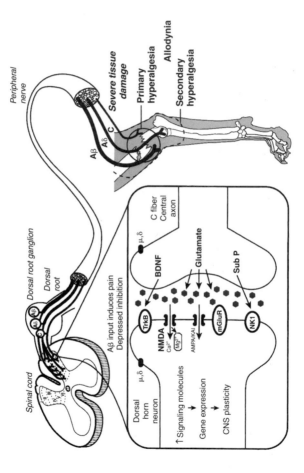

Fig. 2-11 Severe (high-intensity) or chronic painful stimuli activate C fibers, causing the release of glutamate, substance P (Sub P), and brain derived neurotrophic factor (BDNF) at central nerve terminals; this results in the activation of AMPA/KAI, NMDA, NK, and Trk B receptors, producing acute and long-lasting dull, aching, burning pain sensations. Collectively the activation of these receptors increases the activity of a host of signaling molecules that alter gene expression and change the responsiveness (sensitize) of the CNS to subsequent input. Chronic painful stimulation may result in neurochemical changes (neuroplasticity) in the spinal cord such that all stimuli produce pain.

---

the growth of the central terminals of low-threshold mechanoreceptors (Aβ fibers), which normally terminate in lamina IV, into lamina II, the location of C-fiber terminals, providing the anatomic substrate for tactile pain hypersensitivity and spontaneous pain.

• Central sensitization is fundamentally different from peripheral sensitization in that it enables both low-intensity stimuli and low-threshold Aβ sensory fibers to produce pain as a result of changes in sensory processing in the spinal cord.

• Central sensitization, phenotypic switches, and disinhibition are all responsible for increases in the responsiveness of dorsal horn neurons to sensory input (allodynia), receptive field plasticity, continued pain even after amputation (phantom limb pain), and the discomfort and agony experienced by severely injured patients and patients with chronic diseases.

• Wind-up, central sensitization, and the development of a structurally reorganized hyperactive CNS represent a continuum of the pain process, which exists as a consequence of continuous, unrelenting, and untreated pain

• The production of central sensitization within the CNS and, more specifically, the brain may be responsible for memory, or at least the modification of memory. Continued noxious stimuli lasting longer than several hours result in the upregulation of immediate-early genes (c-fos, c-jun), which are regulated by the cyclic adenosine monophosphate (cAMP) response element-binding protein (CREB) and are responsible for activity-dependent plasticity and long-term structural changes (neuroplastic) within the CNS.

Visceral Versus Somatic Pain

Many similarities exist between visceral and somatic pain at the spinal cord level and proceeding cranially. Nociceptive-specific fibers do not appear to be present in the viscera, however. Visceral afferent painful stimuli originating from visceral organs (e.g., gut, liver, spleen, kidney, bladder) are transmitted by Aδ and C fibers along sympathetic and parasympathetic pathways. Parasympathetic, principally vagal, and splanchnic afferent nerve fibers are also responsible for transmitting noxious inputs from visceral organs, including the distal colon (rectum) and bladder. This difference (transmission by sympathetic and parasympathetic pathways) means that most inputs coming from viscera are not perceived. Clamping, burning (cautery), and cutting generally produce no pain when applied to visceral structures. Generalized or diffuse inflammation, ischemia, and mesenteric stretching or dilation (e.g., gastric dilatation-volvulus) may produce severe unrelenting pain. Inflammation and tissue damage are also known to activate a large population of "silent" nociceptors in the gut and bladder, which produce mechanosensitivity in response to otherwise innocuous smooth muscle contractile activity.

- Visceral nociception, unlike somatic nociception, is much more responsive to κ-opioid receptor agonists. The systemic and local administration of the κ-opioid receptor agonist butorphanol may be more effective in treating visceral (colonic, urinary bladder) pain (mg/mg basis) than morphine, a classic μ-opioid agonist.
- Visceral afferent nerve fibers are important in modulating the enteric nervous system, including the gastroesophageal, duodenogastric, colonogastric, rectocolonic, peritoneogastroinitestinal, and voiding reflex loops.
- Reflex regulation of visceral structures also includes motor-secretory and motor-vascular reflexes triggered by extrinsic innervation and axon reflexes, extraspinal and spinal pathways, and splanchnovagal and vagovagal pathways.
- Vagal afferents terminate in the brainstem, and splanchnic afferents proceed through the spinal cord via the spinothalamic and spinoreticular tracts. The nucleus tractus solitarius is the major projection site for vagal and splanchnic afferent inputs, and the dorsal motor nucleus of the vagus nerve also plays a role in the integration of sensory information passing to the PAG and thalamus.

Referred Pain

As the name implies, referred pain is pain involving tenderness, allodynia, and hyperalgesia that is felt in uninjured, intact tissues remote from the presumed causative lesion. Referred pain develops slowly, is generally triggered by deep somatic and visceral rather than superficial injury, and conforms to the "dermatomal rule," whereby pain is often referred to regions derived from the same dermatome. The best examples of referred pain are those associated with stimulation of the visceral afferent nerve fibers and the referral of pain to other muscles, tendons, and joints in the same dermatome. Potential explanations for referred pain include: (1) the peripheral branching of primary sensory nerve fibers to both cutaneous and deep tissues or the branching of primary sensory nerve fibers to both an injured and uninjured referred area, (2) the activation of primary sensory nerve fibers that project to both (left and right) dorsal horns of the spinal cord, and (3) the convergence of primary sensory nerve fibers from different tissue beds on the same population of dorsal horn neurons. The latter explanations emphasize a potential central mechanism in the mediation of referred pain and the potentiation of reflexes from remote tissue regions.

Memory of Pain

In human patients, the perception and memory of pain correlates strongly with the peak intensity of pain but, interestingly, not with its duration. "In primitive life forms whose genome we have inherited, memory subserves only nociception." Furthermore, pain is more likely to occur and be more severe in patients who have a history of injury, suggesting that injury produces central changes that influence nociceptive behavior. The same types of biologic processes and genetic modifications are known to occur in animals in response to painful stimuli. Furthermore, if painful stimuli establish the memory of pain, then therapies that prevent central sensitization and the neuroplastic changes that occur should be beneficial in maintaining or restoring normal pain sensitivity. This argument is the basis for "preemptive" analgesia, in which analgesic therapy administered before a painful event will prevent or reduce subsequent pain and analgesic requirements in comparison with the same analgesic given after a painful event (e.g., surgery). Once hyperexcitability (central sensitization) is established, large doses of analgesic agents are required or the therapy becomes ineffective. In other words, all pain should be treated as early as possible and preemptively when possible.

CONCLUSION

The mechanisms responsible for the production and maintenance of pain are being unraveled. There is no question concerning the role of sensory nerve endings and the nervous system in transducing and transmitting sensations to the brain. Alternative mechanisms regarding pain perception, however, are emerging and suggest that pain can be elicited by the production of inflammatory molecules that travel to the brain through the bloodstream ("humoral" signaling). These molecules increase the concentration of inflammatory signaling molecules in the brain (IL-1β), leading to the enhanced expression of cyclooxygenase-2 and prostaglandin E synthase (two prominent pain inducers) in the cerebrospinal fluid and enhanced pain response and hypersensitivity. The bloodborne inflammatory molecules remain unknown but provide fertile ground for the continued exploration of mechanisms that initiate and transmit painful events and suggest new avenues for the development of pain therapies.

SUGGESTED READINGS

Byers MR, Bonica JJ: Peripheral pain mechanisms and nociceptor plasticity. In Loeser JD, Butler SH, Chapman CR, et al, editors: *Bonica's management of pain,* ed 3. Philadelphia, 2001, Lippincott Williams & Wilkins.

Dray A: Inflammatory mediators of pain, *Br J Anaesth* 75:125-131, 1995.

Fields HL, Heinricher MM, Mason P: Neurotransmitters in nociceptive modulatory circuits, *Annu Rev Neurosci* 14:219-245, 1991.

Fields HL, Basbaum AI: Central nervous system mechanisms of pain modulation. In Wall PD, Melzack R, editors: *Textbook of pain,* ed 4, Edinburgh, 1999, Churchill Livingstone.

Kandel ER: Nerve cells and behavior. In Kandel ER, Schwartz JH, Jessel TM, editors: *Principles of neural science,* ed 3, Norwalk, Conn, 1991, Appleton & Lange.

Koltzenburg M: The changing sensitivity in the life of the nociceptor, *Pain Suppl* 6:S93-S102, 1999.

Levine JD, Reichling DB: Peripheral mechanisms of inflammatory pain. In Wall PD, Melzack R, editors: *Textbook of pain,* ed 4, Edinburgh, 1999, Churchill Livingstone.

Maier SF, Watkins LR: Cytokines for psychologists: implications of bidirectional immune-to-brain communication for understanding behavior, mood, and cognition, *Psychol Rev* 105:83-107, 1998.

Melzack R, Wall PD: Pain mechanisms: a new theory, *Science* 150:971-979, 1965.

Milan MJ: The induction of pain: an integrative review, *Prog Neurobiol* 57:1-164, 1999.

Raja SN, Meyer RA, Ringkamp M, et al: Peripheral neural mechanisms of nociceptor. In Wall PD, Melzack R, editors: *Textbook of pain,* ed 4, Edinburgh, 1999, Churchill Livingstone.

Rexed B: The cytoarchitectonic organization of the spinal cord in the cat, *J Comp Neurol* 96:415-466, 1952.

Ru-Rong J, Woolf CJ: Neuronal plasticity and signal transduction in nociceptive neurons: implications for the initiation and maintenance of pathological pain, *Neurobiol Dis* 8:1-10, 2001.

Sandkuhler J: The organization and function of endogenous antinociceptive systems, *Prog Neurobiol* 50:49-81, 1996.

Snider WD, McMahon SB: Tackling pain at the source: new ideas about nociceptors, *Neuron* 20:629-632, 1998.

Watkins LR: Gial activation: a driving force for pathological pain, *Trends Neurosci* 24:450-455, 2001.

Willis WD, Coggeshall RE: *Sensory mechanisms of the spinal cord,* New York, 1991, Plenum Press.

Willis AD, Westlund KN: Neuroanatomy of the pain system and of the pathways that modulate pain, *J Clin Neurophysiol* 14:2-31, 1997.

Woolf CJ: Excitability changes in central neurons following peripheral damage: role of central sensitization in the pathogenesis of pain. In Willis WD Jr, editor: *Hyperalgesia and allodynia,* New York, 1992, Raven Press.

Woolf CJ, Chong M: Preemptive analgesia: treating postoperative pain by preventing the establishment of central sensitization, *Anesth Analg* 77:362-379, 1993.

Woolf CJ, Costigan M: Transcriptional and posttranslational plasticity and the generation of inflammatory pain, *Proc Natl Acad Sci U S A* 96:7723-7730, 1999.

Woolf CJ, Salter MW: Neuronal plasticity: increasing the gain in pain, *Science* 288:1765-1768, 2000.

Yaksh TL: Spinal systems and pain processing: development of novel analgesic drugs with mechanistically defined models, *Trends Pharmacol Sci* 20:329-337, 1999.

3

Pain and Stress

WILLIAM W. MUIR III

Most people would agree that to ensure animal well-being, we must do what is right for the animal. At a minimum, "what is right" should include the "five freedoms": freedom from hunger and malnutrition, freedom from discomfort, freedom from disease, freedom from injury, and freedom from pain. Stress is the biologic response that an animal exhibits when homeostasis is threatened. No stress occurs unless the animal perceives a threat. Both conscious (e.g., physical restraint, pain) and unconscious (e.g., pain caused by cancer) stressors can elicit a stress response. Historically, most authors have concerned themselves with the body's response to injury and surgical trauma. More recently, however, the importance of the central nervous system (CNS) in modifying the body's response to various stressors (e.g., pain, surgery, and confinement) has become appreciated. Auditory and visual stimuli can produce and potentiate somatosensory input to the CNS, eliciting systemic responses identical to those produced by tissue trauma. This input may be further modified by the animal's memory, evoking predictable behavioral changes characterized by fear, an attempt to either escape or exhibit aggression (fight or flight), or submission. Dogs and cats, like all animals, respond to stressors by exhibiting one or more biologic defense mechanisms targeted toward maintaining homeostasis. Stress then serves a protective role of diverting the body's biologic resources to cope with the stressor. Normally, bodily homeostatic mechanisms function to continually maintain an internal state of well-being. Ineffective responses to stress result in distress, dysfunction, disability, disease, and death (Fig. 3-1).

Whether dogs and cats perceive pain and suffer in the same way that humans do is arguable on the basis of their ability to comprehend pain and the potential for impending doom. Most argue that animals are principally aware of the present with little or no regard for the past or future; they live in "the now." They do not comprehend death. Ultimately, it is the animal's health and interaction with its environment and ongoing external events that determine its well-being. These processes incorporate feeling, perceiving, and awareness and are the simplest of the cognitive processes. In other words, if an animal perceives an event as threatening, its responses will be the same, whether the event is threatening or not. Everyone at some time has probably witnessed the "fight or flight" response in a dog or cat put in a new environment, whether that environment was threatening or not. Therefore it is both ethical and humane to minimize animal stress because all animals react adversely to real or perceived tissue-damaging or life-threatening situations. Both acute and chronic pain are capable of producing a stress response. Pain normally serves a protective function by warning the animal of real or impending tissue damage, but when it is severe, pain can be responsible for temporary periods of "stress-induced analgesia," dramatic increases in neuroendocrine activity, and profound behavioral changes. Even without a painful stimulus, environmental factors (e.g., loud noise, restraint, predators) can produce a state of anxiety or fear that can sensitize and amplify the stress response to a painful stimulus. Distress, an exaggerated form of stress, is present when the biologic cost of stress negatively affects the biologic functions that are critical to the animal's well-being. Therefore pain should be thought of in terms of the stress response that it produces, its potential to produce significant distress, and the degree of animal suffering incurred. In practical terms, the severity and duration of pain determine the location of the patient's pain on the continuum of stress and suffering.

DEFINING TERMS

Pain

Pain is often defined as "an unpleasant sensory and emotional experience associated with actual or potential tissue damage or described in terms of such damage" (see Chapter 4). Pain produces physical or mental uneasiness that ranges from mild discomfort or dull distress to acute, often unbearable, agony. Pain may be generalized or localized, is the consequence of physical injury, and usually produces a desire to avoid, escape, or destroy (autonomy) the factors responsible for

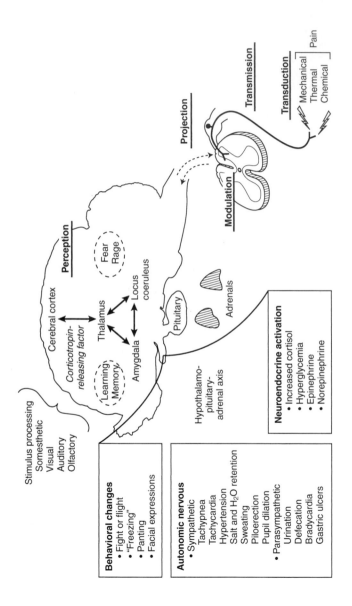

Fig. 3-1 Activation of the neural circuits (transduction, transmission, modulation, projection, perception) responsible for producing pain stimulate the thalamus, locus ceruleus (LC), and amygdala, which induce fear, anxiety, and rage in animals, resulting in behavioral, autonomic, and neuroendocrine changes. Acute pain often produces fear, increased vigilance, and immobilization ("freezing" stance) in some animals, and chronic unrelenting pain can lead to loss of appetite, tissue catabolism, and immunosuppression and can alter learning patterns and memory.

---

producing the pain. Untreated or prolonged painful conditions promote an extended and destructive pain response, characterized by neuroendocrine dysregulation, fatigue, dysphoria, myalgia, abnormal behavior, and altered physical performance.

Stress

Stress consists of the biologic responses of an animal in an attempt to cope with a disruption or threat to homeostasis. A stressor is a physical, chemical, or emotional factor (e.g., trauma, fear) to which an individual fails to make a satisfactory adaptation and that causes physiologic tensions that may be contributory causes of disease.

Distress

Distress is the state produced when the biologic cost of stress negatively affects biologic functions critical to the animal's well-being. Distress also means to cause pain or suffering or to make miserable.

Suffering

Suffering is defined as a perception or feeling of impending destruction or harm; the endurance of or submission to physical or mental affliction, pain, or loss.

BIOLOGIC COMPONENTS OF THE STRESS RESPONSE

The stress response is an adaptive pattern of behavioral, neural, endocrine, immune, hematologic, and metabolic changes directed toward the restoration of homeostasis (Box 3-1).

Most stress is short-lived because of the removal of or short duration of exposure to the stressor. The nature, magnitude, and duration

---

BOX 3-1
Biologic Stress Response

- Behavioral
- Autonomic nervous system
- Neuroendocrine
- Immunologic

- Hematologic
- Metabolic
- Morphologic

BOX 3-2
Systemic Effects of the Stress Response

- Activation of central nervous system (CNS)
    Hypothalamus, amygdala, locus ceruleus (LC)
- Increases in CNS sympathetic output
    Catecholamines
- Endocrine "stress" response
    Pituitary hormone secretion
    Adrenal hormone secretion
- Glucosemia
- Insulin resistance
- Cytokine production
- Acute-phase reaction
- Neutrophil leukocytosis
- Immunologic and hematologic changes

---

of the specific stimulus are important factors in determining the extent of the adaptive responses elicited in the animal. Manipulation of a dog's hip joint or physical restraint of a cat, for example, elicits a relatively brief stress response. During more threatening circumstances, the stress response prepares the animal for an emergency reaction and fosters survival in circumstances of immediate threats (fight or flight). Acute pain is capable of producing a significant stress response in dogs and cats. Pain induced by surgical or accidental trauma evokes responses characterized by activation of the sympathetic nervous system, secretion of glucocorticoids (primarily cortisol), hypermetabolism, sodium and water retention, and altered carbohydrate and protein metabolism (Box 3-2). When stress is se-

---

BOX 3-3
Behavioral Indicators of Stress and Pain

- Appetite
- Activity
- Facial expression
- Appearance
- Attitude

- Vocalization
- Activity
- Posture
- Aggression
- Response to handling

---

vere or allowed to continue for an extended time, it becomes maladaptive, producing distress and the triggering of self-sustaining cascades of neural and endocrine responses that upset the animal's physiologic homeostasis. Severe pain produces behavioral, autonomic, neuroendocrine, and immunologic responses that can lead to self-mutilation, immune incompetence, and gradual deterioration, culminating in death. Prior experience (memory) and current physical status (health, pain state) play an important role in determining the animal's behavioral response and ability to adapt.

BEHAVIORAL INDICATORS OF STRESS AND PAIN

Pain is a stressor, and as such it is responsible for changes in brain function (neural plasticity) that correlate with behavioral modifications, the level of alertness, learning performance, and memory (Box 3-3). Intense stimulation of sensory (somatosensory, visual, acoustic) inputs to the brain activates the locus ceruleus (LC), limbic regions (e.g., hypothalamus, hippocampus, amygdala), and the cerebral cortex, which are involved in adaptive responses to stress. A stress as mild as a cat being confronted by a dog, for example, can double or triple neuronal activity in these stress centers, leading to concurrent activation of a "stress response," which includes behavioral changes. Pain-induced increases in levels of corticotropin-releasing factor (CRF) in the hypothalamus, amygdala, and LC, for example, produce an increased startle response, anxiety, fear, and in some animals, rage. Therefore CRF serves as an excitatory neurotransmitter in the LC, resulting in the release of cortical norepinephrine, dopamine, and 5-hydroxtryptamine (5-HT) and hyperresponsiveness, hyperarousal, vigilance, and agitation. Prolonged

---

BOX 3-4
Common Indicators of Pain in Dogs and Cats

Dogs
- Decreased social interaction
- Anxious expression
- Submissive behavior
- Refusal to move
- Whimpering
- Howling
- Growling
- Guarding behavior
- Aggression; biting
- Loss of appetite
- Self-mutilation

Cats
- Reduced activity
- Loss of appetite
- Quiet/loss of curiosity
- Hiding
- Hissing or spitting
- Excessive licking/grooming
- Stiff posture/gait
- Guarding behavior
- Attempts to escape
- Cessation of grooming
- Tail flicking

---

stress impairs the animal's ability to learn and can change the animal's behavior.

Indicators of pain in dogs and cats can frequently be determined by changes in behavior (Box 3-4). A limp, for example, is an obvious indicator of acute pain or chronic injury. Observation of changes in a dog's or cat's behavior may be the most noninvasive and promising method for determining the severity of an animal's pain and associated stress.

AUTONOMIC NERVOUS SYSTEM

An increase in sympathetic nervous system activity is one of the principal efferent effects initiated by the stress response. Sensory activation of the hypothalamus results in graded increases in CNS sympathetic output, causing increases in heart rate and arterial blood pressure, sweating, piloerection, and pupil dilation. The secretion of catecholamines from the adrenal medulla and the spillover of norepinephrine released from postganglionic sympathetic nerve terminals augment these central effects. Increased concentrations of circulating catecholamines augment glycogenolysis, increase gluconeogenesis, inhibit insulin release, and promote insulin resistance and lipolysis. Skeletal muscle blood flow may be increased out of

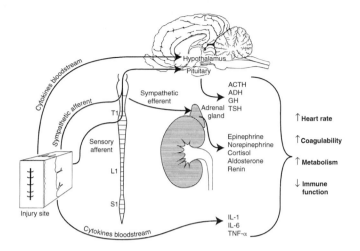

Fig. 3-2 Acute surgical stimulation initiates the release of cytokines (IL 1, IL-6, TNF-α) into the bloodstream and activation of the hypothalamo-pituitary-adrenocorticol (HPA) system axis and sympathetic nervous system. Activation of hypothalamus and pituitary releases adrenocorticotropic hormone (ACTH), vasopressin (or antidiuretic hormone [ADH]), growth hormone (GH), and thyroid-stimulating hormone (TSH). Sympathetic nervous system activation initiates the release of epinephrine, norepinephrine, cortisol, aldosterone, and renin. Together these changes can alter hemodynamics, which elevates heart rate; increase the coagulability of blood predisposing to thrombosis; increase metabolism and caloric requirements; and when exaggerated, depress immune function.

proportion to increases in blood flow to other organ systems, which prepares the animal for fight or flight.

NEUROENDOCRINE AXIS

The neuroendocrine axis can be defined as the biologic interface for afferent sensory input and humoral communication between the CNS and the peripheral glands or organs that are responsible for mobilizing the stress response (Fig. 3-2). Auditory, visual, and somatosensory afferent sensory information is transmitted to the thalamus or directly to the amygdala, activating the hypothalamo-pituitary-adrenocorticol

(HPA) system axis (Table 3-1). This afferent information stimulates the secretion of CRF and vasoactive intestinal peptide (VIP), which in turn stimulate the pituitary gland to release adrenocorticotropic hormone (ACTH), melanocortin, prolactin, vasopressin, thyroid-stimulating hormone (TSH), and growth hormone (GH). The metabolic consequences of these hormonal changes are increased catabolism, the mobilization of substrates to provide energy for tissue repair, and salt and water retention to maintain fluid volume and cardiovascular homeostasis. CRF, ACTH, and corticosterone are all significant modulators of learning and memory processes.

Release of CRF in the Brain

The release of CRF in the brain is one of the major components of the stress response, if not the most important. CRF acts synergistically with vasopressin to stimulate the production of ACTH and β-endorphin, thereby enhancing cell survival and producing analgesic effects, respectively. CRF also stimulates the adrenomedullary release of ACTH and catecholamines. CRF is an excitatory neurotransmitter in the LC, producing increased cortical norepinephrine release and excitation.

Adrenocorticotropic Hormone

ACTH release is stimulated by CRF, catecholamines, vasopressin, and VIP. The primary function of ACTH is to stimulate

---

TABLE 3-1
Neurohumoral Response to Stress

Endocrine Gland	Hormone	Change
Pituitary	ACTH	Increase
	GH	Increase
	Vasopressin	Increase
	TSH	Increase or decrease
Adrenal cortex	Cortisol	Increase
	Aldosterone	Increase
	Catecholamines	Increase
Pancreas	Insulin	Often decreases
	Glucagon	Increase
Thyroid	Thyroxine	Decrease

the adrenal cortex to secrete cortisol, corticosterone, aldosterone, and weak androgenic substances. ACTH also stimulates increased gluco-corticoid production and the adrenomedullary secretion of catechol-amines. ACTH, cortisol, and epinephrine levels are all increased during emergence from anesthesia without surgery, suggesting that anesthesia alone can induce a stress response in animals.

Cortisol

Serum cortisol is commonly measured as an indicator of severity of the stress response in most species. The mortality rate is increased in animals that are not able to increase serum cortisol concentrations. Etomidate, an injectable hypnotic recommended for anesthesia in high-risk cases, is known to increase the mortality rate in very ill human patients as a result of suppression of serum cortisol concentrations. Cortisol stimulates gluconeogenesis, increases proteolysis and lipolysis, facilitates catecholamine effects, and produces antiinflammatory actions.

Catecholamines

Serum concentrations of norepinephrine, epinephrine, and dopamine are increased by CRF. The release of these catecholamines can be responsible for elevations in heart rate, respiratory rate, arterial blood pressure, and cardiac output, leading to an increase in skeletal muscle blood flow that prepares the animal for fight or flight. Epinephrine causes glycogenolysis, gluconeogenesis, inhibition of insulin release, peripheral insulin resistance, and lipolysis.

Glucagon and Insulin

Endogenous endorphins, GH, epinephrine, and glucocorticoids are all capable of stimulating glucagon and insulin (β-adrenergic effect) secretion by the pancreas. More typically, however, surgical procedures increase glucagon secretion and decrease (α effect) insulin secretion, leading to hepatic glycogenolysis, gluconeogenesis from amino acids, glucosemia, and glucosuria.

Other Hormones

A variety of other hormones, including but not limited to GH, TSH, and vasopressin, act together to protect cellular function and restore homeostasis.

Growth Hormone

GH stimulates protein synthesis and inhibits protein breakdown, promotes lipolysis, and produces antiinsulin effects. GH spares glucose for use by the nervous system.

Thyroid Hormones

Thyroxine (T_4) and triiodothyronine (T_3) are secreted into the blood circulation from the thyroid gland during stimulation by TSH. Thyroid hormones stimulate carbohydrate metabolism and heat production and increase and sensitize β-adrenergic receptors in the heart, thereby sensitizing it to the effects of circulating catecholamines.

Vasopressin

Vasopressin, also known as the *antidiuretic hormone,* promotes salt and water retention. Its production and release into the blood circulation in conjunction with increased concentrations of renin (sympathetic effect) increase the circulating blood volume, improving cardiovascular homeostasis.

METABOLISM

The net effect of the majority of the neurohumoral changes produced is an increase in the secretion of catabolic hormones, promoting the production of food substrates from the breakdown of carbohydrates, fats, and protein.

Carbohydrate Metabolism

Hyperglycemia is produced and may persist because of the production of glucagon and relative lack of insulin, although insulin levels may periodically increase. Prolonged hyperglycemia is associated with an increased incidence of wound infection and impaired wound healing.

Fat Metabolism

Lipolytic activity is stimulated by cortisol, catecholamines, and GH, resulting in an increase in circulating glycerol and free fatty acids. Glycerol in turn serves as a source for gluconeogenesis in the liver.

Protein Metabolism

Protein catabolism is a common occurrence and a major concern after severe trauma or extensive surgical procedures. Cortisol increases protein catabolism, resulting in the release of amino acids. These amino acids can be used to form new proteins and to produce glucose and other substrates. Protein supplementation (e.g., glutamine, arginine) during and after surgery results in fewer infections and shorter overall recovery time. Prostaglandins (PGs) (e.g., PGE_2) and cytokines may promote protein catabolism indirectly by increasing the body's energy expenditure.

IMMUNE SYSTEM

Although it is primarily thought of in relation to the identification and destruction of foreign substances, the immune system also functions as a diffusely distributed sense organ that communicates injury-related information to the brain. The immune system can be activated or depressed by stress (Box 3-5). Thus pain, whether accidental or intentional (e.g., surgery), modulates the immune response. The key elements in determining the immune response to pain are its intensity and duration. Chronic pain can produce sustained increases in circulating concentrations of cortisol, epinephrine, norepinephrine, and glucagon, suppressing both the humoral and cellular immune responses. The systemic release of endogenous opioids (endorphin and enkephalin) may contribute to immunosuppression. Mild-to-moderate pain associated with extensive tissue trauma may activate the immune response. The messengers of the immune system are cytokines (e.g., interleukin 1 [IL-1], IL-6, and tumor necrosis factor-α [TNF-α]).

Cytokines

A variety of low-molecular-weight proteins and cytokines are produced from activated leukocytes, fibroblasts, and endothelial cells in

---

BOX 3-5

**Immunologic and Hematologic
Response to Severe Stress**

- Cytokine production
- Acute-phase response
- Neutrophil leukocytosis
- Lymphopenia
- Immune system depression

response to tissue injury. Their role is to protect the body by destroying and removing foreign invaders. They are responsible for the production of a local inflammatory response. When tissue trauma is severe, the excessive production of cytokines can lead to a systemic effect called the *systemic inflammatory response syndrome (SIRS)*. Although pain has never been reported to cause SIRS, it can contribute to its production because it induces similar autonomic and endocrine effects. The major cytokines produced during stress are TNF-α, IL-1, and IL-6.

- IL-1 and IL-6 induce the release of acute-phase (inflammatory) reactants, cause fever, and initiate PG production (e.g., PGE$_2$). IL-1 and IL-6 can stimulate the secretion of ACTH from the pituitary gland and the subsequent release of cortisol.
- TNF-α produces signs of shock, including hypotension, hemoconcentration, hyperglycemia, hyperkalemia, nonrespiratory acidosis, and activation of the complement cascade.

Acute-Phase Response

The acute-phase response can be triggered by severe stress from any cause. The main feature of the acute-phase response is the release of proteins from the liver, which act as inflammatory mediators and scavengers in tissue repair. They include C-reactive protein, fibrinogen, macroglobulin, and antiproteinases. Excessive production of these proteins can contribute to SIRS.

Hematology

The peripheral blood white cell count generally reflects a stress leukogram typified by an elevated number of immature polymorphonuclear leukocytes (left shift) and reduced numbers of lymphocytes.

MORPHOLOGIC CHANGES

Morphologic changes associated with chronic stress or pain are typical of long-term aversive stimuli and include failure to thrive, hair loss or poor coat condition, weight loss, and acceleration of aging.

SUGGESTED READINGS

Carr DB, Goudes LC: Acute pain, *Lancet* 353:2051-2058, 1999.
Carstens E, Moberg GP: Recognizing pain and distress in laboratory animals, *ILAR J* 41(2):62-71, 2000.

Chapman CR, Garvin J: Suffering: the contributions of persistent pain, *Lancet* 353:2233-2237, 1999.

Charney DS, Grillon C, Bremner JD: The neurobiological basis of anxiety and fear: circuits, mechanisms, and neurochemical interactions (part I), *Neuroscientist* 4:35-44, 1998.

Charney DS, Grillon C, Bremner JD: The neurobiological basis of anxiety and fear: circuits, mechanisms, and neurochemical interactions (part II), *Neuroscientist* 4:122-132, 1998.

Clark JD, Rager DR, Calpin JP: Animal well-being I. General considerations, *Lab Anim Sci* 47(6):564-570, 1997.

Clark JD, Rager DR, Calpin JP: Animal well-being II. Stress and distress, *Lab Anim Sci* 47(6):571-585, 1997.

Davis M: The role of the amygdala in fear-potentiated startle: implications for animal models of anxiety, *Trends Pharmacol Sci* 13:35-41, 1992.

Desborough JP: The stress response to trauma and surgery, *Br J Anaesth* 85(1):109-117, 2000.

Weissman C: The metabolic response to stress: an overview and update, *Anesthesia* 73:308-327, 1999.

4

Definitions of Terms Describing Pain

JAMES S. GAYNOR

It is important to have a working understanding of the terminology used to describe pain and analgesia. By knowing the terminology, practitioners can speak intelligently and accurately to one another when discussing cases. The following are definitions, arranged alphabetically, that are commonly used when discussing pain. These terms are used throughout this book.

DEFINITIONS

Acupuncture: The practice of inserting needles at certain points in the skin to achieve specific effects such as pain relief.

Acute pain: Pain that follows some bodily injury, disappears with healing, and tends to be self-limiting.

Allodynia: Pain caused by a stimulus that does not normally cause pain.

Analgesia: The loss of sensitivity to pain.

Anesthesia: Total or partial loss of sensation.

Breakthrough pain: A transient flare-up of pain in the chronic pain setting, which can occur even when chronic pain is under control.

Cancer pain: Pain that can be acute, chronic, or intermittent and is related to the disease itself or to the treatment.

Central sensitization: An increase in the excitability and responsiveness of nerves in the spinal cord.

Chronic pain: Pain that lasts several weeks to months and persists beyond the expected healing time, when nonmalignant in origin.

Epidural: The space above the dura mater.

Hyperalgesia: An increased response to a stimulation that is normally painful (a heightened sense of pain) either at the site of injury (primary) or in surrounding undamaged tissue (secondary, extraterritorial). Stimulated nociceptors respond to noxious stimuli more vigorously and at a lower threshold.

Hyperesthesia: Increased sensitivity to sensation.

Hyperpathia: A painful syndrome characterized by an increased reaction to a stimulus, especially if it is repetitive.

Hypoalgesia: Decreased sensitivity to pain.

Hypoesthesia: Decreased sensitivity to stimulation.

Interventional pain management: Action taken to alter the body's production or transmission of pain signals to the brain. This may involve an invasive procedure to treat or manage pain through an injection of a drug or implantation of a drug delivery device.

Local anesthesia: The temporary loss of sensation in a defined part of the body without loss of consciousness.

Multimodal analgesia: The use of multiple drugs with different actions to produce optimal analgesia.

Myofascial pain: A syndrome of focal pain in a muscle or related tissues, associated with stiffness, muscle spasm, and decreased range of motion.

Neuropathic pain: Pain that originates from injury or involvement of the peripheral or central nervous system (CNS) and is described as burning or shooting, possibly associated with motor, sensory, or autonomic deficits.

Nociception: The transduction, conduction, and CNS processing of nerve signals generated by the stimulation of nociceptors. It is the physiologic process that leads to the perception of pain.

Opioid: A drug that is related naturally or synthetically to morphine.

Pain: *Humans:* An unpleasant sensory and emotional experience associated with actual or potential tissue damage or described in terms of such damage. The inability to communicate in no way negates the possibility that an individual is experiencing pain and is in need of appropriate pain-relieving treatment. *Animals:* An aversive sensation and feeling associated with actual or potential tissue damage.

Pain threshold: The least experience of pain that a patient can recognize.

Pain tolerance level: The greatest level of pain that a patient can tolerate.

Pathologic pain: Pain that has an exaggerated response beyond its protective usefulness. It is often associated with tissue injury incurred at the time of surgery or trauma.

Peripheral sensitization: An increase in the excitability and responsiveness of peripheral nerve terminals.

Physiologic pain: Pain that acts as a protective mechanism that incites individuals to move away from the cause of potential tissue damage or to avoid movement or contact with external stimuli during a reparative phase.

Preemptive analgesia: The administration of an analgesic drug before painful stimulation to prevent sensitization of neurons, or wind-up, thus improving postoperative analgesia.

Regional anesthesia: The loss of sensation in part of the body caused by interruption of the sensory nerves that conduct impulses from that region of the body.

Sedation: CNS depression in which the patient is drowsy but arousable.

Somatic pain: Pain that originates from damage to bones, joints, muscle, or skin and is described by humans as localized, constant, sharp, aching, and throbbing.

Subarachnoid: The space above the pia mater and below the arachnoid mater in which cerebrospinal fluid is found. A subarachnoid injection is also referred to as a *spinal.*

Sympathetic mediated pain: A syndrome in which there is abnormal sympathetic nervous system activity, causing a severe debilitation and often associated with tenderness to a light touch.

Tolerance: A shortened duration and decreased intensity of the analgesic, euphorigenic, sedative, and other CNS-depressant effects, as well as marked elevation in the average dose required to achieve a given effect.

Tranquilization: A state of calmness, mediated through the reticular activating system, in which the patient is relaxed, awake, unaware of surroundings, and potentially indifferent to minor pain.

Visceral pain: Pain that arises from stretching, distension, or inflammation of the viscera and described as deep, cramping, aching, or gnawing, without good localization.

Wind-up: Temporal summation of painful stimuli in the spinal cord. Mediated by C fibers and responsible for "second" pain.

Pain Assessment

5

Pain Behaviors

WILLIAM W. MUIR III AND JAMES S. GAYNOR

- Every animal experiences and demonstrates pain in a unique way. Just because a patient does not display a pain-related behavior, however, does not mean that the patient is not in pain. Although it may be difficult to quantify pain, there are characteristic body positions and behaviors that become recognizable in any animal that is experiencing pain.
- Interactive and unprovoked (noninteractive) behavior assessments may be useful.
- It is important to remember that no behavior by itself is pathognomonic for pain.
- The behavior displayed by an animal depends on many factors, including but not limited to species, age, breed, sex, personality, and the severity and duration of pain (Box 5-1).
- Many animals may display little outward behavior indicative of pain in the presence of humans or other animals, especially potential predators. This behavior may be an innate protective mechanism to prevent a predator from recognizing easy prey.

PAIN BEHAVIORS

Locomotor Activity

Limping and guarding (protecting an injured area from further insult) are clearly the most obvious signs of limb pain, whether long bone, joint, or soft tissue in origin (Figs. 5-1 and 5-2). Limping is a protective behavior to potentially prevent further damage and to decrease pain associated with weight bearing. Stilted gaits, placing excessive weight on the front limbs (hip osteoarthritis), and reluctance to move are also signs of acute or chronic pain.

BOX 5-1

Behavioral and Physiologic Characteristics Associated with Pain in Dogs and Cats

Abnormal Posture
- Hunched-up guarding or splinting of abdomen
- "Praying" position (forequarters on the ground, hindquarters in the air)
- Sitting or lying in an abnormal position
- Not resting in a normal position (e.g., sternal or curled up)
- Statuelike appearance

Abnormal Gait
- Stiff
- Partial or no weight bearing on injured limb
- Slight-to-obvious limp

Abnormal Movement
- Thrashing
- Restless
- Circling

Vocalization
- Screaming
- Whining (intermittent, constant, or when touched)
- Crying (intermittent, constant, or when touched)
- None

Miscellaneous
- Looking, licking, or chewing at the painful area
- Hyperesthesia or hyperalgesia
- Allodynia

Pain-Associated Characteristics That May Also Be Associated with Poor General Health (Medical Problems)
- Restless or agitated
- Trembling or shaking
- Tachypnea or panting
- Weak tail wag
- Low carriage of tail
- Depressed or poor response to caregiver

From Mathew KA: *Vet Clin North Am: Small Anim Pract* 30(4):729-752, 2000.

BOX 5-1
Behavioral and Physiologic Characteristics Associated with Pain in Dogs and Cats—cont'd

Pain-Associated Characteristics That May Also Be Associated with Poor General Health (Medical Problems)—cont'd
- Head hangs down
- Not grooming
- Appetite decreased, picky, or absent
- Dull
- Lying quietly and not moving for hours; does not dream
- Stuporous
- Urinates or defecates and makes no attempt to move
- Recumbent and unaware of surroundings
- Unwilling or unable to walk
- Bites or attempts to bite caregivers

May Also Be Associated with Apprehension or Anxiety
- Restless or agitated
- Trembling or shaking
- Tachypnea or panting
- Weak tail wag
- Low tail carriage
- Slow to rise
- Depressed (poor response to caregiver)
- Not grooming
- Bites or attempts to bite caregiver
- Ears pulled back
- Restless
- Barking or growling (intermittent, constant, or when approached by caregiver)
- Growling or hissing (intermittent, constant, or when approached by caregiver)
- Sitting in the back of the cage or hiding under a blanket (cat)

May Be Normal Behavior
- Reluctant to move head (eye movement only)
- Stretching all four legs when abdomen is touched
- Penile prolapse
- Cleaning (licking) a wound or incision

Continued

BOX 5-1

Behavioral and Physiologic Characteristics Associated with Pain in Dogs and Cats—cont'd

Physiologic Signs That Can Be Associated with Pain
- Tachypnea or panting
- Tachycardia (mild, moderate, or severe)
- Dilated pupils
- Hypertension
- Increased serum cortisol and epinephrine

From Mathew KA: *Vet Clin North Am: Small Anim Pract* 30(4):729-752, 2000.

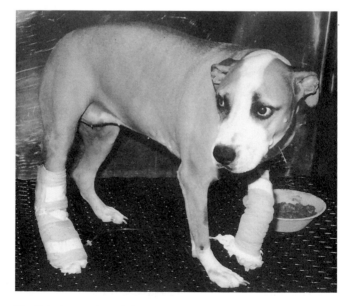

Fig. 5-1 Acute pain. Left foreleg lameness in a dog. Pain causes the dog to lift its left foreleg and walk with a limp.

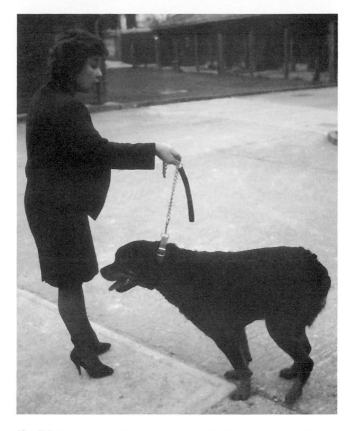

Fig. 5-2 Chronic pain. Severe hip osteoarthritis in a dog. Note that the majority of the dog's weight is being carried on the front legs.

Vocalization

- Vocalization can be associated with painful situations that are mild to severe, depending on the animal's behavior pattern and the environmental circumstances.
- Vocalization is nonspecific. Most practitioners have experienced situations in which animals are anesthetized for minor surgical procedures and wake up vocalizing. Some animals vocalize

postoperatively as a result of emergence delirium associated with recovery from gas anesthesia. This frequently resolves in a short period.
- Some animals will not display many signs of pain until the pain is severe, at which time they may begin to vocalize.
- Vocalization may also be an example of the animal's exhaustion of protective mechanisms (e.g., avoidance, escape) of not displaying pain to potential predators.
- Vocalization in dogs likely manifests as groaning, whining, whimpering, or growling.
- Cats frequently groan, growl, or purr.
- Some animals vocalize postoperatively because of full bladders and the need to urinate. Good nursing practices should not be forgotten when caring for animals in pain.

Altered Facial Expressions and Appearance
Dogs *(Fig. 5-3)*
- Fixed glare, focused
- Glazed appearance
- Oblivious

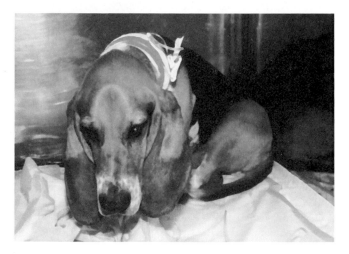

Fig. 5-3 Facial expression. Note the head-down, fixed-gaze, and depressed expression. The dog was oblivious to its environment.

- Depressed
- Ungroomed

Cats *(Fig. 5-4)*
- Furrowed brow
- Squinted eyes (Fig. 5-5)
- Depressed
- Poor hair coat, ungroomed

Body Posture and Activity

Dogs and cats may take on different postures or become reluctant to change position or move, as pain becomes more of a problem.

Reluctance to Move

Animals that are reluctant to move usually have moderate-to-severe pain (Figs. 5-6 to 5-8). This behavior provides protection against movement-induced pain. Usually, slight movement results in some other behavior associated with an abnormal gait (e.g., limping, stilted gait), aggression, or vocalization.

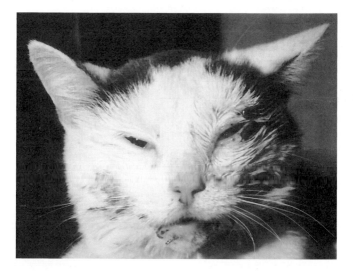

Fig. 5-4 Facial expression. Note the squinted dull eyes and abnormal facial expression.

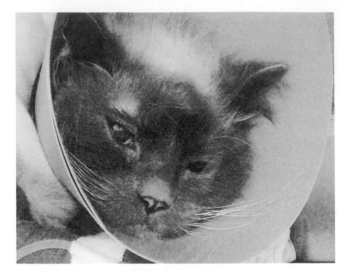

Fig. 5-5 Facial expression. Note the hanging head and squinted eyes.

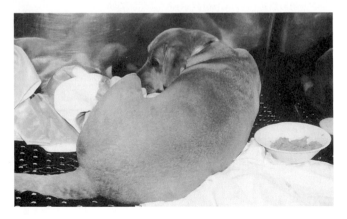

Fig. 5-6 Reluctance to move. Abdominal pain caused this dog to lie facing the back of the cage for hours. Note the depressed expression.

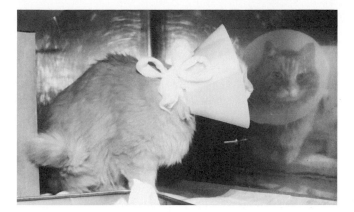

Fig. 5-7 Reluctance to move. Abdominal and bladder pain caused this cat to sit facing the back of the cage for hours.

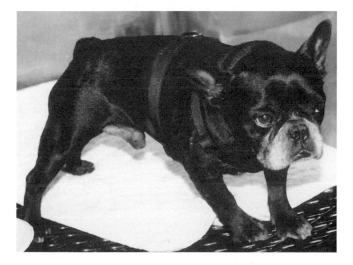

Fig. 5-8 Reluctance to move. Pain caused by trauma to a cervical disk in a dog. Note the statuelike appearance.

Reluctance to Lie Down

Reluctance to lie down is often associated with acute abdominal or thoracotomy pain (Fig. 5-9). Dogs or cats with abdominal pain may sit for hours or assume a "praying" position (Figs. 5-9 and 5-10). Some animals frequently attempt to sit or remain standing for hours. It is common for some animals to fall asleep, slump down, wake up abruptly because of the pain, and then resume their original position (Fig. 5-11).

Changing Positions

Restlessness and frequent changes in body position indicate that an animal is not comfortable. Some dogs may shift from side to side or get up and lie down multiple times (Fig. 5-12). As stated previously, some animals change positions frequently because of a full bladder and may need to have their bladders expressed. Good nursing practices should not be forgotten when caring for animals in pain.

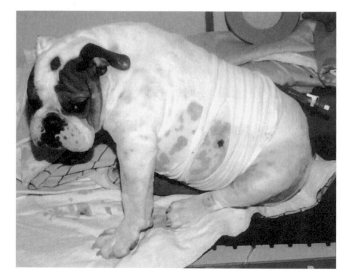

Fig. 5-9 Reluctance to lie down. This dog with traumatic peritonitis would not lie down until exhausted.

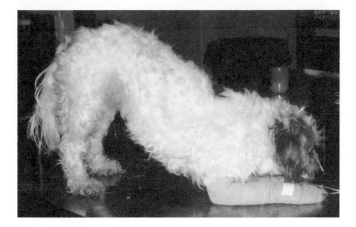

Fig. 5-10 Reluctance to lie down. The so-called praying position characteristic of dogs and cats with abdominal pain.

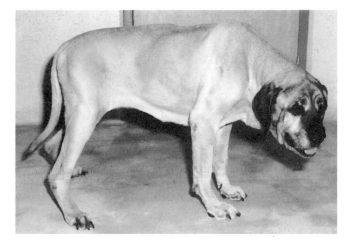

Fig. 5-11 Reluctance to lie down. This dog with chronic bloat and abdominal pain remained standing in one spot until exhausted. Note the head-down, depressed expression.

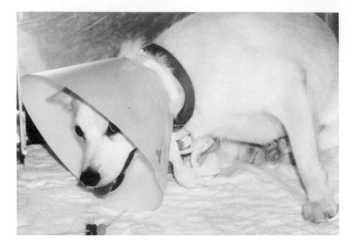

Fig. 5-12 Shifting positions. This dog with abdominal pain would frequently get up and lie down. The dog was careful not to induce more pain, taking several minutes to lie down.

Thrashing
Dogs and cats experiencing severe pain often thrash and are unmanageable. They may become aggressive.

Attitude
- Some animals become submissive or mentally depressed because of acute pain (Fig. 5-13). Depression is more frequently associated with chronic pain, and the animal may be reluctant to move or engage in any activity.
- Dogs and cats may become increasingly aggressive, even those that have never displayed aggression, as their pain becomes more severe (Fig. 5-14).
- Aggression is frequently observed in association with severe acute pain. Often, the slightest manipulation stimulates the patient to attempt to bite the handler.
- Some dogs may become much more timid and fearful.
- Cats are much more likely to hide or attempt to escape (Fig. 5-15).

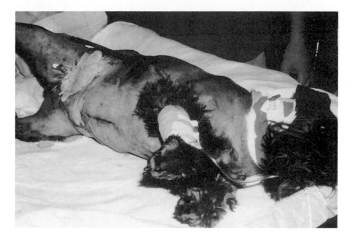

Fig. 5-13 Submissive position. This dog with abdominal trauma demonstrated a submissive posture (on back, rear legs apart, ears flat) when approached.

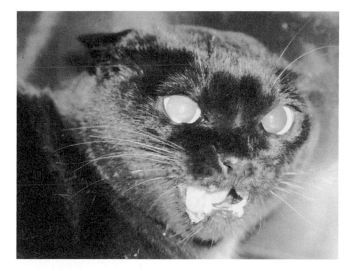

Fig. 5-14 Aggression. Expression of aggression in a cat with a femoral fracture. Note the dilated pupils, flattened ears, and open mouth.

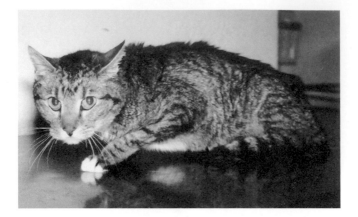

Fig. 5-15 Escape behavior. This cat with chronic pancreatitis attempted to hide or escape when approached. Note the dull, ungroomed hair coat.

Appetite

Anorexia is common in dogs or cats with significant acute or chronic pain. These animals may be misdiagnosed as having some other systemic problem. It is important to determine whether there are concurrent problems that could predispose to anorexia.

Appearance

- Dogs and cats with chronic pain often lose hair coat sheen.
- Cats with chronic pain often fail to groom themselves, resulting in an unkempt appearance (see Fig. 5-15).

Response to Manipulation

- Dogs and cats will frequently respond with purposeful movement and occasionally become aggressive in response to palpation of a painful area. Abdominal splinting or tenseness is often due to abdominal pain, which can be determined only by attempting abdominal palpation. During palpation, animals may try to bite the handler (Fig. 5-16).
- Animals may also become very defensive by protecting the area or by withdrawing to avoid being touched.
- Passive animals may merely freeze or look at the area in question (Figs. 5-17, 5-18, and 5-19).

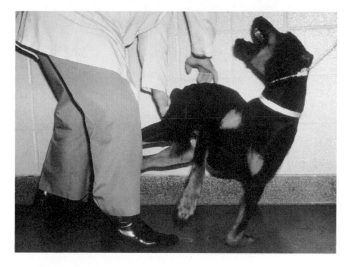

Fig. 5-16 Response to manipulation. This dog became very aggressive any time its pelvis was palpated.

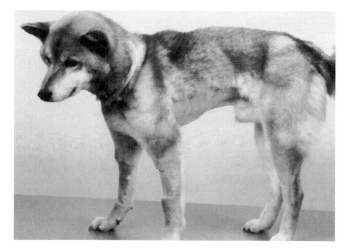

Fig. 5-17 Note the facial expression and tense abdomen in this dog with abdominal pain of unknown origin.

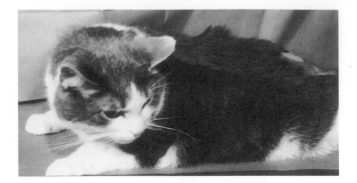

Fig. 5-18 This cat would sit and stare at its rear end. Its tail had been traumatized in an automobile accident.

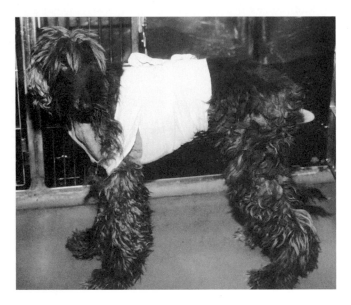

Fig. 5-19 This dog would stare at its left chest wall after a thoracotomy.

Urinary and Bowel Habits

- Dogs and cats experiencing pain commonly lose their house training, presumably because they are too uncomfortable to go outside.
- Dogs and cats may urinate frequently because of painful distention of the bladder or irritation (inflammation) of the bladder or urethra. It is important to remember that animals that have been administered opioids (e.g., morphine, hydromorphone) may be comfortable but still experience urinary retention as a side effect of the drug.
- Cats may also lose their house training as pain increases, which manifests as failure to use the litter box.

SUGGESTED READINGS

Bateson P: Assessment of pain in animals, *Anim Behav* 3:87-107, 1991.

Carstens E, Moberg GP: Recognizing pain and distress in laboratory animals, *ILAR J* 41:62-71, 2000.

Hansen B: Through a glass darkly: using behavior to assess pain, *Semin Vet Med Surg* 12:61-74, 1997.

Mathew KA: Pain assessment and general approach to management, *Vet Clin North Am Small Anim Pract* 30(4):729-752, 2000.

6

Objective, Categoric Methods for Assessing Pain and Analgesia

PETER W. HELLYER

Veterinarians are well trained in assessing organ system function and dysfunction with a wide variety of measurable and quantifiable parameters. For example, changes in blood urea nitrogen (BUN), creatinine, and urine-specific gravity can be used to assess the degree of renal failure and the response to treatment. Unfortunately, no similar set of objective and easily measured parameters is available to assess pain in people or animals. In people, the treatment of acute pain is hampered by a lack of objective criteria with which to measure pain intensity and a reluctance of medical personnel to either ask for or rely on patients' self-reports of pain. Understanding and treating chronic pain in people appropriately is even more complex, requiring an accurate assessment of the amount and type of tissue injury, as well as specific psychosocial, behavioral, and psychologic factors.

In animals, trying to determine the degree of pain and the ability of that animal to cope with its pain can be difficult. In a survey of Canadian veterinarians, Dohoo and Dohoo found that one of the main factors that determined whether veterinarians routinely administered analgesic drugs postoperatively was the veterinarians' perception of the degree of pain felt by animals. The fact that 51.5% of those veterinarians surveyed were considered to be analgesic nonusers (never used analgesics) highlights the clinical importance of being able to recognize pain in the species under a veterinarian's care. In a subsequent survey, animal health technologists in Canada had higher pain perception scores than did veterinarians. A majority (55%) of the animal health technologists surveyed agreed that risks of potent opioids (e.g., morphine, oxymorphone) outweighed the analgesic benefits, suggesting a lack of experience in treating and evaluating dogs and cats for pain. Even among veterinary personnel committed to treating pain, it can at times be frustrating to determine whether the benefits of the analgesic protocol selected (e.g., decreased pain intensity) outweigh the side effects (e.g., sedation, nausea). There is no question that as more studies focus on species-specific pain behaviors, our ability to recognize and treat pain in animals will improve. Nevertheless, the assessment of pain in animals will remain a subjective and inaccurate undertaking for the foreseeable future. Complicating the evaluation of pain is the fact that one set of criteria to measure pain cannot be used to assess all types of pain: acute, chronic, superficial, deep, neuropathic, and so on. One truth remains certain: ignoring pain simply because we have trouble measuring it condemns our patients to undue suffering. Endeavoring to assess and treat pain in animals is a worthwhile and laudable goal of veterinary medicine in spite of current uncertainties.

The evaluation methods described in this chapter are primarily designed to assess acute postoperative and traumatic pain in dogs. These methods can be adapted for cats and other species, provided that the caregiver recognizes that pain behaviors are likely to differ among species. *Importantly, all of the methods described are for the most part subjective and prone to the error of either underestimating or overestimating the degree of pain. Even if the amount of pain is correctly estimated, determining how well the individual animal is coping with the pain may be difficult. In addition, all of the current pain scales are subject to interobserver variability to one degree or another.* Finally, it should be recognized that all of these methods are used to assess the effects of physical pain and that none have been designed to evaluate mental or psychologic dimensions of pain that an animal may be experiencing.

LIMITATIONS OF OBJECTIVE AND CATEGORIC ASSESSMENT OF PAIN

No Established "Gold Standard" to Assess Pain

- There is no "gold standard" with which to assess pain in people, although caregivers can ask human patients whether they are in pain, whether the analgesic treatment has improved pain control, and how well they are coping with the pain.

- Self-reports of pain in people are frequently ignored. Patients who complain of postoperative pain may be viewed as "bad patients."
- No gold standard exists for the assessment of pain in animals or the comparison of one type of scale or measurement instrument with another. Most pain scales have been used to assess acute postoperative pain in dogs and cats. These scales are likely to be ineffective for assessing other types of pain, such as the acute pain and distress caused by pancreatitis, sepsis, or vasculitis. These scales probably are not useful in the assessment of emotional or psychologic pain or in the assessment of chronic pain, such as osteoarthritis or cancer pain.
  1. All of the pain scales used in animals rely on the recognition and/or interpretation of some behavior. The most useful scales rely on the determination of the presence or absence of specific behaviors while minimizing the interpretation of those behaviors.
  2. All pain scales have a subjective component and are subject to observer error and bias.

Physiologic Assessment

- Physiologic data (e.g., changes in heart rate, respiratory rate, arterial blood pressure, pupil dilation) are useful in assessing the response to a noxious (painful) stimulus in the anesthetized animal. For example, physiologic measurements, including heart rate, respiratory rate, rectal temperature, and plasma cortisol and β-endorphin concentrations did not differentiate between cats that underwent surgery (tenectomy, onychectomy) and control cats that were anesthetized and bandaged but had no surgery.
  1. Cardiopulmonary reflexes may obtund the easily recognizable changes in physiologic parameters in response to pain.
  2. Physiologic parameters are not specific enough to differentiate pain from other stressors such as anxiety, fear, or physiologic responses to metabolic conditions (e.g., anemia).
  3. Holton et al found that physiologic parameters were not useful indicators of pain in hospitalized dogs after surgery. Pupil dilation was significantly correlated with the pain score (numeric rating scale) in dogs after surgery. Nevertheless, the authors indicated that pupil size is unlikely to be a useful parameter with which to assess pain in hospitalized dogs.
- Note that some of the pain scales presented in this chapter use physiologic data and some do not. Physiologic parameters are

useful in assessing responses to noxious stimuli in patients under general anesthesia or in conscious patients for transient periods. The longer a conscious patient experiences pain, the less useful are physiologic parameters in assessing the degree of pain.

Behavioral Assessment and Interpretation

- Evaluation of pain in animals relies on behavioral assessment and interpretation of the behaviors by an observer. (Please refer to Chapter 5 for examples of behaviors indicative of pain in dogs.)
- Behavioral changes indicative of pain may be too subtle or take too long to recognize in routine clinical situations. This was verified in the most extensive evaluation to date of pain behaviors in dogs after ovariohysterectomy. Using two evaluation methods, a numeric scoring system and quantitative behavioral measurements, Hardie et al evaluated dogs that had anesthesia only and dogs that had anesthesia plus surgery, with or without analgesia. Surgery resulted in increases in pain score, sedation score, and time spent sleeping and a decrease in greeting behaviors during timed interactions with caregivers. Dogs that received oxymorphone (preoperatively and 6, 12, and 18 hours later) had a faster return to more normal greeting behaviors than did dogs that had surgery and placebo. Quantitative behavioral measurements were able to differentiate between dogs that had surgery and were administered oxymorphone from placebo-treated dogs, whereas the numeric scoring system was not.
- Sporadic observation of animal behavior may not reveal signs of pain. Except in the most severe circumstances, the signs of pain may be "masked" by behavior that is stereotypical of the species being observed. For instance, dogs may wag their tails and greet an observer at the cage door in spite of being in pain. (Hardie et al observed a faster return to greeting behaviors in dogs that had surgery and were administered oxymorphone as compared with dogs that were administered placebo.) Cats may simply hide in the back of their cages and demonstrate no behaviors that would suggest to a casual observer that they are in pain. Flock animals, such as sheep, may be startled when an observer approaches and attempt to conceal any signs of pain by staying bunched up with the rest of the flock (personal observations).
- Behavioral changes indicating pain may not be what we expect. A cat sitting quietly in the back of the cage after surgery may be in pain; however, pain would not be recognized if the caregiver

had expected to see more active signs of pain, such as pacing, agitation, or vocalizing.

1. Unfamiliarity with normal behaviors typical of a particular species or breed makes recognition of pain-induced behaviors difficult or impossible.
2. Species-specific pain scales have not been developed, except for rats.
3. Pain tolerance of individual animals within a species may vary markedly. A genetic predisposition to pain tolerance may explain some of the variability observed in clinical patients.

GUIDELINES FOR USE OF PAIN SCALES

Purpose of Assessment Method

- Regardless of the scale or method used to assess pain, the caregiver must recognize the limitations of the scale and the purpose for which the scale was developed. For example, if a scale includes lack of grooming and unkempt appearance as a criterion for pain, it is unlikely that a caregiver could draw any reasonable conclusions about grooming in the immediate postoperative period. Thus lack of grooming would not be expected to be a helpful criterion during the first 12 to 24 hours after surgery. Likewise, inactivity is an extremely difficult, if not impossible, parameter to assess if the animal is never let out of its cage and allowed to explore its surroundings.

- The evaluation of acute surgical and traumatic pain in dogs and cats has received a fair amount of attention in recent years. Many of the criteria commonly used, such as vocalizing, trying to escape, and thrashing, are not applicable to chronic pain. In addition, clinical criteria used to assess chronic pain, such as lack of exercise, lack of grooming, inappetence, and weight loss, are not incorporated into these scales for reasons already mentioned. In general, responses to acute surgical and traumatic pain are likely to be more marked and readily recognizable than clinical signs associated with chronic pain.

- The clinical signs of pain and discomfort associated with acute, nonsurgical diseases (e.g., pancreatitis, pleuritis, vasculitis) might not be recognizable when pain scales developed for acute surgical pain are used. For example, how does one assess the discomfort and suffering associated with constant vomiting, fever-induced myalgia, or abdominal pain and cramping? If a dog vomits 5, 10, or 20 times an hour, are there simply concerns about stopping the vomiting and rehydrating the patient or might there be concerns regarding abdominal pain and discomfort associated with the vomiting? What does a clinical sign such as pressing or banging the head on the side of the cage indicate in a dog with acute septic peritonitis? Does the clinical sign indicate the development of secondary neurologic symptomatology, or does it represent the desperate attempts of the animal to cope with its pain and suffering? Assessing this type of patient with a standard pain scale developed to evaluate a dog after surgery would likely give it a score that would be too low to prompt analgesic therapy. Thus care must be taken so that overreliance on a particular pain scale does not preclude the use of good clinical judgment and assessment of the patient.

- Cancer pain may have components of acute pain (e.g., pain caused by expansion of a tumor or by surgical, radiation, or chemotherapy treatment) and components of chronic pain. Thus assessment of cancer pain requires the caregiver to use methods that can detect behavioral changes associated with both acute and chronic pain. An increase in pain-related behaviors may indicate the progression of disease and prompt additional diagnostic and therapeutic interventions, as well as changes in analgesic therapy.

- Evaluating the degree of lameness of the affected limb(s) is often used to assess chronic orthopedic pain. In addition, observations of owners are essential to detect more subtle signs of chronic pain, such as lack of activity, change in attitude or interaction with family members, and changes in appetite. Response to therapy, such as increased activity after administration of a nonsteroidal antiinflammatory drug, may provide important information regarding the role that pain has played in behavioral changes that may even surprise owners.

Guide to Therapy

- The purposes of any pain scale are to help guide analgesic, medical, or surgical treatment and to provide diagnostic and prognostic information regarding the onset of healing and the resolution of tissue injury (Box 6-1).
- Pain scales may be used to ensure that individual animals are comfortable during the recuperative phase after surgery, trauma,

---

BOX 6-1

Key Points Related to Pain Scales

1. Pain scales should be used to ensure that pain is assessed and treated in every patient.
2. Pain scales are an adjunct to good physical examinations and thorough patient evaluation.
3. All pain scales have their limitations.
4. Individual behaviors indicative of pain should frequently prompt analgesic therapy, regardless of pain score.
5. Effective analgesic therapy should result in a low pain score and an animal that appears comfortable.

---

invasive diagnostic procedures, or illness. This is particularly important in animals that are unlikely to demonstrate overtly recognizable signs of pain, such as cats or "stoic" dogs.

- Pain scales may encourage the frequent evaluation of patients that are likely to be in pain, ensuring that pain does not go unrecognized or undertreated.
  1. Many human hospitals in the United States are now required to monitor pain as one of the patient's vital signs.
  2. An institutional commitment for the treatment of pain is required to ensure that pain is not overlooked or ignored.
- Pain scales should not be used to deny analgesic therapy to an animal that is likely to be in pain after some procedure. Rather, the pain scale should be used to determine whether analgesic therapy needs to be increased or can be tapered off.
  1. Do not use rigid minimum scores to prompt therapy.
  2. Individual behaviors suggestive of animal pain or distress should overrule results of a pain score.
  3. If the procedure is likely to be painful, but the pain score is too low to prompt treatment, try a test dose of analgesic and observe the patient's response.
- Critically ill or compromised animals may not be able to demonstrate behaviors required to prompt treatment according to the pain scale.
  1. Consider low-dose opioid therapy in the animal likely to have pain that is slightly obtunded. Increased awareness of

surroundings, but not agitation, suggests a beneficial effect of analgesic therapy.
- If unsure that the patient is in pain but tissue trauma has occurred, treat for pain conservatively and observe results.

Frequency of Observations

Acute Surgical and Traumatic Pain

- The health status of the animal, extent of surgery or injuries, and anticipated duration of analgesic drug administration determine the frequency and interval of evaluations.
- In general, evaluations should be made at least hourly for the first 4 to 6 hours after surgery, provided that the animal has recovered from anesthesia, has stable vital signs, and is resting comfortably.
- Animals not recovering as anticipated from anesthesia or surgery and critically ill animals require more frequent evaluations until their conditions have stabilized.
- Patient response to analgesic therapy and expected duration of action of analgesic drug(s) will help to determine the frequency of evaluations. For example, if a dog is resting comfortably after the postoperative administration of morphine, it may not need to be reassessed for 2 to 4 hours.
- Animals should be allowed to sleep after analgesic therapy. Vital signs often can be checked without unduly disturbing a sleeping animal. In general, animals are not wakened to check their pain status.
- Continuous, undisturbed observations, coupled with periodic interactive observations (e.g., open the cage, palpate wound) are likely to provide more information than occasional observations of the animal through the cage door. Unfortunately, continuous observations are not practical in most clinical situations. In general, the more frequent the observations, the more likely it is that subtle signs of pain will be detected.

SUBJECTIVE AND SEMIOBJECTIVE PAIN SCALES FOR ACUTE SURGICAL AND TRAUMATIC PAIN

Preemptive Scoring System

- The preemptive scoring system is a subjective scoring system based on the amount of pain an individual believes the animal will experience after a given procedure.

BOX 6-2
Preemptive Scoring System

Minor Procedures: No Pain or Temporary Pain
Physical examination, restraint
Radiography
Suture removal, cast application, bandage change*
Grooming
Nail trim

Minor Surgeries: Minor Pain
Suturing, debridement
Urinary catheterization
Dental cleaning
Ear examination and cleaning
Abscess lancing
Removing cutaneous foreign bodies

Moderate Surgeries: Moderate Pain
Ovariohysterectomy, castration, cesarean section
Feline onychectomy
Cystotomy
Anal sacculectomy
Dental extraction
Cutaneous mass removal
Severe laceration repair

Major Surgeries: Severe Pain
Fracture repair, cruciate ligament repair
Thoracotomy, laminectomy, exploratory laparotomy
Limb amputation
Ear canal ablation

Preemptive scoring system used to anticipate the amount of pain induced by surgical procedures. Modified from *A roundtable discussion: rethinking your approach to sedation, anesthesia, and analgesia,* Lenexa, Kan, 1997, Veterinary Medicine Publishing. The pain categories are only a "best guess" of the amount of pain a certain procedure induces. In general, the more tissue trauma, the greater the pain. Individual animals may have more or less pain than the category suggests.
*Setting of fractures and some bandage changes can be quite painful.

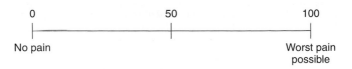

Fig. 6-1 Visual analog scale *(VAS)* used to estimate an animal's current pain status. The scale is a 100-mm line representing the entire spectrum of pain, from no pain to the worst pain possible. The observer draws a line that best represents the animal's estimated pain.

- Preemptive scoring systems assign a degree of pain (none, mild, moderate, severe) based on the procedure performed and the amount of tissue trauma involved (Box 6-2).
- In general, the greater the amount of tissue trauma, the greater the assigned level of pain.
- Preemptive scoring systems are useful in planning perioperative analgesic strategies. Procedures inducing moderate-to-severe pain often require the use of multiple analgesic drugs and techniques to adequately manage pain.
- Preemptive scoring systems are not useful in determining the degree of pain felt by an individual patient or in assessing response to therapy.
- Individual patients may experience more or less pain than predicted by the preemptive pain scale.

Visual Analog Scale
- The visual analog scale (VAS) is a semiobjective scoring system.
- The VAS is typically a straight, horizontal line, 100 mm in length, bracketed with descriptors of pain intensity (e.g., no pain, worst pain possible) on either end of the line (Fig. 6-1).
- The patient draws a vertical line across the scale that best represents his or her degree of pain. The patient may be asked to assess the pain at the current time or the worst pain that occurred since the last assessment.
- The VAS has been used extensively for people and is generally completed by the patient experiencing the pain. The scale avoids the use of imprecise descriptive terms and provides many points from which to choose. In people, bracketing the VAS with terms

such as *no relief of pain* and *complete relief of pain* may provide more clinically useful information, since patients do not all start with the same degree of pain.

1. The use of the VAS may result in greater variability of pain scores than use of a simple descriptive scale.
2. The VAS may erroneously appear to be a more sensitive scale compared with other scales, resulting in overinterpretation or excessive confidence in the results.
3. The advantages of the VAS are primarily ease of use and its ability to provide a general sense of whether pain is getting worse or improving.
4. A disadvantage of a standard VAS used to rate pain intensity is that pain is a multidimensional experience and pain intensity is only one aspect of that experience.

- Key disadvantages of the VAS in veterinary medicine occur primarily because the scale relies on an observer to identify and interpret pain behaviors.

1. Observer bias may play a key role in assessment of pain, leading to the possibility of overdiagnosing or underdiagnosing pain.
2. In people, at least one study has shown that an individual's score must move at least 13 mm along the 100-mm scale for a change in acute, traumatic pain to be clinically significant. Even if there is a 50% change in the VAS score, it is not known whether that represents an adequate degree of pain relief unless the patient is asked. The sensitivity of the VAS has not been determined in animals; therefore changes in VAS score should be interpreted in light of overall patient appearance.
3. Variability of visual acuity among observers may affect the accuracy of the VAS.
4. Observer variability, when more than one observer evaluates an animal, affects the accuracy of the VAS.

Simple Descriptive Scale

- The simple descriptive scale (SDS) is a semiobjective scoring system.
- The SDS usually consists of four or five categories or descriptions of pain intensity (Box 6-3). Each description is assigned a number, which becomes the patient's pain score. This scale dif-

---

BOX 6-3
Simple Descriptive Scale

1. No pain   3. Moderate pain
2. Mild pain   4. Severe pain

---

fers from the preemptive scoring system in that the SDS assigns a score based on observation of the animal and not the nature of the procedure performed.
- Advantages of the SDS are that it is simple to use and the results are not affected by visual acuity (no drawing of a line required).
- Disadvantages of the SDS are that it is not a sensitive scale for assessment of pain (consists of only four or five categories); therefore it may overestimate or underestimate the degree of pain and the efficacy of analgesic therapy.
- Observer bias may play a key role in determining the pain score.

Numerical Rating Scale
- The numerical rating scale (NRS) is a semiobjective scoring system.
- The NRS consists of multiple categories with which to evaluate the patient, with descriptive definitions of pain for each category (Table 6-1). The NRS generally uses categories that are assigned whole numbers, and the importance of each category is not weighted.
- The NRS prompts the observer to evaluate certain aspects of the patient that might otherwise go unnoticed (e.g., appearance of the eyes, interactive behaviors, physiologic parameters).
- Advantages of the NRS include a more thorough patient evaluation than what is prompted by the VAS or SDS, an easy method for tabulating the score, and numerous categories on which to base an assessment of patient comfort.
- Disadvantages of the NRS include lack of accuracy and little improvement over the SDS.
  1. Categories are generally scored by whole numbers, suggesting that equal differences exist between categories when in fact this may not be true.

TABLE 6-1

Pain Score Evaluation Form Used by the Colorado State University Veterinary Teaching Hospital

Observation	Score	Patient Criteria
Comfort	0	Asleep or calm
	1	Awake; interested in surroundings
	2	Mild agitation; obtunded and uninterested in surroundings
	3	Moderate agitation; restless and uncomfortable
	4	Extremely agitated; thrashing
Movement	0	Normal amount of movement
	1	Frequent position changes or reluctance to move
	2	Thrashing
Appearance	0	Normal
	1	Mild changes: eyelids partially closed; ears flattened or carried abnormally
	2	Moderate changes: eyes sunken or glazed; unkempt appearance
	3	Severe changes: eyes pale; enlarged pupils; "grimacing" or other abnormal facial expressions; guarding; hunched-up position; legs in abnormal position; grunting before expiration; teeth grinding
Behavior (unprovoked)	0	Normal
	1	Minor changes
	2	Moderately abnormal: less mobile and less alert than normal; unaware of surroundings; very restless
	3	Markedly abnormal: very restless; vocalizing; self-mutilation; grunting; facing back of cage

Numeric rating scale used to assess pain in dogs and cats. Adapted from Hellyer PW, Gaynor JS: *Comp Cont Educ* 20:140-153, 1998.

IT IS NOT THE INTENT OF THIS FORM TO REQUIRE THAT ANIMALS PROVE THEY ARE IN PAIN BEFORE THERAPY IS INITIATED. Instead, this form is intended to aid in the evaluation of dogs and cats that may be in pain after surgery or trauma. The exact score that will indicate that treatment for pain is appropriate will vary from individual to individual. Animals that are expected to be in moderate-to-severe pain, based on the surgical procedure performed, should be treated BEFORE assessment indicates severe pain. Many animals will receive analgesics before pain is detected based on this scoring system. Regardless of score, if there is evidence that the animal is in pain, a test dose of analgesic should be administered and changes in behavior noted.

TABLE 6-1

Pain Score Evaluation Form Used by the Colorado State University Veterinary Teaching Hospital—cont'd

Observation	Score	Patient Criteria
Interactive behavior	0	Normal
	1	Pulls away when surgical site is touched; looks at wound; mobile
	2	Vocalizing when wound is touched; somewhat restless; reluctant to move but will if coaxed
	3	Violent reaction to stimuli; vocalizing when wound is not touched; snapping, growling, or hissing when approached; extremely restless; will not move when coaxed
Vocalization	0	Quiet
	1	Crying; responds to calm voice and stroking
	2	Intermittent crying or whimpering; no response to calm voice and stroking
	3	Continuous noise that is unusual for this animal
Heart rate	0	0%-15% above presurgical value
	1	16%-29% above presurgical value
	2	30%-45% above presurgical value
	3	>45% above presurgical value
Respiration rate	0	0%-15% above presurgical value
	1	16%-29% above presurgical value
	2	30%-45% above presurgical value
	3	>45% above presurgical value
Total score (0-24) _____		

2. In spite of numerous categories, pain in animals may go undiagnosed. For example, a dog with severe abdominal pain may not receive a high enough number to be considered in pain when a scale designed to assess surgical pain is used.

3. In the postsurgical period, the NRS may be too insensitive to detect differences between animals that receive analgesics and those that go untreated. Thus the NRS may only be able to identify those animals with extreme pain that overtly demonstrate pain behaviors and would have been identified otherwise.

BEHAVIORAL PAIN SCALES FOR ACUTE SURGICAL AND TRAUMATIC PAIN

Behavioral and Physiologic Responses Scale

- The University of Melbourne Pain Scale (UMPS) is a scale based on specific behavioral and physiologic responses. The UMPS includes multiple descriptors in six categories of parameters or behaviors related to pain (Table 6-2).
- Advantages of the UMPS may include increased accuracy over the preemptive scoring system, VAS, SDS, or NRS and an ability to weight the importance of certain behaviors or parameters.
  1. Multiple factors evaluated increase the sensitivity and specificity of the UMPS.
  2. The UMPS relies on behavioral observations, thereby limiting interpretation and observer bias.
  3. The UMPS evaluates changes in behavior or demeanor, adding to the sensitivity of the scale.
- Disadvantages of the UMPS include limited validation to date. The specific types of patients and procedures in which the UMPS would be expected to be accurate have not been elucidated.
  1. The UMPS may not be sensitive enough to detect small changes in pain behaviors, particularly if patient evaluations are performed only periodically.
  2. The UMPS was designed to evaluate dogs after surgery. The accuracy of the scale for other uses or for use with cats has not been established.
  3. The UMPS requires some knowledge of the demeanor (mental status) of the dog before anesthesia and surgery. Although the veterinary staff usually knows this, the dog's actual men-

TABLE 6-2

University of Melbourne Pain Scale
(Behavioral Assessment Scale)

Category	Descriptor	Score
1. Physiologic data		
a.	Physiologic data within reference range	0
b.	Dilated pupils	2
c. Choose only one	Percentage increase in heart rate relative to preprocedural rate	
	>20%	1
	>50%	2
	>100%	3
d. Choose only one	Percentage increase in respiratory rate relative to preprocedural rate	
	>20%	1
	>50%	2
	>100%	3
e.	Rectal temperature exceeds reference range	1
f.	Salivation	2
2. Response to palpation (choose only one)	No change from preprocedural behavior	0
	Guards/reacts* when touched	2
	Guards/reacts* before touched	3
3. Activity (choose only one)	At rest: sleeping	0
	At rest: semiconscious	0
	At rest: awake	1
	Eating	0
	Restless (pacing continuously, getting up and down)	2
	Rolling, thrashing	3

Modified from Firth AM, Haldane SL: *J Am Vet Med Assoc* 214:651-659, 1999.

The pain scale includes six categories. Each category contains descriptors of various behaviors that are assigned numeric values. The assessor examines the descriptors in each category and decides whether a descriptor approximates the dog's behavior. If so, the value for that descriptor is added to the patient's pain score. Certain descriptors are mutually exclusive (e.g., a dog cannot be in sternal recumbency and standing at the same time). These mutually exclusive descriptors are grouped together with the notation "choose only one." For the fourth category, mental status, the assessor must have completed a preprocedural assessment of the dog's dominant/aggressive behavior to establish a baseline score. The mental status score is the absolute difference between preprocedural and postprocedural scores. The minimum possible total pain score is 0 points; the maximum possible pain score is 27 points.

*Includes turning head toward affected area; biting, licking, or scratching at the wound; snapping at the handler; or tense muscle and a protective (guarding) posture.

Continued

TABLE 6-2

University of Melbourne Pain Scale (Behavioral Assessment Scale)—cont'd

Category	Descriptor	Score
4. Mental status (choose only one)	Submissive	0
	Overtly friendly	1
	Wary	2
	Aggressive	3
5. Posture		
a.	Guarding or protecting affected area (includes fetal position)	2
b. Choose only one	Lateral recumbency	0
	Sternal recumbency	1
	Sitting or standing, head up	1
	Standing, head hanging down	2
	Moving	1
	Abnormal posture (e.g., prayer position, hunched back)	2
6. Vocalization† (choose only one)	Not vocalizing	0
	Vocalizing when touched	2
	Intermittent vocalization	2
	Continuous vocalization	3

Modified from Firth AM, Haldane SL: *J Am Vet Med Assoc* 214:651-659, 1999.

The pain scale includes six categories. Each category contains descriptors of various behaviors that are assigned numeric values. The assessor examines the descriptors in each category and decides whether a descriptor approximates the dog's behavior. If so, the value for that descriptor is added to the patient's pain score. Certain descriptors are mutually exclusive (e.g., a dog cannot be in sternal recumbency and standing at the same time). These mutually exclusive descriptors are grouped together with the notation "choose only one." For the fourth category, mental status, the assessor must have completed a preprocedural assessment of the dog's dominant/aggressive behavior to establish a baseline score. The mental status score is the absolute difference between preprocedural and postprocedural scores. The minimum possible total pain score is 0 points; the maximum possible pain score is 27 points.

†Does not include alert barking.

tal status when truly comfortable at home will probably not be known. In other words, the mental status of the dog after surgery will be compared with an already altered mental status that exists simply because the dog is in a veterinary hospital and away from familiar surroundings.

Behavioral Response Scale

- The Glasgow Composite Pain Tool is a scale based on specific behavioral signs believed to represent pain in the dog (Box 6-4).
  1. The behaviors included in the scale were derived from a questionnaire sent to veterinarians.

BOX 6-4
The Glasgow Composite Pain Tool

The questionnaire is made up of a number of sections, each of which has several possible answers. Please tick the answers that you feel are appropriate to the dog you are assessing. If more than one answer is appropriate, then tick all that apply. Approach the kennel and ensure you are not wearing a laboratory coat or theater "greens," since the dog may associate these with stress and/or pain. While you approach the kennel, look at the dog's behavior and reactions. From outside the dog's kennel, look at the dog's behavior and answer the following questions.

Look at the Dog's Posture; Does It Seem . . .
Rigid ☐   Neither of these ☐
Hunched or tense ☐

Does the Dog Seem to Be . . .
Restless ☐   Comfortable ☐

If the Dog Is Vocalizing, Is It . . .
Crying or whimpering ☐   Screaming ☐
Groaning ☐   Not vocalizing/none of these ☐

If the Dog Is Paying Attention to Its Wound, Is It . . .
Chewing ☐   Ignoring its wound ☐
Licking, looking, or rubbing ☐

From Holton L, Reid J, Scott EM, et al: *Vet Rec* 148:525-531, 2001.

Continued

BOX 6-4
The Glasgow Composite Pain Tool—cont'd

Now approach the kennel door and call the dog's name. Then open the door and encourage the dog to come to you. From the dog's reaction to you and behaviors when you were watching him/her, assess his/her character.

Does the Dog Seem to be . . .
Aggressive ☐   Quiet or indifferent ☐
Depressed ☐   Happy and content ☐
Disinterested ☐   Happy and bouncy ☐
Nervous, anxious, or fearful ☐

Now look at the dog's response to stimuli. If the mobility assessment is possible, open the kennel and put a lead on the dog. If the animal is sitting down, encourage it to stand and then come out of the kennel. Walk slowly up and down the area outside the kennel. If the dog was standing up in the kennel and has undergone a procedure that may be painful in the perianal area, ask the animal to sit down.

During This Procedure Did the Dog Seem to Be . . .
Stiff ☐   None of these ☐
Slow or reluctant to rise or sit ☐   Assessment not carried out ☐
Lame ☐

The next procedure is to assess the dog's response to touch. If the animal has a wound, apply gentle pressure to the wound using two fingers in an area approximately 2 inches around it. If the position of the wound is such that it is impossible to touch, then apply the pressure to the closest point to the wound. If there is no wound, apply the same pressure to the stifle and surrounding area.

When Touched Did the Dog . . .
Cry ☐   Growl or guard wound ☐
Flinch ☐   None of these ☐
Snap ☐

From Holton L, Reid J, Scott EM, et al: *Vet Rec* 148:525-531, 2001.

BOX 6-4
The Glasgow Composite Pain Tool—cont'd

Definitions of expressions used in the Glasgow Composite Pain Tool for dogs.

Posture

Rigid: Animal lying in lateral recumbency, legs extended or partially extended in a fixed position.

Hunched: When animal is standing, its back forms a convex shape with abdomen tucked up, or, back in a concave shape with shoulders and front legs lower than hips.

Tense: Animal appears frightened or reluctant to move, overall impression of tight muscles. Animal can be in any body position.

Normal body posture: Animal may be in any position, appears comfortable, muscles relaxed.

Comfort

Restless: Moving bodily position, circling, pacing, shifting body parts, unsettled.

Comfortable: Animal resting and relaxed, no avoidance or abnormal body position evident or settled, remains in same body position, at ease.

Vocalization

Crying: Extension of the whimpering noise, louder and with open mouth.

Whimpering: Often quiet, short, high-pitched sound, frequently closed mouth (whining).

Groaning: Low moaning or grunting deep sound, intermittent.

Screaming: Animal making a continual high-pitched noise, inconsolable, mouth wide open.

Attention to Wound Area

Chewing: Using mouth and teeth on wound area, pulling stitches.

Licking: Using tongue to stroke area of wound.

Looking: Turning head in direction of area of wound.

Rubbing: Using paw or kennel floor to stroke wound area.

Ignoring: Paying no attention to the wound area.

Continued

BOX 6-4

The Glasgow Composite Pain Tool—cont'd

Demeanor

Aggressive: Mouth open or lip curled showing teeth, snarling, growling, snapping, or barking.

Depressed: Dull demeanor, not responsive, shows reluctance to interact.

Disinterested: Cannot be stimulated to wag tail or interact with observer.

Nervous: Eyes in continual movement, often head and body movement, jumpy.

Anxious: Worried expression, eyes wide with whites showing, wrinkled forehead.

Fearful: Cowering away, guarding body and head.

Quiet: Sitting or lying still, no noise, will look when spoken to but does not respond.

Indifferent: Not responsive to surroundings or observer.

Content: Interested in surroundings, has positive interaction with observer, responsive and alert.

Bouncy: Tail wagging, jumping in kennel, often vocalizing with a happy and excited noise.

Mobility

Stiff: Stilted gait, also slow to rise or sit, may be reluctant to move.

Slow to rise or sit: Slow to get up or sit down but not stilted in movement.

Reluctant to rise or sit: Needs encouragement to get up or sit down.

Lame: Irregular gait, uneven weight bearing when walking.

Normal mobility: Gets up and lies down with no alteration from normal.

Response to Touch

Cry: A short vocal response. Looks at area and opens mouth, emits a brief sound.

Flinch: Painful area is quickly moved away from stimulus either before or in response to touch.

Snap: Tries to bite observer before or in response to touch.

Growl: Emits a low prolonged warning sound before or in response to touch.

Guard: Pulls painful area away from stimulus or tenses local muscles in order to protect from stimulus.

None: Accepts firm pressure on wound with none of the aforementioned reactions.

From Holton L, Reid J, Scott FM, et al; *Vet Rec* 148:525-531, 2001.

2. The expressions used to describe pain behaviors were reduced to specific words and phrases and validated by using a variety of statistical methods.

- Advantages of this scale include limited interpretation and bias by the observer.
    1. The Glasgow Composite Pain Tool has increased accuracy over the preemptive scoring system, VAS, SDS, and NRS.
    2. Observers identify whether a behavior is present.
    3. Terms used to describe individual behaviors are specifically defined, thereby decreasing uncertainty in use of the scale.
    4. Physiologic data are not included, making the scale easier to use than the UMPS and perhaps more accurate.
- Disadvantages of the scale are limited validation in actual animal studies and a lack of a numeric scoring system that would allow for comparison of scores over time.

RECOMMENDED PAIN SCALE

- A modified pain scale is presented in Box 6-5. This scale is a composite scale derived from the UMPS and the Glasgow Composite Pain Tool. This composite scale was developed as part of a study evaluating pain after routine surgery in dogs and cats (unpublished observations).
    1. Behaviors are identified as either present or absent.
    2. Physiologic data are not included, with the exception of dilated pupils.
    3. Salivation and vomiting are included as indicators of nausea and as occasional signs of pain. Regardless of the cause, frequent vomiting undoubtedly decreases the comfort of the patient.
- The modified scale provides a record for tracking the frequency of behaviors indicative of pain. The frequency of pain behaviors should be low or decreasing with effective analgesic therapy. If a numeric score is desired, behaviors can be assigned the number located in parentheses.
- Advantages of this scale are ease of use and minimal interpretation required. Specific descriptors for individual behaviors are provided, which decreases interobserver variability.
- Disadvantages of this scale include lack of validation by clinical studies comparing it with other scales and an arbitrary numeric scale when a specific score is required.

BOX 6-5

Modified Pain Scale Recommended for the Evaluation of Acute Postsurgical Pain in Dogs and Cats

Time: _____ _____

Posture:
Normal	(0)	_____	_____
Rigid	(1)	_____	_____
Hunched	(2)	_____	_____
Tense	(2)	_____	_____
Abnormal body posture	(3)	_____	_____
Define: _____			
Guarding affected area	(4)	_____	_____

Does the Dog or Cat Seem to Be:
At rest	(0)	_____	_____
Comfortable	(0)	_____	_____
Restless	(1)	_____	_____
Uncomfortable	(2)	_____	_____
Rolling, thrashing	(3)	_____	_____

Dilated Pupils? (Yes: 1; No: 0) _____ _____

Salivation? (Yes: 1; No: 0) _____ _____

Vomiting? (Yes: 1; No: 0) _____ _____

If Yes, Number of Times/5 Min _____ _____

Vocalization:
Not vocalizing	(0)	_____	_____
Barking (If abnormal for this dog: 1)		_____	_____
Crying or whimpering	(2)	_____	_____
Groaning, hissing	(3)	_____	_____
Screaming	(4)	_____	_____

Modified from the University of Melbourne Pain Scale and the Glasgow Composite Pain Tool. See Table 6-3 for definition of terms. When using this scale, observe dog or cat for presence or absence of specific behaviors and monitor for improvement in pain behaviors over time. If a specific score is desired, assign numbers in parentheses and add up to obtain overall pain score. The numeric scoring system has not been validated at this time.

BOX 6-5

Modified Pain Scale Recommended for the Evaluation of Acute Postsurgical Pain in Dogs and Cats—cont'd

Mental Status:

Aggressive _____ _____

Obtunded _____ _____

Disinterested _____ _____

Nervous/anxious/fearful _____ _____

Happy/content _____ _____

Happy/bouncy _____ _____

Submissive _____ _____

Change in mental status? _____ _____
(Yes: 1; No: 0)

Walking:

Assessment not carried (0) _____ _____
out/too sedated

Will not walk/stand _____ _____

Note: _____

None of these (0) _____ _____

Stiff (1) _____ _____

Ataxic (1) _____ _____

Slow or reluctant (2) _____ _____
to rise or sit

Lame (2) _____ _____

Palpation: When Touched Did the Dog or Cat . . .

None of these (0) _____ _____

Look toward wound (1) _____ _____

Anxious (1) _____ _____

Cry (2) _____ _____

Flinch (?) _____ _____

Snap/bite/hiss (3) _____ _____

Growl or guard wound (3) _____ _____

SUGGESTED READINGS

A roundtable discussion: rethinking your approach to sedation, anesthesia, and analgesia, Lenexa, Kan, 1997, Veterinary Medicine Publishing.

Cambridge AJ, Tobias KM, Newberry RC, et al: Subjective and objective measurements of postoperative pain in cats, *J Am Vet Med Assoc* 217:685-689, 2000.

106Dohoo SE, Dohoo IR: Factors influencing the postoperative use of analgesics in dogs and cats by Canadian veterinarians, *Can Vet J* 37:552-556, 1996.

Dohoo SE, Dohoo IR: Attitudes and concerns of Canadian animal health technologists toward postoperative pain management in dogs and cats, *Can Vet J* 39:491-496, 1998.

Ferrell BR, Dean GE, Grant M, et al: An institutional commitment to pain management, *J Clin Oncol* 13:2158-2165, 1995.

Firth AM, Haldane SL: Development of a scale to evaluate postoperative pain in dogs, *J Am Vet Med Assoc* 214:651-659, 1999.

Hansen BD, Hardie EM, Carroll GS: Physiological measurements after ovariohysterectomy in dogs: what's normal? *Appl Anim Behav Sci* 51:101-109, 1997.

Hardie EM, Hansen BD, Carroll GS: Behavior after ovariohysterectomy in the dog: what's normal? *Appl Anim Behav Sci* 51:111-128, 1997.

Hellyer PW, Gaynor JS: How I treat: acute postsurgical pain in dogs and cats, *Compend Contin Educ* 20:140-153, 1998.

Holton L, Reid J, Scott EM, et al: Development of a behaviour-based pain scale to measure acute pain in dogs, *Vet Rec* 148:525-531, 2001.

Holton LL, Scott EM, Nolan AM, et al: Comparison of three methods used for assessment of pain in dogs, *J Am Vet Med Assoc* 212:61-66, 1998.

Holton LL, Scott EM, Nolan AM, et al: Relationship between physiological factors and clinical pain in dogs scored using a numerical rating scale, *J Small Anim Pract* 39:469-474, 1998.

Mathews KA: Pain assessment and general approach to management, *Vet Clin North Am Small Anim Pract* 30:729-755, 2000.

McQuay HJ, Moore RA: Methods of therapeutic trials. In Wall PD, Melzack R, editors: *Textbook of pain,* ed 4, Edinburgh, 1999,Churchill Livingstone.

Melzack R, Katz J: Pain measurement in persons in pain. In Wall PD, Melzack R, editors: *Textbook of pain,* ed 4, Edinburgh, 1999, Churchill Livingstone.

Mogil JS: The genetic mediation of individual differences in sensitivity to pain and its inhibition, *Proc Natl Acad Sci U S A* 96:7744-7751, 1999.

Roughan JV, Flecknell PA: Behavioral effects of laparotomy and analgesic effects of ketoprofen and carprofen in rats, *Pain* 90:65-74, 2001.

Salmon P, Manyande A: Good patients cope with their pain: postoperative analgesia and nurses' perceptions of their patients' pain, *Pain* 68:63-68, 1996.

Smith JD, Allen SW, Quandt JE: Changes in cortisol concentration in response to stress and postoperative pain in client-owned cats and correlation with objective clinical variables, *Am J Vet Res* 60:432-436, 1999.

Todd KH, Funk KG, Funk JP, et al: Clinical significance of reported changes in pain severity, *Ann Emerg Med* 27:485-489, 1996.

Turk CD, Okifuji A: Pain: assessment of patients' reporting of pain: an integrated perspective, *Lancet* 353:1784-1788, 1999.

PART THREE

Pain Management

7

Pharmacologic Principles and Pain

Pharmacokinetics and Pharmacodynamics

WILLIAM W. MUIR III AND RICHARD A. SAMS

Although the administration of drugs to animals is an everyday occurrence, knowledge of the general principles governing the development of drug doses and dosage regimens while avoiding drug toxicity is often incomplete or absent. Clinical pharmacology is the study of drug administration and drug effects in sick or injured animals as opposed to experimental animals. For example, if it is known that renal elimination of a drug is diminished during renal failure, then the dose of that drug must be reduced accordingly. Familiarity with the sciences of pharmacokinetics and pharmacodynamics is a prerequisite to understanding clinical pharmacology. At first glance, these sciences are seemingly undecipherable, since they are based on a quagmire of confusing terms, mathematical formulas, and complex computer-based models—each claiming to more accurately reflect drug disposition. Regardless of the math, knowledge of the basic principles that have evolved from pharmacokinetic and pharmacodynamic modeling of drug disposition and effect is essential to a rational understanding of drug therapy and the selection of therapeutic regimens that are safe and efficacious. This last statement is extremely important for drugs that are used for the treatment of pain because of the potential for many analgesic drugs to produce addiction, tolerance, and toxicity.

1. Fundamental principles described by clinical pharmacology
   a. Factors affecting drug absorption and distribution
   b. Mechanism of drug elimination and excretion
   c. Dose routes and calculation of dosage regimens
   d. Relationships between drug concentration and effect

111

Fig. 7-1 A, Plasma-concentration time curve for a drug varies, depending on the route of administration. **B,** The Cp for morphine decreases rapidly after intravenous administration to dogs. **C,** The Cp for sustained-release morphine increases more gradually and is sustained as a peak value for a longer period after oral administration. **D,** The Cp for the transcutaneous administration of fentanyl (fentanyl patch; 75 μg/hr) in dogs increases very slowly before it reaches steady-state concentrations (up to 24 hours). The drug's effects are expected to parallel the Cp. (From Dohoo SE, Tasker RAR: *Can J Vet Res* 61:251-255, 1997; Egger CM, Duke T, Archer J, et al: *Vet Anesth* 27:159-166, 1998.)

PHARMACOKINETICS

Pharmacokinetics is a quantitative approach to the study of the disposition of drugs or drug metabolites in the body (Fig. 7-1). Most frequently, the time course of a drug elimination is determined from blood or plasma, although other media such as cerebrospinal fluid (CSF), tears, urine, feces, and saliva are occasionally monitored as indicators of therapeutically relevant drug concentrations. Drug concentration versus time profiles are used to derive pharmacokinetic models that mathematically describe the distribution of the drug into theoretic body compartments. These compartments (central [blood volume] and peripheral [muscle, skin, bone, fat]) do not necessarily correspond to any physiologically relevant space (e.g., extracellular water) but have become a standard means of communicating a drug's concentration-time profile in the plasma.

- Physiologically based pharmacokinetic modeling is a quantitative attempt to exactly model drug disposition in the body in terms of physiologically identifiable compartments and thereby predict tissue concentrations within specific organs, tissues, and fluids. This latter approach provides minimal additional clinically relevant information and therefore will not be discussed further.
- The most commonly used and clinically applicable pharmacokinetic model is termed *first order,* meaning that the rate of drug elimination from the plasma depends on the concentration of the drug in the plasma (one exponential term [Fig. 7-2]). In other words, the rate of drug elimination from the plasma decreases as the concentration in the plasma decreases. A plot of the log concentration of a first-order drug elimination versus time curve produces a straight line (see Fig. 7-2). More complex multiple compartment models are used when the plot of the drug log concentration versus time curve is not linear (Fig. 7-3).

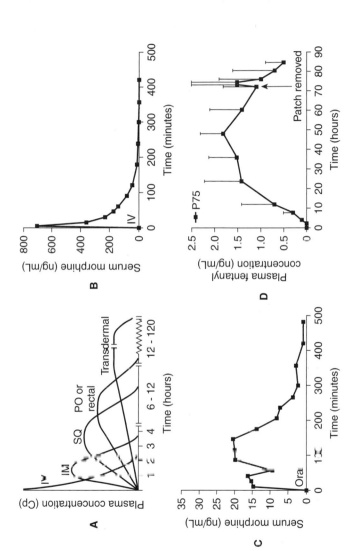

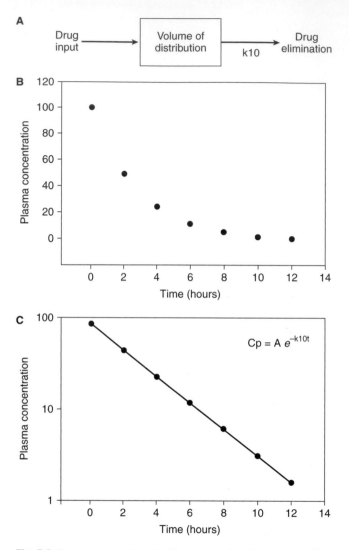

Fig. 7-2 One-compartment model of intravenous drug disposition. **A,** Pharmacokinetic models are used to describe drug disposition (drug concentration versus time profiles). **B,** The disposition of many drugs can be described by a first-order or one-compartment mode (e.g., ketoprofin), in which the rate of drug elimination depends on the drug Cp (i.e., the rate of decrease in Cp decreases as Cp decreases). **C,** A plot of the log concentration of Cp is a straight line.

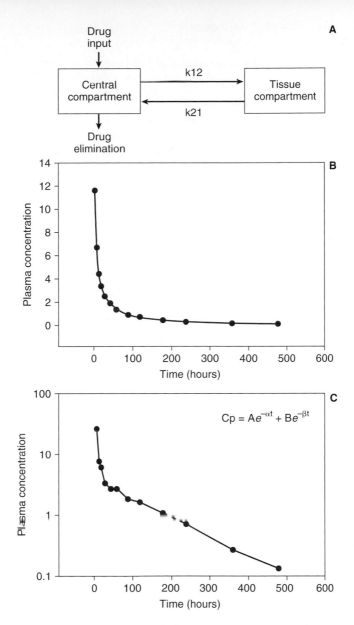

Fig. 7-3 Two-compartment model of intravenous drug disposition. **A,** Multiple compartment models are used when **B,** a plot of the Cp versus time and **C,** log of Cp versus time curves show curvature. Two-compartment models are common for many drugs (opioids, α_2-agonists).

- The rates of drug absorption, distribution, and elimination (metabolism and excretion) are used mathematically to derive pharmacokinetic variables (volume of distribution [V_d], clearance, half-life) from which therapeutic drug concentrations, "standard doses," and dosage regimens can be determined.
- The more rapidly a drug is delivered to the tissue at which the drug acts, the more rapid is the equilibration between drug in plasma and the tissue. This is largely a function of perfusion (i.e., the rate of drug delivery to the tissue by the blood). Low tissue binding (affinity) for a drug (e.g., nonspecific tissue binding) increases the time needed for equilibration because more of the drug must be delivered to the tissue to bring it to equilibrium with the plasma. Limitations to diffusion of the drug to the active site also delay equilibration.

FACTORS AFFECTING DRUG ABSORPTION AND DISTRIBUTION

Drugs administered by routes other than the intravenous route (e.g., transcutaneous, subcutaneous, intramuscular, oral) must be absorbed into the body so that they can be distributed to the target site. Drugs that are administered intravenously are dependent on the injection technique used (bolus, incremental injection, infusion) and factors that promote (increased tissue blood flow) or limit (high protein binding) their distribution to the target site.

Absorption

A drug must pass through several different membranes to reach its site of action. The nature of the membranes determines the rate of passage of the drug through them (diffusion), and consequently, the rate at which the drug response occurs. The rate of passage of a drug through a membrane can range from zero (i.e., no movement of drug across the membrane) to the rate of blood flow to the membrane (i.e., the drug moves across the membrane as fast as it is delivered to it). Biologic membranes are composed of a bimolecular layer of lipid molecules coated by a protein layer on each surface. Hydrophilic drugs have a difficult time crossing lipid (hydrophobic) membranes. Many biologic membranes appear to contain pores that permit passage of small molecules. Some biologic membranes have mechanisms that transport specific molecules across the membrane. Examples of various transport mechanisms include diffusion, ultrafiltration, and carrier-mediated transport.

Diffusion
The following are determinants of rates of diffusion across biologic membranes.
- Concentration gradient: The concentration difference across a biologic membrane determines the direction of diffusion (high concentration to low concentration) and its rate (i.e., the rate of diffusion is directly proportional to the concentration difference).
- *Lipophilicity* is a term used to describe the solubility of the drug in fatty or oily solutions and is measured by determining the oil/water partition coefficient *(P = lipophilicity)*. The oil/water partition coefficient of a drug is a major determinant of its rate of diffusion across biologic (lipid/hydrophobic) membranes. The rate of diffusion across a membrane increases linearly with log P up to a maximum value and then declines for many drugs; for gastrointestinal absorption after oral administration, the optimal value is log P = 0.5 to 2.0; for other membranes, the optimal value may be different. The lipophilicity is determined by the number and type of different chemical substituents that are attached to the primary chemical molecule (Table 7-1).

TABLE 7-1
Relative Lipophilicity of Drugs

Drug	Key Chemical Substituents	Relative P
Most NSAIDs	COO^-, COOH	Poor
Promazine, xylazine	NH_2	
Morphine	OH	Intermediate
Lidocaine, bupivacaine	$NHCH_2 H_5$	
Oxymorphone	=O	Good
Butorphanol	CH_2- cyclobutyl	
Fentanyl	CH_3, $N(CH_3)_2$	
Naloxone	$CH_2CH=CH_2$	Excellent
Barbiturates	C_6H_5	

P, Lipophilicity.

$$[Drug]_{oil}:[Drug]_{water}$$

$$P = \frac{[Drug]_{oil}}{[Drug]_{water}}$$

- Membrane characteristics (anatomic and structural characteristics) and the permeability of different membranes may vary considerably. For example, most capillary membranes are highly permeable, but capillary membranes of the brain contain glial cells that are much less permeable to the diffusion of less lipophilic molecules. (The blood-brain barrier is not a barrier to the diffusion of lipophilic molecules because they readily diffuse through the membrane.) Drugs that are highly lipophilic readily diffuse into the various tissue compartments (e.g., extracellular space, intracellular space, CSF). The epidural or intrathecal administration of analgesic drugs provides a good example of the practical importance of lipophilicity. Highly lipid-soluble drugs (e.g., fentanyl, oxymorphone) rapidly diffuse out of the epidural space or CSF into surrounding tissues, producing a relatively short duration of analgesic effects. Morphine is less lipid soluble than fentanyl and oxymorphone and therefore produces a much longer duration of analgesic effects when administered by the epidural route.
- Small molecules (e.g., electrolytes, water, ethanol) appear to diffuse through membranes via aqueous pores. Very large molecules do not readily diffuse through membranes.

Ultrafiltration
Water and relatively small molecules (molecular weight [MW] <10,000 daltons) are forced through certain membranes (e.g., glomerular filtration) by the hydrostatic pressure of the blood. Drug molecules bound to plasma proteins are not filtered because the proteins are too large to pass through the membrane.

Carrier-Mediated Transport
Many membranes possess specialized transport mechanisms that regulate the movement of drugs and other molecules across cell membranes. These transport mechanisms generally use a carrier molecule and may (active transport) or may not (facilitated transport) require energy. Carrier-mediated transport is particularly important for the transfer of drugs across the renal tubules, biliary tract, gastrointestinal tract, and the blood-brain barrier.

- Carrier-mediated transport may or may not limit diffusion but does show the characteristics of saturation. Competitive inhibition of transport may occur if a second molecule binds to the carrier, thereby interfering with the transport of the first molecule.
- Active transport is usually coupled to an energy source such as adenosine triphosphate (ATP) and can transport molecules against an electrochemical gradient (e.g., transport of essential nutrients from the gastrointestinal tract against a concentration gradient). It is usually specific and competitive.
  1. Specificity: The transport mechanism is usually specific for a single substance or a group of closely related substances (e.g., transport of anions from the blood to the renal tubule in the nephron).
  2. Competitive: The transport process is competitively inhibited by other molecules also transported by the system (e.g., probenecid competitively inhibits transport of various penicillins in the renal tubules).
- Facilitated transport promotes the equilibration of the transported substance (e.g., transport of a molecule in the direction of its electrochemical gradient).

Distribution

The distribution of a drug to the active site is governed by four factors: *drug binding and ionization, perfusion,* and *diffusion* (discussed previously). Once a drug enters the blood, it is distributed throughout all the tissues of the body as a percentage of total blood flow or cardiac output. The body's tissues can be categorized based on the percentage of the cardiac output they receive into vessel-rich groups (e.g., heart, lung, brain, liver, kidney), muscle groups, fat groups, and vessel-poor groups (e.g., tendons, ligaments, joint spaces) for descriptive purposes. Skin can be either a vessel-rich or vessel-poor group tissue, depending on temperature. Vessel-rich group tissues receive the majority (greatest percentage) of the cardiac output and are expected to receive the greatest amount of drug in the shortest period. A decrease in cardiac output prolongs the time necessary for drug distribution, and as a result of compensatory homeostatic responses, alters drug distribution. Animals in shock, for example, have a greater percentage of their cardiac output (and therefore any intravenously administered drug) delivered to the heart, lungs, and brain. Distribution depends on total blood flow to the tissue of interest, drug binding to proteins within the blood, the ionic nature of the molecule, and factors that may facilitate or limit the permeability of the drug into tissues (see "Absorption").

Blood Flow Rate

Drugs are delivered rapidly to highly perfused tissues and slowly to poorly perfused tissues. The rate of diffusion of a drug across a membrane depends on its rate of delivery to the tissue if the drug rapidly passes through the membrane; this is known as *blood-flow rate-limited diffusion.*

* The rate of diffusion of a drug across a membrane depends on the membrane permeability characteristics if the membrane is a barrier to drug passage; this is known as *membrane-limited diffusion.*

Protein Binding

Many drugs bind reversibly to macromolecules such as plasma proteins (e.g., albumen, α_1-acid glycoprotein) and tissue proteins (Drug + Protein = Drug-Protein Complex). A bound drug is not free to diffuse or interact with receptors; some active transport processes strip bound drugs from binding sites.

* Drug protein binding in the blood reduces the concentration of *free drug* available for diffusion across membranes; therefore the rate of diffusion across the membrane is decreased when a drug is extensively bound.
* At equilibrium, the concentration of free drug is the same on both sides of the membrane; the concentration of the total drug (bound and unbound) may be quite different on the two sides of the membrane, depending on how much of it is bound to proteins.

Differential Ionization

Ionized substances do not *diffuse* across biologic membranes. There are pH differences across many biologic membranes (e.g., the pH of gastric contents ranges from about 2 to 3 and that of plasma is 7.4). These differences lead to accumulation of more total drug (i.e., ionized plus nonionized) on that side of the membrane where the drug is more ionized.

* The partitioning (tissue to plasma ratio [$R_{T/P}$] of a drug between two regions of differing pH is described by the Henderson-Hasselbach equation:

$$R_{T/P} = \frac{(1 + \text{antilog } [pKa - pH_T])}{(1 + \text{antilog } [pKa - pH_P])}$$

where pH_T and pH_P are the pH values of a tissue and plasma, respectively, and pKa is the dissociation constant of the drug. Although the pH of the plasma is maintained within very narrow limits, the pH of various tissues can vary considerably.

DRUG ELIMINATION

Two principal mechanisms, metabolism and excretion, determine drug elimination from the body. The liver and kidneys are the two major organs of elimination for most drugs, although the plasma (Hoffman elimination) and lungs are potential sites for the elimination of some drugs and inhaled gases (nitrous oxide [N_2O]) and vapors (inhalant anesthetics). The metabolism of drugs and other foreign substances is a protective mechanism that usually results in decreased lipophilicity (consequences: less protein binding, smaller V_d, higher rate of renal excretion) in some cases. Drug metabolism can result in the activation of drug effects (e.g., prodrugs: parecoxib) or toxicity.

Metabolism in the Liver

Most metabolism in the liver is mediated by the cytochrome P_{450} enzyme system, which is a heterogeneous group of enzymes. Synthesis of some of these enzymes is induced by exposure to other substances, including drugs such as phenobarbital and rifampin, and some of these enzymes are inhibited by exposure to certain inhibitors such as chloramphenicol. The capacity of the cytochrome P-450 enzyme system is very high; therefore drugs at therapeutic concentrations rarely saturate the system. Consequently the rate of metabolism is generally proportional to drug concentration; however, in cases of poisoning, the enzyme system may be saturated, and the rate of metabolism may be slower than expected.

- The anatomic position of the liver requires that substances absorbed from the gastrointestinal tract pass through it before reaching the systemic circulation; if the substance is rapidly and extensively metabolized by the liver, then the substance will undergo extensive *first-pass metabolism* (Fig. 7-4) and only a small fraction of the dose will reach the systemic circulation unchanged (e.g., isoxsuprine, propranolol, morphine, lidocaine). First-pass metabolism alters the design of dosage regimens.
- Major metabolic pathways in mammals include the following:
  1. Phase I pathways: Oxidation, reduction, hydrolysis. (Esterases are also found in plasma.)

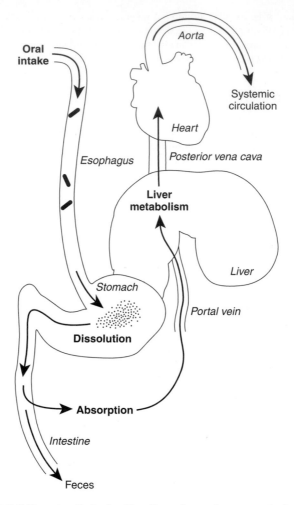

Fig. 7-4 First-pass elimination. The effects of many drugs are markedly reduced (e.g., oral opioids) or rendered biologically inactive by metabolism in the liver or by biliary excretion during first passage through the liver.

2. Phase II pathways: Conjugation (e.g., reaction of a drug or phase I metabolite with glucuronic acid). Note that glucuronic acid conjugation is deficient in cats. Differences between species are frequently due to the absence of a particular enzyme system in one species; for example, in cats the ability to conjugate most substances with glucuronic acid is absent.

3. Spontaneous decomposition occurs in the plasma at physiologic pH and near-normal temperature by means of a base-catalyzed reaction (Hoffmann elimination). In this reaction, protons (H^+) are cleaved from the α-carbon atom of the molecule, resulting in subsequent metabolism and inactive byproducts (e.g., etomidate, atracurium).

Excretion of Drugs and Drug Metabolites

Excretion of drugs and drug metabolites involves the kidneys, biliary mechanisms, and other routes (sweat and saliva).

Renal Excretion

Renal excretion is the most important route of *excretion;* it involves three mechanisms: glomerular filtration, tubular secretion, and passive reabsorption.

- *Glomerular filtration* of unbound drug. (Highly bound drugs such as the nonsteroidal antiinflammatory drugs [NSAIDs] are not excreted by glomerular filtration.)
- *Tubular secretion* of anions (e.g., NSAIDs, penicillins, cephalosporins, glucuronic acid conjugates) and cations (e.g., cimetidine) by active processes.
- *Passive reabsorption* of lipophilic drugs. (The pH of urine can have profound effects on the extent of tubular reabsorption.)

Biliary Excretion

Biliary excretion is an active process usually restricted to drugs or metabolites above a species-specific molecular size; drug conjugates are frequently secreted in the bile.

- *Enterohepatic cycling* involves the intestinal reabsorption of a drug excreted into the intestine from the liver through the bile.

Other Routes of Excretion

Excretion of drugs occurs in sweat and saliva.

ROUTES OF DRUG ADMINISTRATION

The advantages and disadvantages of various specific routes of drug administration are described in more detail elsewhere in this text (see Chapter 8). From a pharmacokinetic viewpoint, a drug can be administered by intravenous and extravascular routes with conventional or modified (prolonged release) delivery systems.

Intravenous Bolus Dose

An intravenous bolus dose refers to the rapid injection of the total dose of the drug in solution directly into a vein; the dose is usually expressed in terms of mass (e.g., mg or g) or mass per unit of body weight (bw) (e.g., mg/kg bw).

Intravenous Infusion

Intravenous infusion is slow, continuous injection of the dose of a drug directly into a vein; the dose is usually expressed in terms of mass and time (e.g., mg/min or g/hr) or mass per unit of bw per unit of time (e.g., μg/kg bw/min). A variety of commercially available infusion pumps are available for the infusion of drugs.

Extravascular Administration

Extravascular administration is administration of a dosage form by a route other than the vascular system (e.g., oral, rectal, intramuscular, subcutaneous, intraarticular, transcutaneous).

Prolonged-Release Dosage Forms

These are dosage forms designed to release the drug at a slow rate (e.g., slow-release tablets, liposome-encapsulated); note that prolonged-release dosage forms designed for use in humans may not release the drug at the desired rate in other species.

PHARMACOKINETIC CONCEPTS

Pharmacokinetic concepts are essential to an understanding of peak drug effect and the duration of drug action. The basic concepts include volume of distribution, clearance, and half-life. These are the data from which loading dose, maintenance dose, and dosing interval are initially determined. Additional concepts such as mean resonance time and bioavailability are used to adjust and refine initial calculations.

Volume of Distribution

The V_d is the apparent degree of dilution of a drug within the body. The word *apparent* is used because some drugs are bound to tissues, resulting in V_d much larger than the total volume of body water. Simply explained, if 10 mg of drug were injected into the body and the plasma concentration (Cp) was 0.002 mg/ml, then the V_d would be 5000 ml (5 L). The V_d of morphine is 6.1 L/kg in the dog and 1.35 L/kg in the cat. The V_d of lidocaine is 4.9 L/kg in the dog and 3.6 L/kg in the cat. These examples emphasize species differences and the much smaller V_d of morphine in the cat compared with that in the dog. The V_d calculated during the elimination phase is described by the relationship between the amount of drug injected into the body and the Cp of the drug at that time:

$$V_d = \frac{\text{Amount injected into body}}{Cp}$$

The V_d calculated at steady-state equilibrium (V_{dss}) defines the extent of drug dilution at the peak of drug distribution and is a more accurate assessment than V_d for drugs that appear to equilibrate with multiple body compartments. The V_{dss} is calculated as:

$$V_{dss} = \frac{\text{Dose}}{AUC?}$$

- Units of V_d are volume (e.g., ml or L) or volume per unit of bw (e.g., ml/kg bw).
- A large V_d implies extensive distribution of the drug to tissues, whereas a small V_d implies more limited distribution to tissues. Phenylbutazone has a V_d of 180 ml/kg bw in the horse; isoxsuprine has a V_d of 10 L/kg bw in the horse.
- The lower limit for V_d is the plasma volume; there is no upper limit, but values of 5 to 10 L/kg bw for lipophilic (e.g., propranolol) or highly tissue-bound (e.g., digoxin) drugs are not uncommon.
- The *mean resonance time (MRT)* is a term used to describe the average time that molecules of drug injected into the body stay in the body or the time it takes for 63.2% of a drug injected into the body to be eliminated. The MRT can be used to calculate V_{dss}.

$$V_{dss} = \frac{\text{Dose}}{AUC \times MRT}$$

Clearance

Plasma clearance (CL) is the volume of biologic fluid (blood, plasma) that is completely freed (cleared) of drug by all routes of elimination. Units for clearance are flow (e.g., ml/min) or flow per unit of bw (e.g., ml/min/kg bw). These units (ml/min/kg) emphasize that clearance is not the amount of drug being removed from the body but the amount of biologic fluid "cleared" of drug. Clearance can be calculated as the rate of elimination of the drug by all routes divided by the Cp of the drug:

$$CL = \frac{\text{Rate of elimination}}{Cp}$$

- The lower limit for clearance by an organ of elimination is zero. The upper limit is the plasma flow to the organ. Individual organ clearances can be added together for the total body clearance:

$$CL_T = CL_H + CL_R + CL_{other}$$

where CL_T is the total clearance, CL_H is the hepatic clearance, CL_R is the renal clearance, and CL_{other} represents the sum of all other clearance processes.

- The total clearance is considered the most useful pharmacokinetic parameter because it is a direct indicator of organ function and can be used to predict the average concentration or steady-state concentration of drug in the blood or plasma. For example, if the plasma clearance is 0.1 ml/min/kg and the rate of drug administration is 0.1 μg/kg/min, then the average drug concentration of the plasma is 1.0 μg/ml (0.1 μg/min/kg divided by 0.1 ml/min/kg). Knowing the total clearance provides the ability to adjust the drug dose rate during administration (impaired drug clearance) and drug interactions.

- The total clearance of all of the elimination processes in the body is calculated by dividing the dose administered by the total area under the Cp versus time curve (AUC) from the time of dosing until drug concentrations can no longer be measured (CL = Dose/AUC). In other words, if the target steady-state Cp and clearance for a drug are known, then the dose rate can be calculated by: Dose rate = Cp × CL. For example, if the target Cp is 80 μg/ml and the clearance is 0.125 ml/min/kg, then the dose rate will be 10 μg/min/kg (80 μg/ml × 0.125 ml/min/kg) or 3.6 mg every 6 hours.

Half-Life

The elimination half-life ($t_{1/2}$) is the time required for the Cp of the drug to decrease to 50% of an earlier value (Box 7-1). The units for half-life are expressed as time (minutes, hours).

- The half-life of a drug can also be used to determine the time required for a drug administered by infusion to reach a steady-state Cp (Box 7-2).
- The $t_{1/2}$, total clearance, and V_d are related by the following equation:

$$t_{1/2} = \frac{0.693 \times V_d}{CL}$$

- Changes in total clearance or V_d alter the $t_{1/2}$. For example, reduced renal clearance resulting from renal disease or toxicity decreases total clearance and increases the $t_{1/2}$.

BOX 7-1
Estimated Time for Drug Removal

1 half-life—50% eliminated
2 half-lives—75% eliminated
3 half-lives—87.5% eliminated
3.3 half-lives—90% eliminated
4 half-lives—93.75% eliminated
5 half-lives—97% eliminated

BOX 7-2
Estimated Time Required to Reach Steady State

1 half-life—50% of steady-state
2 half-lives—75% of steady state
3 half-lives—87.5% of steady state
3.3 half-lives—90% of steady state

Bioavailability

The term *bioavailability (F)* is generally taken to mean the amount of drug that reaches the systemic circulation after being administered by a nonintravenous route. For example, the bioavailability of many opioids is relatively low in dogs after oral administration because of erratic absorption and metabolism by the liver (first-pass effect) before the drug reaches the systemic circulation.

Bioequivalence

Bioequivalence is a term that is used when two products (drugs) are compared. Two drugs are considered to be bioequivalent when the Cp versus time profiles and pharmacologic, therapeutic, and toxic effects are the same after administration of equal doses. Although the peak and trough Cps of two drugs may not necessarily be exactly the same, they are considered to be bioequivalent when the maximum and minimum Cps and the time required to produce a predetermined response are the same.

Calculation of Dosage Regimens

The ability to estimate and calculate drug dosage schedules and regimens is critical to producing an appropriate therapeutic effect and avoiding adverse effects and toxicity.

Maintenance Dose

The maintenance dose is the dose administered throughout a dosage regimen to maintain effective drug concentrations (Fig. 7-5). The maintenance dose (MD) is equal to the desired Cp times the total body clearance.

$$MD = Cp \times CL$$

• For example: calculate the maintenance dose for a drug with a V_d of 2000 ml/kg bw and clearance of 20 ml/min/kg bw to be administered to a 22-lb dog to achieve a steady-state plasma drug concentration of 2 μg/ml:

$$MD = 2 \ \mu g/ml \times 20 \ ml/min/kg \ bw$$

$$MD = 40 \ \mu g/min/kg \ bw$$

$$MD = 40 \ \mu g/min \times 10 \ kg = 400 \ \mu g/min$$

or (60 min × 6 hr × 40 μg/min/kg) 14.4 mg every 6 hr

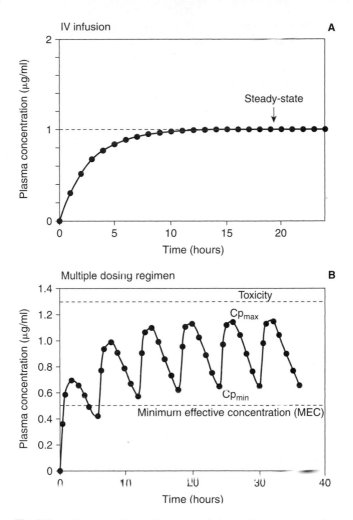

Fig. 7-5 A, Drugs administered intravenously by continuous rate infusion (CRI) reach a steady-state value that can be predicted by their half-lives (i.e., 90% of steady-state in 3.3 half-lives). **B,** The Cp varies between a Cp_{max} and Cp_{min} when drugs are administered at regular intervals (hours). Fluctuations between Cp_{max} and Cp_{min} at steady state increase as the dosing interval increases and can be predicted by the drug's half-life. The Cp_{max} is equal to two times the Cp_{min} when the dosing interval is equal to the drug's half-life.

- The time required to reach steady-state drug concentrations is determined by the terminal half-life of the drug (50% of final value in one half-life; 75% in two half-lives; 87.5% in three half-lives; 90% in 3.3 half-lives, see Box 7-2). Delay in achieving desired plasma drug concentrations may be critical for certain drugs (e.g., transcutaneous fentanyl patch).

Loading Dose

The loading dose (LD) is administered at the start of a dosage regimen to achieve effective drug concentrations rapidly. The LD is equal to the desired or target Cp multiplied by the V_d:

$$LD = Cp \times V_d$$

- Example: calculate the loading dose for a drug with a V_d of 2000 ml/kg bw and clearance of 20 ml/min/kg bw to be administered to a 22-lb dog to achieve a Cp of 2 μg/ml:

$$LD = 2 \ \mu g/ml \times 2000 \ ml/kg \ bw$$

$$LD = 4000 \ \mu g/kg \ bw \times 10 \ kg \ bw$$

$$LD = 40,000 \ \mu g \times 1 \ mg/1000 \ \mu g = 40 \ mg$$

Note: The value of the clearance term was provided but was not needed for this calculation.

Dosing Interval

The dosing interval is the period between doses in a multiple dosage regimen. An infinitely small dosing interval is a continuous rate infusion (CRI). The time taken to achieve 90% steady-state Cp during CRI is 3.3 half-lives. A drug with a 2.5-hour half-life would take approximately 8.25 hours to reach 90% of its final steady-state Cp if administered by CRI (see Fig. 7-5). Fluctuations between the maximum plasma concentration (Cp_{max}) and minimum plasma concentration (Cp_{min}) at steady state increase as the dosing interval increases (see Fig. 7-5). $Cp_{max} = 2 \times Cp_{min}$ when the dosing interval equals the half-life.

- For example: calculate the maximum dosing interval for a drug with a V_d of 2000 ml/kg bw and a clearance of 20 ml/min/kg bw if we want Cp_{max} to be no more than twice Cp_{min}.

$$Dosing \ interval = t_{1/2} = 0.693 \times V_d/CL =$$
$$0.693 \times (2000 \ ml/kg \ bw)/(20 \ ml/min/kg \ bw)$$
$$Dosing \ interval = 69.3 \ min$$

PHARMACODYNAMICS

Pharmacodynamics is the quantitative approach to describing the relationship between drug concentration and effect. Pharmacologic effects require that drug molecules be bound to constituents of cells or tissues to produce an effect. Other than the inhalant anesthetics (e.g., isoflurane, sevoflurane), which are believed to produce their effects by interacting with and structurally altering membrane lipids, most drugs produce their effects by binding to membrane proteins. Most drugs exert their effects by combining with various regulatory proteins, including enzymes (NSAIDs), carrier molecules, ion channels (local anesthetics), and "receptors" (opioids, α_2-agonists). The term *receptor* is commonly used to mean any macromolecule (generally a protein) with which the drug combines to produce its effects. Drug concentration at the receptor site is not commonly measured but is assumed to be related to the concentration of drug in blood or plasma. The drug concentration at the receptor site, however, may not be identical to its concentration in blood because of a number of factors, including drug binding to plasma and tissue proteins, ion trapping of the drug, and slow passage of the drug through membranes. Equilibration of drug between the plasma and the receptor site generally produces a predictable relationship between Cp and effect (dose-effect relationship). The clinical goal is to develop and administer a therapeutic regimen that establishes and maintains an effective plasma drug concentration for as long as is necessary.

Receptor Pharmacology

Drug receptors are really receptors for endogenous substances (e.g., endorphins, enkephalins for opioid receptors). Many different types of drug receptors in the body, when occupied by drugs, are capable of producing a myriad of cellular effects, including analgesia (Table 7-2). The pharmacologic response that follows drug (ligand) occupation of receptors is proportional to the number or fraction of occupied receptors. Analgesia is produced when a ligand attaches to the receptor, either initiating or preventing its activation.

Agonist

An agonist is a drug that binds to and activates a receptor and produces a biologic effect (Fig. 7-6). Drugs that produce the maximal response possible are called *full agonists* (i.e., the intrinsic activity is 1).

TABLE 7-2

Receptor Agonists and Antagonists Known to Produce Analgesia

Receptor Agonists/Antagonists	Receptor Subtypes
Receptor Agonists	
Opioid	μ, κ, δ
α_2	α_{2A}, α_{2B}, α_{2D}
Cannabinoid	$CB_{1,2}$
Receptor Antagonists	
Prostaglandin	EP_{1-4}
Histamine	H_1
Calcium	N and L type
Tachykinin	NK_1
NMDA	NR_1
AMPA	iGluR1-3

NMDA, N-methyl-D-aspartate; *AMPA,* α-amino-3-hydroxy-5-methyl-4-isoxazole propionic acid.

Antagonist

An antagonist is a drug that binds to a receptor and produces no biologic effect. Drug antagonists block, interfere with, or reverse the effects of agonists. A pure antagonist is assumed to produce no agonistic effects and has an intrinsic activity of zero.

- Competitive receptor antagonists compete for the receptor site. Their effects are said to be surmountable or reversible because they can be overcome by a higher dose of the agonist. Competitive antagonists shift the dose-effect curve to the right (e.g., atropine, most opioid and α_2-antagonists [opioid: nalorphine, naloxone, nalmefene; α_2: tolazoline, yohimbine, atipamezole]).
- Noncompetitive receptor antagonists produce an effect that cannot be overcome by increasing concentrations of the agonist (e.g., phenoxybenzamine, an α_1-antagonist]). Effects of noncompetitive receptor antagonists are irreversible until the drug is completely eliminated.
- Physiologic antagonism is not receptor mediated but is a term used to describe the production of an effect that is opposite to that which is not wanted (e.g., dopamine administration to raise blood pressure).

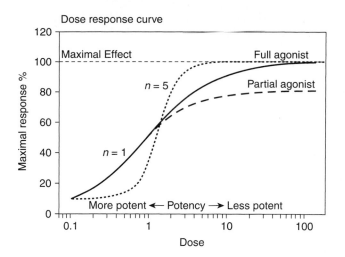

Fig. 7-6 The dose-response curve can be thought of in terms of the Cp-effect relationship and relates the drug concentration to the effect produced. Drugs that act at receptor sites (e.g., opioids, α_2-agonists) are called *full agonists* when they produce the maximal response possible (e.g., morphine, hydromorphone, fentanyl) and *partial agonists* when they produce less than the maximal effect (e.g., buprenorphine). Drugs that produce a maximal effect at lower Cp or doses are more potent than drugs that require higher Cp. The shape of the Cp-effect curve (N) is important for estimating the drug's therapeutic range and is important in the development of pharmacokinetic-pharmacodynamic models.

Partial Agonist

A partial agonist is a drug that interacts with a receptor but produces less than the maximum effect (see Fig. 7-6). A partial agonist produces less than full agonist effects (i.e., intrinsic activity is between 0.0 and 1.0) and is by definition less efficacious than a full agonist. Partial agonists may also act as partial antagonists.

Intrinsic Activity

The term *intrinsic activity* refers to the maximal possible effect that can be produced by a drug. Intrinsic activity is determined by the drug-receptor relationship for a drug that acts on receptors. Receptor pharmacology assumes that a drug's effect is proportional to the number of receptors occupied, implying that a greater effect is produced by occupation of more receptors and that a maximal effect can be produced without occupation of all the drug's receptors. Low-efficacy opioids (e.g., butorphanol) or partial agonists (e.g., buprenorphine) must by definition occupy more receptors to produce a given effect than higher-efficacy opioids (e.g., fentanyl) and are said to produce a "ceiling effect" in which higher doses of the drug do not produce a greater degree of analgesia because all the receptors are occupied. Intrinsic efficacy for opioids is as follows: fentanyl > hydromorphone > morphine > buprenorphine > butorphanol > nalbuphine.

Potency

Drug potency depends on the drug's affinity for the receptor (i.e., tendency for the drug to bind to the receptor) and efficacy (i.e., ability to produce an effect). Potency is the intensity of effect produced for a given drug dose. Two drugs can be equiefficacious (i.e., produce the same maximal response) but vary in potency (dose required to produce the response). The drug that requires the larger dose to produce the desired effect is said to be less potent.

Spare Receptors

The term *spare receptors* or *receptor reserve* is used to describe situations in which a drug produces a maximal effect by occupying only a small fraction of the total number of receptors, leaving the remaining receptors as spares or in reserve. More potent drugs (high intrinsic activity) occupy a smaller number of receptors than less potent drugs to produce a given effect and therefore have a larger receptor reserve.

Racemic Mixtures

Some drug molecules have two or more three-dimensional structures. Drugs that have the same chemical formula but two different structures are termed *isomers* of one another. Isomers that have different structures as a result of the interchange of any two groups around a central carbon atom are termed *enantiomorphs*. A drug that has an asymmetrical carbon atom (an asymmetrical center is termed a *center of chirality*) and exists as an equimolar mixture of optical (mirror image) isomers is called a *racemic mixture*. The two components of racemic mixtures may have similar or different receptor effects. Medetomidine is a racemic mixture of dexmedetomidine and levomedetomidine. Levomedetomidine is believed to be pharmacologically inactive.

Pharmacodynamic Models

As stated previously, pharmacodynamics is the study of the relationship between drug concentration and effect. Pharmacokinetics and pharmacodynamics share drug concentration as a common feature, which allows them to be combined to describe the dose-effect relationship. The most commonly used and simplest model for describing the dose-effect relationship over a range of drug concentrations is derived from the Hill equation, which relates the drug effect to the maximum drug effect (E_{max}), drug (plasma) concentration (Cp), and the drug concentration required to produce 50% of the maximum effect (EC_{50}):

$$E = \frac{E_{max} \times Cp}{EC_{50} + Cp}$$

- This equation usually produces a hyperbolic or sigmoid drug concentration–effect curve, which permits the estimation of drug effects at differing drug doses and provides insight into the pharmacodynamics of the drug. The shape of the hyperbolic drug concentration–effect curve can be modified by adding a constant parameter (N) if necessary (see Fig. 7-6):

$$E = \frac{E_{max} \times Cp^{N}}{EC_{50} + Cp^{N}}$$

Pharmacokinetic-Pharmacodynamic Models

Pharmacokinetic-pharmacodynamic models are valuable in designing drug dosage regimens, particularly when the desired effect is known. In addition, information obtained from these models is valuable in defining the drug's therapeutic index and lethal dose (Fig. 7-7).

Median Effective Dose

The median effective dose (ED_{50}) is the dose of drug required to produce a predetermined specified effect in 50% of treated animals.

Median Lethal Dose

The median lethal dose (LD_{50}) is the dose of drug required to cause death in 50% of treated animals.

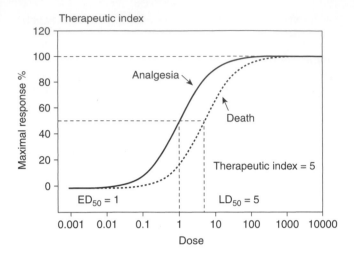

Fig. 7-7 The therapeutic index of a drug is determined by dividing the LD_{50} by the ED_{50} and provides a measure of the margin of safety for that drug.

Therapeutic Index

The therapeutic index (TI) is a measure of the margin of safety of a drug and is determined by dividing the LD_{50} by the ED_{50}.

$$TI = \frac{LD_{50}}{ED_{50}}$$

The TI may vary depending on the predetermined pharmacologic endpoint desired (e.g., analgesia versus sedation). In many instances, the ED_{50} increases while the LD_{50} stays the same, resulting in a decrease in the TI.

DRUG INTERACTIONS

The ability of one drug to alter the effects of another, thereby producing a different drug effect, is frequently encountered and often expected during clinical drug therapy. Drug interactions can be pharmacokinetic or pharmacodynamic in origin and may produce beneficial, untoward, or toxic effects. Pharmacokinetic drug interactions occur when one drug alters the Cp and therefore the effects of another drug. Infusions of lidocaine, for example, are known to slow the metabolism and elimination of drugs in the liver (opioids, α_2-agonists), thereby intensifying and prolonging their effects. A relatively recent and troubling drug interaction is that produced by the monoamine oxidase (MAO) inhibitor anipryl, which is used to control aggression in dogs and is known to interfere with the metabolism of the opioid agonist meperidine in dogs. Pharmacodynamic drug interactions occur when one drug alters a second drug's effects without changing the second drug's Cp or elimination (pharmacokinetics). The opioid antagonist naloxone, for example, is administered to reverse unwanted or toxic effects produced by prior opioid (morphine, hydromorphone) administration.

Pharmacokinetic Drug Interactions

Pharmacokinetic drug interactions occur when one drug alters the concentration and therefore the effects of another. Most pharmacokinetic drug interactions occur when one drug changes another drug's absorption, distribution, metabolism, excretion, or protein binding. (Protein-bound drugs are inactive.)

Pharmacodynamic Drug Interactions

Pharmacodynamic drug interactions occur when one drug alters the effects of another drug without altering its Cp. The most common causes of pharmacodynamic drug interactions include the various types of drug antagonism (competitive, noncompetitive), *potentiation, additivity,* and *supraadditivity (synergism).* Elaborate mathematical and statistical methods have been developed to determine whether various drug mixtures produce additive or synergistic effects. The *isobologram* is derived by comparing the effects of two drugs alone and in combination at several fixed dosages or ratios, and in its simplest form, illustrates when the drug combination being analyzed is additive, antagonistic, or synergistic (Fig. 7-8).

Additivity

Additivity or summation occurs when one drug's effects are simply additive to those of another drug. For example, if two drugs that produce analgesia are mixed together and administered, the analgesia produced is the sum of each drug's individual analgesic activity. This is generally the case when two full opioid agonists (e.g., morphine

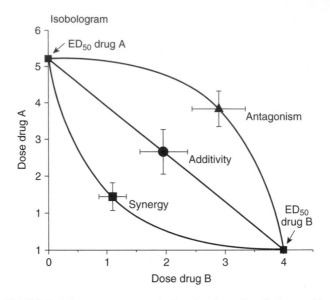

Fig. 7-8 Isobolograms are one method used to determine whether combinations of drugs are additive, synergistic, or antagonistic. The ED_{50} values for two drugs are plotted on the X and Y axes. The line that connects them is the line of additivity: a dose of drug A that produces a 25% effect and a dose of drug B that produces a 25% effect should produce a 50% effect. If lower doses than anticipated produce a 50% effect, the drug combination is said to be synergistic (concave curve), and if higher doses are required to produce the 50% effect, then the drugs are antagonistic (convex curve).

and fentanyl) are mixed together and administered. The drug dosages need not be the same because of differences in drug potency.

Potentiation

Potentiation or synergism occurs when a mixture of two or more drugs produces a greater response than expected (i.e., greater than the sum of their individual effects; see Fig. 7-8). The ability of acepromazine, a drug with little or no analgesic effects, to increase the analgesic effects of opioids (e.g., morphine, oxymorphone) is an excellent example of drug-induced potentiation or synergism. Clinically, drug synergism can be expected when two or more drugs are mixed together and produce their effects by different pharmacologic mechanisms. Various combinations (e.g., NSAIDs and opioids; opioids and α_2-agonists; opioids and local anesthetics; opioid and dissociative anesthetics) frequently demonstrate synergistic effects. Synergistic drug combinations must be administered very carefully, however, because additional unwanted and potentially toxic effects may also be potentiated (e.g., respiratory depression, bradyarrhythmias).

CLINICAL ISSUES

Therapeutic regimens, although dependent on and guided by the pharmacokinetic and pharmacodynamic principles discussed previously, must be designed and adjusted to effectively treat disease on the basis of the severity or intensity of the disease. This last statement has significant clinical relevance because drugs that act by the same or similar mechanisms of action (opioids) are frequently administered together, and drugs that are known to possess the highest intrinsic efficacy do not always produce adequate clinical effects (clinical efficacy) in patients with severe disease. Furthermore, chronic drug use can produce a variety of altered physiologic states that may be responsible for changes in a drug's pharmacokinetic and pharmacodynamic behavior. Drug tolerance and physical dependence are among the two most common problems encountered in veterinary practice.

Clinical Efficacy

Clinical efficacy refers to a drug's ability to produce a clinically beneficial therapeutic effect, regardless of that drug's intrinsic activity (maximal effect) and the dose required to produce that effect (potency). *Analgesic drugs are only as good as the pain being treated.* Fentanyl, for example, may be totally ineffective in the treatment of severe pain produced by a herniated disk. This last example has extremely important clinical implications for the administration of analgesic drugs because it implies that the severity of the disease, or in this case, the intensity of pain determines the drug's clinical efficacy. When the intensity of pain increases, the effectiveness of any given drug will decrease, and in the case of opioids, more receptors will need to be occupied to produce a therapeutic effect. Eventually, a point is reached at which no matter how many receptors are occupied, analgesia cannot be produced. In other words, the intensity of the pain dictates which analgesic drugs should be used first. Low-efficacy opioids (e.g., codeine, butorphanol, pentazocine) may be adequate for the treatment of most causes of mild-to-moderate pain and can be used in combination with higher-efficacy opioids (e.g., morphine, oxymorphone) to enhance analgesic effects but are totally ineffective and attenuate the analgesic effects of higher-efficacy opioids when used to treat severe pain. The degree of analgesia produced by an opioid is therefore determined by the intensity of pain and the intrinsic activity of the opioid. If an opioid produces analgesic effects when administered alone, an additive drug interaction will take place when it is administered with another opioid. If, however, an opioid fails to produce an analgesic effect when administered in large doses, it may antagonize or reduce the effects of a second opioid.

Tolerance

Tolerance is said to occur when the patient requires increasing drug doses over time to maintain a desired effect. Drug tolerance can develop acutely (within hours) or chronically (over days, weeks, months) and may be attributed to pharmacokinetic (e.g., liver enzyme induction and increased clearance) or pharmacodynamic (altered cellular metabolism reducing the drug's effects) changes. One potential mechanism for opioid tolerance is *receptor desensitization* caused by a decrease in functional opioid receptors secondary to chronic opioid administration. Regardless of cause, the development of drug tolerance presents a significant problem in the treatment of pain, generally requiring that drug therapy be discontinued for a period and that alternative analgesic therapies be implemented.

- Drugs that require occupancy of a smaller number of receptors to produce an effect and are therefore more potent (e.g., fentanyl) are less likely to produce tolerance than less potent drugs (e.g., codeine, butorphanol, meperidine).

Physical Dependence

Physical dependence is a pharmacologic property of a drug characterized by the development of untoward effects when that drug is acutely withheld or antagonized. The development of excitement, aggression, and seizures in a dog after the acute administration of naloxone to reverse the central nervous system and respiratory effects of an opioid (e.g., oxymorphone) is one example of physical dependence.

SUGGESTED READINGS

Abram SE, Mampilly GA, Milosavljevic D: Assessment of potency and intrinsic activity of systemic versus intrathecal opioids in rats, *Anesthesiology* 87:127-134, 1997.

Dohoo S, Tasker RAR, Donald A: Pharmacokinetics of parenteral and oral sustained-release morphine sulphate in dogs, *J Vet Pharmacol Ther* 17:426-433, 1994.

Egger CM, Duke T, Archer J, et al: Comparison of plasma fentanyl concentrations by using three transdermal fentanyl patch sizes in dogs, *Vet Anesth* 27:159-166, 1998.

Holford NHG, Sheiner LB: Understanding the dose-effect relationship: clinical application of pharmacokinetic-pharmacodynamic models, *Clin Pharmacokinet* 6:429-453, 1981.

Morgan D, Cook CD, Smith MA, et al: An examination of the interactions between the antinociceptive effects of morphine and various μ-opioids: the role of intrinsic efficacy and stimulus intensity, *Anesth Analg* 88:407-413, 1999.

Solomon RE, Gebhart GF: Synergistic antinociceptive interactions among drugs administered to the spinal cord, *Anesth Analg* 78:1164-1172, 1994.

Tallarida RJ: Statistical analysis of drug combination for synergism, *Pain* 49:93-97, 1992.

Woolf CJ, Chong N: Preemptive analgesia: treating postoperative pain by preventing the establishment of central sensitization, *Anesth Analg* 77:362-379, 1993.

8

Drugs Used to Treat Pain

WILLIAM W. MUIR III

The pharmacologic approach to the treatment of pain has evolved from a long history of folk remedies, herbal medicine, and more recently, the synthesis of chemical compounds specifically designed to activate or depress a wide variety of receptors or ion channels that are known or believed to be responsible for producing pain. Regardless of the significant scientific and technologic advances that have been made during the last decade, few if any drugs can be considered to produce excellent or even good analgesia for extended periods in dogs and cats without the risk of significant side effects or toxicity. Inadequate or unavailable scientific data, limited formulations, and an astonishing absence of controlled clinical trials further limit the chronic use of many drugs in dogs and cats. In general, currently popular drugs that have demonstrated some efficacy in the treatment of pain (nociceptive, neuropathic, idiopathic) fall into one of four broad categories: opioids, nonsteroidal antiinflammatory drugs (NSAIDs), α_2-agonists, and local anesthetics. Each group of drugs is more or less efficacious, depending on the type of pain being treated. To this list can be added an ever-increasing number of adjunctive medications known to alter either central or peripheral neuronal activity (e.g., neuroleptics [tranquilizers], anticonvulsants, antidepressants, topical preparations) or produce antiinflammatory effects (e.g., glucocorticosteroids). This chapter provides a general overview of the drugs available for the treatment of pain, emphasizing the most clinically relevant aspects of each drug group. Other chapters in this text describe and discuss the pharmacology of specific representatives of each drug group, emphasizing the drug mechanism of action, relevant pharmacology and pharmacokinetics, toxicity, and potential drug interactions (Table 8-1).

TABLE 8-1

Principal Analgesic Drugs

Drug	Relative Efficacy		Practical Issues
	Chronic Use	Acute Use	
Opioids	+/−	+ +	Tolerance
NSAIDs	+ +	+/−	Efficacy, toxicity
α₂-Agonists	−	+	Sedation
Local anesthetics	−	+ + +	Loss of motor control, toxicity

+, Efficacious; −, minimal efficacy.

OPIOIDS

The term *opioid* is preferred to the older name *narcotic,* since by definition narcotics include drugs that induce sleep, but most opioid analgesics do not induce sleep. Simply stated, opioids are any one of a growing number of natural or synthetic compounds that produce morphinelike effects by acting on opioid receptors, with the principal desired effect being the production of analgesia. From a pharmacologic perspective, opioids are of three different types: opioid agonists that act at three or four clinically relevant opioid receptor subtypes; opioid antagonists that are in general devoid of agonist activity and are used clinically to antagonize or reverse opioid effects; and opioid agonist-antagonists and partial agonists that produce morphinelike effects but are generally less toxic (although often less effective) than morphine.

Opioids vary in their receptor specificity, potency, and efficacy at the different opioid receptors (μ, κ, δ, σ), resulting in a wide variety of clinical effects, depending on the opioid administered, the dose, and the species to which the drug is administered (e.g., dog, cat) (Box 8-1). Opioid agonists have a relatively high affinity for μ and κ receptors and are noted for their ability to produce analgesia and sedation (e.g., morphine, meperidine, oxymorphone). Opioid antagonists block or reverse the effects of opioid agonists by combining with opioid receptors and producing minimal or no effects. Opioid agonists-antagonists and partial agonists act by combining with opioid receptors and producing partial or complete activation of the receptor, depending on the receptor (μ, κ, δ, σ) being activated. Opioid

```
┌─────────────────────────────────────────────────────────────┐
│                         BOX 8-1                               │
│                 Opioid Receptor Subtypes                      │
│                 ─────────────────────────                     │
│ Receptor Subtype                                              │
│ μ     Supraspinal, spinal, and peripheral analgesia; minimal  │
│          to mild sedation; respiratory depression;            │
│          bradycardia; ileus; urine retention; temperature     │
│          reduction                                            │
│ κ     Supraspinal, spinal (?), and peripheral analgesia;      │
│          minimal sedation, respiratory depression, and        │
│          bradycardia                                          │
│ δ     Supraspinal, spinal, and peripheral analgesia; minimal  │
│          sedation, respiratory depression, and bradycardia;   │
│          ileus, urine retention; temperature reduction        │
│ σ     Excitement-delirium, tachycardia, hypertension          │
└─────────────────────────────────────────────────────────────┘
```

agonists-antagonists and partial agonists may act as antagonists for opioid agonists because of their relatively high affinity for opioid receptors and comparatively low potential for toxicity.

Pharmacologic Considerations

As suggested in Table 8-2, different opioids produce varied pharmacologic effects based on their ability to combine with and activate the various opioid receptor subtypes. The prevalence and location of the various receptor subtypes in the different species, effects caused by opioid receptor selectivity, molecular size and shape, and the influence of various disease processes ultimately determine the opioid's pharmacologic properties in any given animal. Methadone, for example, is known to act primarily at μ-opioid receptors but is also known to partially inhibit N-methyl-D-aspartate (NMDA) receptors in the spinal cord.

Central Nervous System

Opioids relieve or reduce pain by combining with opioid receptors in the central nervous system (CNS) and periphery. They are generally considered to be the most effective of all analgesic medications but vary widely in their analgesic potency and clinical efficacy when used to treat different types of pain (e.g., superficial, visceral, deep). Fentanyl, for example, is at least 100 times more potent than morphine and produces excellent clinical analgesia when administered at what would be considered extremely small (μg/kg) doses

TABLE 8-2
Selectivity for Opioid Receptor Subtypes

Drug	μ	κ	δ	σ
Agonists				
Morphine	+++	++	++	−
Meperidine	++	+	++	−
Methadone	+++	+	++	−
Codeine	+	+	+	−
Oxymorphone	+++	+	+	−
Fentanyl	++++	−	+	−
Partial/Mixed Agonists				
Butorphanol	++	(++)	−	++
Pentazocine	+	(++)	+	++
Nalbuphine	+	(++)	(++)	+
Buprenorphine	(+++)	−	−	−
Antagonists				
Naloxone	+++	++	++	−
Naltrexone	+++	++	++	−
Atypical Opioid				
Tramadol	+	?	?	−

+, Mild effect; ++, moderate effect; +++, pronounced effect; ++++, very pronounced effect; ( ), partial agonist effects, ?, unknown; −, little or no effect.

compared with most opioid analgesics (e.g., morphine, oxymorphone, butorphanol [mg/kg]).

Most opioid agonists produce minimal to moderate sedation when administered at recommended dosages as single-drug therapy. However, they are capable of producing profound CNS and respiratory depression or arrest when administered with tranquilizers (neuroleptanalgesia) or injectable or inhalant anesthetics or when administered to patients with head trauma or seizures or to patients who are depressed and debilitated. When sedated, most dogs and cats demonstrate increased responsiveness to sound. Some dogs will react wildly and aggressively to loud or high-pitched noises. Increased dosages of opioids can produce nervousness, agitation, increased locomotor activity, dysphoria, and occasionally hyperthermia (cats). Cats are particularly susceptible to the neuroexcitatory effects of opioids. Early experience with morphine suggested that opioids produced excitement and mania in cats (morphine mania). This response is now known to be due to species differences and a relative drug overdose. Seizures can be triggered on rare occasions and have been attributed to drug metabolites or preexisting CNS disorders. Aged pets may be particularly susceptible to the CNS and behavioral effects of opioids, with some animals demonstrating indifference, malaise, and disorientation. Others may become timid or aggressive when approached. The development of "release of suppressed behavior," manifesting as aggression, must be considered when any drug that alters CNS activity is administered. Changes in behavior and the development of aggression have been attributed to central neurochemical mechanisms involving both opioid and dopamine receptors.

Nausea and vomiting (in dogs and cats) and panting (in dogs) are acute phenomena that are frequently observed after intramuscular opioid administration. Opioids are known to stimulate the chemoreceptor trigger zone (CTZ) and reset thermoregulatory centers in the hypothalamus, resulting in a slight fall in body temperature. Vomiting may be considered an advantage if the dog or cat has recently eaten and is being considered as a candidate for surgery. Vomiting and retching, however, are problematic if the patient is believed to have a pharyngeal, esophageal, or gastric foreign body. Panting is a common clinical sign after the administration of an opioid to dogs but does not provide adequate ventilation because only dead-space gas is moved in and out of the upper airways. Dogs and cats that have received opioids as preanesthetic medication may require manual or mechanical ventilation to achieve adequate ventilation and avoid respiratory acidosis during anesthesia. Shivering is common after anesthesia because body temperature may be decreased. Shivering increases postoperative oxygen and caloric requirements, which could become important in older, very young, and small patients. Shivering may also be a sign of inadequate analgesia. Some opioids (e.g., meperidine) decrease the incidence of shivering by a mechanism independent of the drug's analgesic effects.

Most opioids depress the cough reflex by a central mechanism. Cough suppression is produced at subanalgesic doses and is prominent with less effective opioids (e.g., codeine) and opioid agonists-antagonists (e.g., butorphanol). Cough suppression may lead to the accumulation of mucous secretions in the airways of patients recovering from anesthesia, predisposing them to upper airway obstruction.

Opioids generally produce pinpoint pupils (miosis) in dogs as a result of CNS stimulation of parasympathetic segments of the oculomotor nerve. This response can be inhibited by prior administration of anticholinergic drugs (e.g., atropine, glycopyrrolate). The pupil dilates (mydriasis) in cats as a result of stimulation of CNS sympathetic pathways.

Respiratory System

Opioids are notorious for their respiratory depressant effects in depressed or anesthetized animals. Opioids increase the concentration of carbon dioxide necessary to produce an initial increase in rate and depth of breathing (increase in respiratory threshold) and depress the ventilatory response to increasing inspired concentrations of carbon dioxide (decrease in respiratory sensitivity). Clinically, both effects predispose patients to hypoventilation and the development of respiratory acidosis. Although of significant clinical relevance, respiratory depression is not a frequently reported problem in dogs and cats administered opioids as compared with humans. The best explanation for this difference is that most opioids do not produce the same degree of euphoria and CNS depression in dogs or cats as they do in humans. In other words, the severity of opioid-induced respiratory depression in dogs and cats is directly related to the amount of CNS depression produced. As long as the patient remains conscious, it is unlikely that respiratory depression will become problematic. Respiratory depression in patients administered tranquilizers or sedatives in conjunction with opioids before anesthesia is of greater concern, and in these patients, ventilation should be closely monitored.

Chest wall rigidity, or "woody chest syndrome," can occur in dogs or cats administered large or repeated doses of opioids (e.g., fentanyl). Increased thoracic and abdominal muscle rigidity may be related to the CNS excitation caused by larger doses of opioids, and when severe, can result in increases in body temperature and interfere with breathing.

Cardiovascular System

Other than bradycardia and occasional bradyarrhythmias, opioids produce relatively few if any clinically significant cardiovascular effects in dogs and cats when administered at recommended doses. First-degree (prolonged PR interval), second-degree (P interval not followed by a QRS interval), and rarely, third-degree (no relationship between P and QRS complexes) atrioventricular block can occur, which is attributed to a vagally mediated increase in parasympathetic tone and is therefore responsive to anticholinergic therapy.

Opioids produce clinically insignificant effects on the force of cardiac contraction (inotropy), arterial blood pressure, and cardiac output unless administered as a rapid intravenous bolus. Some opioids (e.g., morphine, meperidine) are noted for producing histamine release (in cats) or splanchnic sequestration of blood (in dogs), which could exacerbate hypotension. The clinical impact of these effects, however, remains to be demonstrated. Histamine release in cats is signaled by increased redness of the ears and paws, which results from increased blood flow.

Other Organ Systems

Gastrointestinal System

Opioids delay gastric emptying and prolong intestinal transit time. Gastric and intestinal smooth muscle tone are increased producing "ropy guts," which are particularly evident after the administration of an opioid to puppies or kittens. Increases in intestinal smooth muscle tone are caused by centrally mediated increases in vagal tone and activation of opioid receptors throughout the gastrointestinal tract. The onset of opioid-induced gastrointestinal effects may result in defecation and a period of diarrhea in dogs. This is followed by a decrease in propulsive peristaltic activity and absorption of water from the intestinal tract, predisposing the patient to constipation, a condition that becomes more prominent when opioids are administered for several days. Opioids increase esophageal, biliary, duodenal, and anal sphincter tone, making it difficult to perform endoscopic examinations, particularly of the duodenum. Opioids should be avoided in patients believed to have an obstructed biliary tract or biliary neoplasm.

Genitourinary System

Opioids inhibit the voiding reflex and increase external urethral sphincter tone, resulting in urine retention. Urine retention can be an important postsurgical consideration in dogs and cats that have undergone prolonged surgical procedures or abdominal surgery or in those with preexisting bladder dysfunction. Although popular because of their analgesic and sedative effects, most opioids decrease uterine contractions, thereby prolonging labor. This issue may be of little consequence if a cesarean section is performed. Respiratory depression of the fetus is of potential concern, however, and can be treated with opioid antagonists or doxapram.

Clinical Issues

Opioids are controlled substances, making their clinical use problematic because of strict ordering, storage, and record-keeping requirements. These bureaucratic issues aside, opioids are the most effective therapy for pain from all causes. They are least effective, however, in the treatment of pain caused by nerve injury and other forms of neuropathic pain (e.g., spinal cord compression). The routine clinical use of opioids for analgesia or as preanesthetic medication must be considered within the framework of the patient's medical problems, the severity of the patient's pain, and the potential for anesthesia. Low doses of opioid agonists-antagonists (e.g., butorphanol), for example, can be additive with opioid agonists (e.g., oxymorphone). Opioid antagonist effects, however, are to be expected when large or repeated doses of an opioid agonist-antagonist (e.g., butorphanol, pentazocine) or partial agonist (e.g., buprenorphine) are administered to a patient that has received an opioid agonist (e.g., morphine, oxymorphone). Furthermore, not all opioid effects can be antagonized. The administration of the partial agonist buprenorphine, for example, after administration of an opioid agonist (e.g., morphine, oxymorphone) can lead to increased respiratory depression in some patients. Finally, diseases (liver, renal, CNS) and drugs (anesthetics) that prolong opioid metabolism and elimination may be responsible for prolonged drug effects, resulting in extended periods of depression and unconsciousness.

NONSTEROIDAL ANTIINFLAMMATORY DRUGS

NSAIDs represent a diverse group of chemical compounds that are currently the most popular analgesic drugs used in small animal veterinary practice (Box 8-2). In addition to *analgesia* they are noted for their *antiinflammatory* and *antipyretic* effects. NSAIDs act by nonspecifically inhibiting various isoforms of arachidonate cyclooxygenase synthase (COX), which are responsible for the production of prostaglandins (e.g., PGE_2) from arachidonic acid. Prostaglandins produce their algesic, proinflammatory, and pyretic effects by activating prostaglandin receptors throughout the body.

BOX 8-2
Nonsteroidal Antiinflammatory Drugs

Salicylic Acids
Aspirin

Para-Aminophenol
Acetaminophen

Fenamic Acids
Flunixin meglumine

Pyrazolones
Dipyrone
Phenylbutazone

Propionic Acids
Carprofen
Ketoprofen
Naproxen
Ibuprofen

Oxicams
Piroxicam
Meloxicam

Acetic Acids
Ketorolac
Etodolac

There are at least two types of COX: COX-1 and COX-2. COX-1, or "housekeeping" COX, is primarily involved in cell signaling and maintaining tissue homeostasis. Inhibition of COX-1 is believed to be responsible for the majority of acute and chronic toxicities of NSAIDs. COX-2, sometimes referred to as *inducible COX,* is induced in inflammatory cells and is the principal enzyme responsible for the production of inflammatory mediators. Most NSAIDS that are currently available inhibit both COX-1 and COX-2 isoenzymes. The recent availability of relatively specific COX inhibitors (e.g., COX-2; rofecoxib, celecoxib) offers the potential to provide improved analgesic and antiinflammatory effects for extended periods without interfering with the normal physiologic role (housekeeping functions) that prostaglandins have throughout the body. The nonsedating, analgesic, and low-toxicity profile of newer NSAIDs (e.g., carprofen, etodolac) has helped allay traditional concerns about gastrointestinal and renal toxicity, blood clotting abnormalities, and efficacy. Future NSAIDs hold the promise of greater specificity for inhibition of COX-2 or the various prostaglandin receptors, improved convenience (oral and parenteral preparations), a long duration of action (administration once a day), and less toxicity.

Pharmacologic Considerations

Regardless of their diverse chemical structure and selectivity for COX-1 or COX-2, most NSAIDs produce relatively subtle therapeutic differences. NSAIDs that primarily affect COX-1 (e.g., aspirin, ibuprofen) are somewhat of an exception to the previous statement, based on their ability to inhibit platelet aggregation. Because it is not easy to determine the extent to which pain and inflammation are dependent on either COX-1–mediated or COX-2–mediated effects, it is difficult to select the one best NSAID. Since the majority of proinflammatory prostaglandins are believed to be produced by the induction of COX-2, it is reasonable to conclude that drugs producing more specific COX-2 effects would be more effective in producing analgesic, antiinflammatory, and antipyretic effects, but this conclusion remains speculative. Similarly, NSAIDs that interfere with normal homeostatic activity (COX-1 effects) would be more likely to produce toxicity. Clinically, these conclusions turn out to be generally true in that COX-2 inhibitors are often more effective and less toxic than COX-1 inhibitors. Nevertheless, veterinarians should not hesitate to try an alternative NSAID if the one currently selected does not prove to be of therapeutic benefit. It is also important to remember that NSAIDs can produce toxicity by mechanisms that are independent of COX inhibition.

Central Nervous System

NSAIDs are noted for producing important CNS effects that alter the animal's level of consciousness or behavior. Peripheral analgesia, although primarily due to the local inhibition of prostaglandin production, may also be due to the inhibition of prostaglandin generation in the spinal cord and brain. NSAIDs are synergistic with opioids and reduce the amount of opioid required to produce effective analgesia.

Neurons within the hypothalamus that are responsible for regulating body temperature are affected by prostaglandins, resulting in an increase in the setpoint and in fever. NSAIDs return the setpoint to normal by inhibiting prostaglandin production.

Respiratory System

NSAIDs are not known to produce clinically relevant effects on the respiratory system. They may, however, improve respiratory function in animals with respiratory- and inflammatory-mediated bronchoconstrictive diseases. On rare occasions, NSAIDs have been incriminated in the production of acute asthma-like signs. The mechanism for this is unclear, but it has been suggested that leukotriene (e.g., LTC-4, LTD-4) production may increase when arachidonate metabolism is diverted from the COX pathway. Increased production of LTC-4 and LTD-4 causes airway hyperreactivity and bronchial contractions.

Cardiovascular System

NSAIDs do not produce significant cardiovascular effects.

Inhibition of prostaglandin production secondary to infection, trauma, or a generalized systemic inflammatory response can help prevent vasodilation, edema, and platelet consumption.

Some NSAIDs, particularly those that possess significant COX-1 selectivity (e.g., aspirin), are noted for their inhibitory effect on platelet aggregation, resulting in the potential for prolonged bleeding times and the development of edema at sites of tissue injury.

NSAIDs occasionally cause fluid retention in patients with heart failure.

Other Organ Systems

Gastrointestinal System

Prostaglandins play an important role in the development of a protective gastric barrier to intraluminal acidity, sustaining secretory activity and maintaining normal gut motility. The use of NSAIDs predisposes to gastric ulceration, particularly in animals with gastrointestinal disease.

Genitourinary System

Prostaglandins play an important role in maintaining normal renal tubular function. The use of NSAIDs may promote renal blood flow and produce diuretic effects in some animals.

Clinical Issues

NSAIDs are weak analgesics. Although most effective for treating pain caused by inflammation or trauma, they rarely eliminate all pain and are relatively ineffective for treating severe pain. Gastrointestinal, renal, or liver toxicity and the potential for excessive bleeding are potential problems associated with the clinical use of NSAIDs. These issues are particularly important in very young or old animals and in animals that are immunocompromised or have preexisting cardiovascular, renal, or liver disease. The potential for altered platelet function and blood dyscrasias should be considered if NSAIDs are to be administered chronically. Significant differences between drugs and their metabolism by different species (dogs versus cats) emphasize the importance of strictly adhering to dose recommendations and dosing schedules if toxicity is to be prevented.

α_2-AGONISTS

α_2-Agonists were initially developed for use as antihypertensive agents (e.g., clonidine) in humans and for their sedative, muscle relaxant, and analgesic effects in animals (Box 8-3). Moderate-to-excellent analgesia can be produced, but only with an associated degree of sedation. Like the opioids, α_2-agonists produce the majority of their clinically relevant pharmacologic effects by activating a variety of α_2-receptor subtypes (e.g., α_{2A}, α_{2B}, α_{2C}, α_{2D}) in the CNS and periphery. The discovery of a receptor-based mechanism has led to the identification and synthesis of α_2-receptor antagonists (e.g., yohimbine, tolazoline, atipamezole). Based on differences in chemical structure, some α_2-agonists are capable of activating imidazoline receptors (I_1, I_2) and producing direct effects (e.g., xylazine). The diversity in chemical structure, receptor specificity, and receptor density and location among the various α_2-agonists has led to considerable differences in drug dosages and effects of α_2-agonists among and within species. Notorious for the frequency, scope, and severity of their cardiovascular side effects, α_2-agonists must be administered with caution to very young, aged, or debilitated patients

---

BOX 8-3

α_2-Agonists

- Xylazine
- Detomidine
- Medetomidine
- Dexmedetomidine
- Romifidine

and are contraindicated in most patients with cardiovascular diseases. Future α_2-agonists will be designed to activate specific receptor subtypes, ideally limiting their CNS depressant actions and decreasing the frequency of side effects.

Pharmacologic Considerations

More than any other group of drugs with analgesic effects, the clinical use of α_2-agonists centers on their CNS (sedative), cardiovascular, and respiratory effects. In addition to the production of analgesia, consideration must be given to the potential for the development of profound sedation with unexpected or aggressive behavioral changes, significant bradycardia, and respiratory depression. The potential for drug interactions (particularly with anesthetics) and amplification of toxic side effects is high.

Central Nervous System

α_2-Agonists produce sedative and analgesic effects by activating both presynaptic and postsynaptic α_2-receptors in the CNS. Sedation in dogs and cats is attributed to activation of the CNS α_{2A}-receptor subtype in areas of the brain that are responsible for awareness, arousal, and vigilance. Activation of α_1-receptors may play some part in the pharmacology of most α_2-receptor agonists because most currently available α_2-receptors can activate α_1-receptors. Increased and potentially toxic doses of most α_2-agonists produce an initial period of reduced or poor sedation attributed to activation of CNS α_1-receptors. Like other calming drugs (e.g., phenothiazines), α_2-agonists are capable of eliciting a release of "suppressed behavior." Dogs or cats that appear sedated may become suddenly aroused and aggressive if disturbed. Many dogs, cats, and especially horses seem to demonstrate increased sensitivity to sound and initial tactile contact.

Activation of α_2-receptors in the brain and spinal cord decreases pain-related neurotransmitters and interferes with sensory transmission. α_2-Agonists also act peripherally at α_2-receptors to produce analgesia, and some α_2-agonists (e.g., xylazine) produce local anesthetic effects.

Vomiting is a common side effect in dogs, and especially in cats, after the intravenous administration of an α_2-agonist. Activation of α_2-receptors within the CTZ is responsible for nausea and retching.

All α_2-agonists impair the control of body temperature through CNS-mediated dose-dependent effects on temperature thresholds for sweating, vasoconstriction, and shivering. These effects predispose dogs and cats to hypothermia, particularly during the postoperative period. However, α_2-agonists are also an effective treatment for shivering. Occasionally the administration of α_2-agonists is responsible for triggering hyperthermia secondary to intense peripheral vasoconstriction and an inability to dissipate heat. Hyperthermia is more likely to occur in hot, humid environments.

Respiratory System

α_2-Agonists produce a dose-dependent decrease in breathing rate and volume that parallels the degree of CNS depression. Pronounced CNS depression is associated with increases in respiratory center threshold and decreases in respiratory center sensitivity (decreased response to Pco_2) to carbon dioxide. Both effects combine to produce significant respiratory acidosis and hypoxemia in some patients. Clinical doses generally produce mild respiratory acidosis, which is of little consequence unless the patient becomes unconscious or is administered an anesthetic.

α_2-Agonists cause marked relaxation of the upper airway muscles of the pharynx and larynx, which can result in irregular breathing patterns, inspiratory dyspnea, and upper airway obstruction, particularly in brachycephalic breeds.

Cardiovascular System

The α_2-agonists are capable of producing extensive and at times profound cardiovascular effects. Chief among these are effects on heart rate and rhythm. Sinus bradycardia and bradyarrhythmias are common after the administration of α_2-agonists. First-degree and second-degree atrioventricular block are the most common bradyarrhythmias to occur, although third-degree atrioventricular block and sinus arrest with ventricular escape beats are occasionally observed. Atrioventricular block and decreases in heart rate are caused by the combined effects of decreases in CNS sympathetic output and increases in vagally mediated parasympathetic tone, indicating that the administration of an anticholinergic (e.g., atropine, glycopyrrolate) may be effective in preventing or inhibiting bradycardia and atrioventricular block. It is important to remember that the administration of an anticholinergic to dogs or cats that have been given an α_2-agonist makes them more susceptible to the development of ventricular arrhythmias, including ventricular fibrillation. Therefore anticholinergics and α_2-agonists should not be administered to patients with preexisting ventricular arrhythmias, myocardial contusion, or any other cause of ventricular electrical instability. Some α_2-agonists (e.g., xylazine) transiently sensitize the heart to catecholamine-induced arrhythmias, especially during halothane anesthesia. The clinical relevance of this effect, however, has not been established, and this effect has not been observed during isoflurane or sevoflurane anesthesia.

Arterial blood pressure (ABP) usually increases transiently and then decreases from baseline values after the administration of an α_2-agonist. The early period of vasoconstriction and hypertension is initiated by stimulation of peripheral vascular α_1- and α_2-receptors and is partly responsible for the development of bradyarrhythmias because of an increase in baroreceptor reflex activity and vagal tone. The long-term decrease in arterial blood pressure parallels decreases in CNS sympathetic output and heart rate.

Cardiac output decreases almost immediately after the administration of an α_2-agonist, primarily because of decreases in heart rate (CO = HR × Stroke Volume; where CO is cardiac output and HR is heart rate). The short-term and long-term decreases in cardiac output also can be attributed to vasoconstriction (increased afterload) and decreases in CNS sympathetic output, resulting in a decrease in cardiac contractile force and stroke volume.

Other Organ Systems

Gastrointestinal System

Vomiting and retching are common consequences of α_2-agonist administration in dogs and cats. Lower doses and subcutaneous administration help minimize this side effect, which is mediated by α_2-receptor effects in the CTZ in the CNS. α_2-Agonists produce immediate and pronounced decreases in gastrointestinal motility in dogs and cats, which can last for several hours. Gastrointestinal stasis is caused by stimulation of α_2-receptors in the gut and increases in serum gastrin concentration. This effect is somewhat dose-dependent but is believed to be responsible for postoperative ileus, gas accumulation, and potentially, the development of "bloat" in dogs.

Endocrine System

α_2-Receptors modulate the release of insulin by the pancreas, causing a transient decrease in serum insulin levels and an increase in serum glucose levels, resulting in glycosuria. This effect is mediated by α_2-receptor modulation of insulin secretion by beta cells in the pancreas.

Genitourinary System

α_2-Agonists promote diuresis both by their glucosuric effects and direct actions on the renal tubules to decrease renal tubular salt and water absorption. Labor can be delayed or prolonged as a result of sedative and muscle relaxant effects.

Clinical Issues

Although potentially useful as analgesics for minor medical or surgical procedures or as preanesthetic medication for general anesthesia, the α_2-agonists produce too many side effects to be considered as routine therapy for all but healthy dogs and cats. They may have considerable benefit as analgesics when administered into the epidural or subarachnoid space, but these routes of administration and others await detailed clinical evaluation.

LOCAL ANESTHETICS

All local anesthetics block the initiation and conduction of electrical activity (action potentials) in nerves (Table 8-3). Small-diameter (C, Aδ) nerve fibers are blocked first in preference to large myelinated fibers (Aβ), thereby producing analgesia (i.e., loss of sensory function) and varying degrees of paralysis (i.e., loss of motor function). More specifically, local anesthetics block sodium ion channels in neuronal cells and other tissues, thereby preventing an influx of sodium ions, membrane depolarization, and creation of a propagated action potential. Nonspecific membrane effects similar to those produced by inhalant anesthetics may be partially responsible for their CNS and analgesic effects. Analgesia is a direct result of sodium ion channel blockade and membrane stabilization. Local anesthetics are most frequently used to produce analgesia by administering them at specific sites (topical, local) or on nerves (regional).

TABLE 8-3
Local Anesthetic Drugs

Drug	Route of Administration
Lidocaine	IV, T, I, NB, E, S
Bupivacaine	I, NB, E, S
Mepivacaine	I, NB, E, S
Ropivacaine	I, NB, E, S
Cetacaine	T
Mexiletine	PO

IV, Intravenous (systemic or regional); *T,* topical; *I,* infiltration; *NB,* nerve-block; *E,* epidural; *S,* spinal; *PO,* oral.

Pharmacologic Considerations

Although noted for their local analgesic effects, most local anesthetic drugs produce mild CNS depressant (anesthetic-sparing), antiarrhythmic, antishock, and gastrointestinal promotility effects. Significant differences exist among the various local anesthetics with regard to their metabolism, elimination, and potential to produce toxicity in dogs, cats, and horses. Cats and horses, for example, are much more susceptible to the neurotoxic side effects of local anesthetics than dogs.

Central Nervous System

Local anesthetics, as their name implies, produce analgesia by suppressing or blocking electrical activity in both sensory and motor nerves. Their preferential blocking of small unmyelinated nerves suggests that appropriate (small) doses should limit motor dysfunction, but this has been difficult, if not impossible, to take advantage of clinically.

Low doses of local anesthetics produce negligible effects on the CNS. Mild sedation may occur as a result of membrane-stabilizing effects, a generalized decrease in neuronal activity, and a centrally mediated decrease in sympathetic tone. Most local anesthetics potentiate the effects of injectable (e.g., thiopental, propofol) and inhalant anesthetics (e.g., halothane, isoflurane, sevoflurane), resulting in a decrease in the amount of anesthetic required (anesthetic sparing) to produce surgical anesthesia.

Large doses of local anesthetics are capable of producing CNS stimulation typified by nervousness, excitement, agitation, disorientation, nystagmus, and convulsions. These effects are believed to be caused by the inhibition of inhibitory processes within the CNS, and when severe, can result in death caused by respiratory paralysis.

Respiratory System

Local anesthetics produce minimal if any significant effects on the respiratory system other than those associated with their effects on the CNS.

Large volumes of solutions containing local anesthetic drugs have the potential to produce respiratory paralysis when administered by epidural or spinal (subarachnoidal) routes. The migration of the local anesthetic cranially to the C6 nerve roots can paralyze the diaphragm, resulting in hypoventilation and apnea.

Cardiovascular System

Therapeutic doses of local anesthetics produce minimal cardiovascular effects in otherwise healthy dogs and cats. Heart rate may increase as a result of sympathetic suppression and arteriolar dilatation.

A large dose or rapid intravenous administration of local anesthetic drugs decreases cardiac output, arterial blood pressure, and heart rate. A reduction in cardiac output is caused by decreases in CNS sympathetic output, myocardial contractile force, and venous return. These effects are more prominent in stressed or sick animals that are dependent on sympathetic nervous system activity for maintaining homeostasis.

Local anesthetics possess antiarrhythmic activity but have the potential to produce sinus bradycardia and bradyarrhythmias with associated hypotension when administered too rapidly by the intravenous route. Local anesthetics should not be administered to dogs or cats with high-grade (two or more blocked P waves) second-degree or third-degree atrioventricular block, since they can cause further depression of conduction and suppress ventricular escape beats, leading to cardiac arrest.

Other Organ Systems

Gastrointestinal System

High sympathetic tone can cause complete gut stasis and can be responsible for the development of ileus in the postsurgical patient. Local anesthetics promote gastrointestinal motility by suppressing sympathetic tone.

Hematopoietic System

Some local anesthetics (e.g., benzocaine, dibucaine) can produce methemoglobinemia. This is particularly important in puppies and cats of all ages.

Clinical Issues

The biggest clinical issues associated with currently available local anesthetics are their lack of selectivity for sensory nerve fibers, their potential to cause motor paralysis, and the unavailability of effective oral preparations. Local anesthetics produce good-to-excellent analgesia when administered topically or injected locally but at the expense of a loss of motor function (temporary paralysis when administered epidurally), which can become problematic in some surgical patients (cesarean section, fracture repair) and may induce untoward behavioral responses in others. The systemic infusion of lidocaine produces clinically relevant analgesia when administered adjunctively with inhalant (e.g., isoflurane, sevoflurane) or injectable (e.g., ketamine, propofol) anesthetics, opioids, or α_2-agonists whose analgesic effects are potentiated. Mexiletine ("oral lidocaine") can be used as an alternative to injectable lidocaine for this purpose. Toxicity (CNS and cardiovascular) is most likely to occur after accidental intraarterial injection, after bolus injections of large doses, during high infusion rates, or when multiple bolus injections of smaller doses are administered over a short period. Cimetidine and other drugs that modify liver metabolism can prolong the elimination of local anesthetics and increase the potential for toxicity.

NONTRADITIONAL ANALGESICS FOR THE TREATMENT OF PAIN

A growing number of drugs representing widely diverse chemical families are being used increasingly as adjunctive and adjuvant therapy for the treatment of acute, but more commonly, chronic pain (Tables 8-4 and 8-5). Corticosteroids, local anesthetics, anticonvulsants, and several behavior-modifying drugs (e.g., clomipramine) are capable of producing adjuvant analgesic activity. Anticonvulsants and behavior-modifying drugs (e.g., tricyclic antidepressants, clomipramine) may be efficacious for treating chronic pain syndromes, particularly neuropathic pain. Many drugs used to enhance calming and produce muscle relaxation before surgery (e.g., acepromazine,

TABLE 8-4

Adjuvant Analgesic Drugs

Drug Category	Concerns
Corticosteroids Prednisone Prednisolone Dexamethasone	Tissue edema, immune suppression
Local Anesthetics Lidocaine Mexiletine	CNS toxicity, CV depression
Tranquilizers/Muscle Relaxants Acepromazine Chlorpromazine Diazepam Midazolam	CNS depression, hypotension
Anticonvulsants Gabapentin Phenytoin Carbamazepine	Disorientation, depression
Antidepressants Amitriptyline Clomipramine	Behavioral changes, anticholinergic effects
Calcium Antagonists Diltiazem	Bradycardia, hypotension
Sympatholytics Propranolol Atenolol Prazosin	Bradycardia, hypotension
Miscellaneous Drugs Codeine Dextromethorphan Tramadol Clonidine Ketamine Magnesium salts ($Mg^{-2}SO_4^{-2}$)	Disorientation, depression

CV, Cardiovascular.

TABLE 8-5

Adjuvant Analgesic Drugs

Drug	Dosage in Dogs	Dosage in Cats
Corticosteroids		
Prednisone	1.0-2.2 mg/kg PO	1-2 mg/kg PO
Prednisolone	1.0-2.2 mg/kg PO	1-2 mg/kg PO
Dexamethasone	0.10-0.15 mg/kg SC, PO	0.10-0.15 mg/kg SC, PO
Local Anesthetics		
Lidocaine	2-4 mg/kg IV bolus then 25-75 µg/kg IV infusion	0.25-1.0 mg/kg IV bolus then 10-40 µg/kg IV infusion
Mexiletine	4-10 mg/kg PO	—
Tranquilizers/Muscle Relaxants		
Acepromazine	0.025-1.13 mg/kg IV, SC, IM	0.05-2.25 mg/kg IM, SC, IV, PO
Chlorpromazine	0.05-0.50 mg/kg SC, IM; 0.8-4.4 mg/kg PO	0.5 mg/kg IM, IV; 2-4 mg/kg PO
Diazepam	2-5 mg/kg IV; 0.5-2.2 mg/kg PO	2-5 mg/kg IV; 0.5-2.2 mg/kg PO
Midazolam	0.066-0.22 mg/kg IV, IM	0.066-0.22 mg/kg IV, IM
Anticonvulsants		
Gabapentin	300-1200 mg	—
Phenytoin	20-35 mg/kg PO	2-3 mg/kg PO
Carbamazepine	Not recommended	—
Antidepressants		
Clomipramine	1-3 mg/kg PO	1-5 mg/kg PO
Calcium Antagonists		
Diltiazem	0.5-1.5 mg/kg PO	1.75-2.5 mg/kg PO
Sympatholytics		
Propanolol	0.125-1.10 mg/kg PO	0.4-1.2 mg/kg PO
Atenolol	0.25-1.0 mg/kg PO	2-3 mg/kg
Prazosin	1 mg/15 kg PO	—

PO, Oral; *SC,* subcutaneous; *IV,* intravenous; *IM,* intramuscular.

TABLE 8-5
Adjuvant Analgesic Drugs—cont'd

Drug	Dosage in Dogs	Dosage in Cats
Miscellaneous Drugs		
Codeine	1-2 mg/kg PO	—
Dextromethorphan	0.5-2 mg/kg PO, SC, IV	—
Tramadol	5-10 mg/kg IV (experimental dosage)	5-10 mg/kg IV (experimental dosage)
Clonidine	10 μg/kg IV	10 μg/kg IV
Ketamine	0.5 mg/kg	0.5 mg/kg
	2-5 μg/kg/min	2-10 μg/kg/min
Magnesium salts ($Mg^{-2}SO_4^{-2}$)	5-15 mg/kg	5-15 mg/kg

---

diazepam) produce adjunctive analgesic effects when combined with inhalant (e.g., isoflurane, sevoflurane) or injectable (e.g., ketamine, propofol) anesthetics, opioids, or α_2-agonists. The potential to produce significant drug interactions and side effects and to enhance the toxicity of the primary analgesic drug presents a risk. The coadministration of acepromazine and opioids, for example, may improve overall analgesic effectiveness by two to three times but also increases the potential for increased respiratory depression and the development of significant respiratory acidosis. To date, there are no controlled clinical trials demonstrating the efficacy or safety of most if not all of the drugs considered to be useful for producing adjuvant analgesia. Ideally, future studies will fill this void.

SUGGESTED READINGS

Booth DM: *Small animal clinical pharmacology and therapeutics,* Philadelphia, 2001, WB Saunders.

Hobbs WR, Rall RW, Verdoorn TA: Hypnotics and sedatives. Ethanol. In Hardman JG et al, editors: *Goodman & Gillman's the pharmacological basis of therapeutics,* ed 9, New York, 1996, McGraw-Hill.

Muir WW: Pain. In Muir WW, Hubbell JAE, Skarda RT, et al: *Handbook of veterinary anesthesia,* ed 3, St Louis, 2000, Mosby.

Reisine T, Pasternak G: Opioid analgesics and antagonists. In Hardman JG et al: *Goodman & Gillman's the pharmacological basis of therapeutics,* ed 9, New York, 1996, McGraw-Hill.

9

Opioids

ANN E. WAGNER

DEFINITION

An *opioid* can be defined as any natural or synthetic drug that has
opiate-like activities, exerting its effects by interacting with opiate
receptors of cell membranes (Box 9-1).

Analgesic Efficacy

Opioids, which characteristically *produce analgesia without loss of
proprioception or consciousness,* are currently the most efficacious
systemic means of controlling acute or postoperative pain.

Other Effects

In addition to their analgesic effects, opioids may cause side effects
(see "Side Effects/Toxicity").

Opiate Receptors

- *Function:* Opiate receptors mediate the various effects of opioids (Box 9-2).
- *Classification:* The location, identification, and actions of various opiate receptors are subject to ongoing investigation, and
  consequently, the classification of opioid drugs and receptors
  presented here may not reflect the latest findings. (For instance,
  there may actually be seven subtypes of the μ receptor; see also
  "Relevant Pharmacology.")
- *Locations*
  1. Central nervous system: Traditionally, it was believed that
     opiate receptors were located only in the central nervous sys-
     tem, particularly in the brain and in the dorsal horn of the

---

BOX 9-1
Definitions

- A pure opioid *agonist* binds to one or more types of receptor and causes certain effects, such as analgesia or respiratory depression (e.g., morphine).
- An opioid is considered a *partial agonist* if its binding at a given receptor causes an effect that is less pronounced than that of a pure agonist (e.g., buprenorphine).
- An opioid *antagonist* binds to one or more types of receptor but causes no effect at those receptors. By competitively displacing an agonist from a receptor, the antagonist effectively "reverses" the agonist's effect (e.g., naloxone).
- An opioid *agonist-antagonist* binds to more than one type of receptor, causing an effect at one but no effect or a less pronounced effect at another (e.g., butorphanol).

BOX 9-2
Classification of Opiate Receptors and Their Effects

μ-1	Supraspinal analgesia
μ-2	Respiratory depression
	Bradycardia
	Physical dependence
	Euphoria
μ-3	Hyperpolarization of peripheral nerves induced by inflammation/immune response
κ	Analgesia
	Sedation
	Miosis
δ	Modulation of μ receptor activity

---

spinal cord, where impulses from peripheral nerves are modulated before being transmitted to higher centers.
2. Peripheral tissues: Although recent studies suggest that opioid receptors and activities also occur in some peripheral tissues, the clinical applications of these findings have yet to be fully evaluated.

PROTOTYPE AND MEMBERS

Agonists

Morphine *

> **DESCRIPTION:** *Morphine is the principal alkaloid derived from opium and the prototype opioid agonist to which all others are compared (Table 9-1). For many reasons, morphine is generally considered the primary analgesic in small animal practice.*
>
> **ANALGESIC EFFICACY:** *Although other opioids may be more potent, to date, none is more effective than morphine at relieving pain.*
>
> **MAIN EFFECT:** *Analgesia without loss of sensation or proprioception.*
>
> **POSSIBLE SIDE EFFECTS**

1. Depression of the respiratory center, resulting in decreased minute volume and increased arterial carbon dioxide tension.
2. Depression of the cough center.
3. Stimulation of the vomiting center and increased intestinal peristalsis, which may cause defecation shortly after administration, along with stimulation of gastrointestinal sphincters, which can lead to eventual constipation.
4. Increased antidiuretic hormone, with urine production decreased by up to 90%.
5. Histamine release: Morphine should be administered slowly and in conservative doses if given intravenously because of the potential for histamine release, which may occur within 1 minute and persist for at least 60 minutes.
6. Cardiovascular effects: Morphine generally causes minimal depression of cardiac contractility but can cause bradycardia, which is generally responsive to anticholinergic agents.
7. Excitement/dysphoria: Morphine may cause excitement or dysphoria in some animals, with dogs generally being less affected than cats and horses.

> **DURATION:** *Analgesic effects of morphine may last up to 4 hours, an advantage in the management of acute pain associated with trauma or surgery.*

---

*Morphine, Morphine Sulfate Injection, Elkins-Sinn, Cherry Hill, New Jersey.

TABLE 9-1

Comparative Potencies, Suggested Dosages, and Dosing Frequencies of Common Opioid Analgesics

Opioid Analgesic	Relative Potency	Dog Dose (mg/kg)	Cat Dose (mg/kg)	Comments
Morphine	1	0.5-2 q2-4h	0.2-0.5 q3-4h	Oral tablets and suspension also available
Morphine, sustained release (oral)		2-5 q12h	?	Use caution when given IV (histamine release)
Oxymorphone	10	0.05-0.4 q2-4h	0.02-0.1 q3-4h	Minimal to no histamine release
Hydromorphone	10-15	0.05-0.2 q2-6h	0.05-0.1 q2-6h	Minimal to no histamine release
Methadone	1-1.5	1-1.5	?	Not available in U.S.
Meperidine	0.1	3-5 q1-2h	3-5 q1-2h	Not recommended for IV use (histamine release)
Fentanyl	100	*Loading:* 2-5 µg/kg *CRI:* 2-5 µg/kg/hr (pain management); 10-45 µg/kg/hr (surgical analgesia)	*Loading:* 1-3 µg/kg *CRI:* 1-4 µg/kg/hr (pain management); 10-30 µg/kg/hr (surgical analgesia)	Constant rate infusion required for sustained effect

CRI, Constant-rate infusion.

Drugs may be administered intravenously (IV), intramuscularly (IM), and subcutaneously (SQ/SC) unless otherwise stated. Dosages are mg/kg unless otherwise stated. Required dosages and duration of analgesia will vary from individual to individual; these are guidelines only.

Continued

TABLE 9-1

Comparative Potencies, Suggested Dosages, and Dosing Frequencies of Common Opioid Analgesics—cont'd

Opioid Analgesic	Relative Potency	Dog Dose (mg/kg)	Cat Dose (mg/kg)	Comments
Sufentanil	1000	5 µg/kg loading; 0.1 µg/kg/min	?	Unpredictable sedation, may require tranquilizer
Alfentanil	10	?	?	Rapid onset, short duration (10 min?)
Remifentanil	50	*Loading:* 4-10 mg/kg *CRI:* 4-10 µg/kg/hr (pain management); 20-60 µg/kg/hr (surgical analgesia)	?	Extremely rapid elimination
Butorphanol	3-5	0.1-0.4 q1-4h	0.1-0.4 q2-6h	
Butorphanol, oral		0.5-2 q6-8h	0.5-1 q6-8h	
Buprenorphine	25	0.005-0.02 q8-12h	0.005-0.02 q8-12h; 0.01-0.02 PO, tid, qid	May be difficult to antagonize
Nalbuphine	1	0.5-1 q4h	0.2-0.4 q4h	
Pentazocine	0.25-0.5	1-3 q2-4h	1-3 q2-4h	

CRI, Constant-rate infusion; *PO,* by mouth (per os).

Drugs may be administered intravenously (IV), intramuscularly (IM), and subcutaneously (SQ/SC) unless otherwise stated. Dosages are mg/kg unless otherwise stated. Required dosages and duration of analgesia will vary from individual to individual; these are guidelines only.

COST: *Morphine is inexpensive enough that cost should not be an excuse for inadequate treatment of pain.*

Oxymorphone*

DESCRIPTION: *A semisynthetic opioid.*
ANALGESIC EFFICACY AND DURATION: *Similar to morphine.*
OTHER EFFECTS

1. Oxymorphone does not cause histamine release; therefore it is safer for intravenous (IV) administration than morphine.
2. Clinical impression suggests that oxymorphone may be less likely to produce excitement than morphine.
3. More likely to induce panting than morphine. Panting results from a resetting of the thermoregulatory center, so the animal "thinks" it needs to cool off despite a normal or low body temperature.

COST: *Oxymorphone is approved for use in dogs and cats but is considerably more expensive than morphine.*

Hydromorphone†

DESCRIPTION: *A semisynthetic opioid.*
ANALGESIC EFFICACY: *Nearly the same efficacy and potency as oxymorphone. Hydromorphone may actually produce better analgesia in cats than does morphine.*
DURATION: *Similar to morphine and oxymorphone in duration.*
COST: *Currently, it is considerably less expensive than oxymorphone, so it has been recommended as a lower-cost alternative to oxymorphone.*
OTHER COMMENTS: *Although hydromorphone can induce some histamine release, the effect is apparently mild and unlikely to cause vasodilation and hypotension, so IV administration is considered relatively safe. Hydromorphone produces less sedation than morphine or oxymorphone in dogs and cats.*

---

*Oxymorphone, P/M Oxymorphone HCl Injection, Mallinckrodt, St. Louis, Missouri.
†Hydromorphone, Hydromorphone HCl, Wyeth-Ayerst, Philadelphia, Pennsylvania.

Methadone*

DESCRIPTION: *A synthetic opioid.*
ANALGESIC EFFICACY: *Similar to morphine.*
DURATION: *2 to 6 hours.*
OTHER COMMENTS: *Methadone may have N-methyl-D-aspartate (NMDA) receptor antagonist activity, which may add another dimension to its analgesia and may help prevent development of opioid tolerance.*

Meperidine†

DESCRIPTION: *A synthetic opioid, about one tenth as potent as morphine. Because of its short duration and possible cardiovascular effects, meperidine is less satisfactory for long-term analgesia than morphine.*
ANALGESIC EFFICACY: *Similar to morphine.*
DURATION: *Appears to be of much shorter duration in animals, with analgesia lasting generally less than 1 hour.*
OTHER COMMENTS

1. Negative inotropy: Unlike other opioids, meperidine reportedly may have significant negative inotropic effects.
2. Histamine release: Like morphine, meperidine can induce histamine release. For this reason, IV administration is not recommended

Fentanyl‡

DESCRIPTION: *A short-acting synthetic opioid.*
ANALGESIC EFFICACY: *Similar to morphine. Fentanyl can decrease the minimum alveolar concentration (MAC) requirement for inhaled anesthetics by up to 63%.*
DURATION: *Fentanyl's effects last only about 30 minutes after a single injection. For clinical application, its duration is commonly extended by administering it as a constant-rate infusion, both*

---

*Methadone, Dolophine HCl, Eli Lilly, Indianapolis, Indiana.
†Meperidine, Meperidine HCl, Astra, Westborough, Massachusetts.
‡Fentanyl, Fentanyl Citrate Injection, Abbott Laboratories, North Chicago, Illinois.

intraoperatively to augment surgical analgesia and reduce the requirement for inhalation anesthetics (10 to 45 μg/kg/hr) and postoperatively for pain management (2 to 5 μg/kg/hr). Despite its supposed short duration, there is a great deal of individual variation in recovery time from fentanyl infusions.

OTHER COMMENTS

1. The use of fentanyl intraoperatively may be especially advantageous in patients with compromised cardiac function, because (unlike inhaled anesthetics) it causes minimal cardiovascular depression or hypotension, while contributing to significant reduction in the MAC requirement.
2. Experimental findings and clinical impression suggest that tolerance to fentanyl can occur, perhaps as soon as 3 hours after administration is begun.

Sufentanil*

DESCRIPTION: *A synthetic opioid about 1000 times as potent as morphine.*
DURATION: *About half as long as that of fentanyl.*
OTHER COMMENTS: *Currently, sufentanil is not commonly used for pain management in animals.*

Alfentanil†

DESCRIPTION: *A synthetic opioid about 25 times as potent as morphine.*
DURATION: *Shorter in duration than fentanyl.*
OTHER COMMENTS: *Currently, alfentanil is not commonly used for pain management in animals.*

Remifentanil‡

DESCRIPTION: *Remifentanil is another synthetic opioid that is about half as potent as fentanyl and is unique among opioids in that it is*

---

*Sufentanil, Sufenta, Taylor Pharmaceuticals, San Clemente, California.
†Alfentanil, Alfenta, Taylor Pharmaceuticals, San Clemente, California.
‡Remifentanil, Ultiva, GlaxoWellcome, Research Triangle Park, North Carolina.

metabolized by nonspecific esterases that occur in blood and tissues throughout the body (mainly in skeletal muscle). This gives remifentanil the clinical advantage of extremely rapid clearance that does not depend on liver or kidney function.

DURATION: *Because of this rapid clearance, constant-rate infusion is required for sustained analgesia. Recovery is generally expected to occur within 3 to 7 minutes after termination of an infusion.*

OTHER COMMENTS: *Remifentanil may be useful in situations in which intense analgesia is needed for a short or variable period.*

Carfentanil*

DESCRIPTION: *Synthetic opioid approximately 10,000 times more potent than morphine.*

OTHER COMMENTS: *Used mainly for capture of wild and feral animals; not normally used in pain management.*

Agonist-Antagonists
Butorphanol†

DESCRIPTION: *A synthetic opioid believed to exert its effects mainly at κ receptors, producing varying degrees of analgesia and sedation with minimal cardiopulmonary depression. It has minimal effect at μ receptors, and consequently, is labeled a μ-receptor antagonist.*

ANALGESIC EFFICACY: *Butorphanol appears to be a less effective analgesic than morphine and other pure μ-agonist opioids.*

1. Plateau or ceiling effect: Although at low doses butorphanol's analgesic potency is about three times that of morphine, doses greater than about 0.8 to 1 mg/kg are associated with a plateau or ceiling effect, such that no further enhancement of analgesia occurs.
2. Butorphanol appears to be more effective for mild-to-moderate pain, and for visceral pain, than for severe or somatic pain.

DURATION: *The duration of butorphanol's analgesia is debatable and probably varies depending on the species, degree of pain, and route of administration. Some studies suggest a duration of less*

*Carfentanil, Wildnil, Wildlife Pharmaceuticals, Fort Collins, Colorado.
†Butorphanol, Torbugesic, Fort Dodge Animal Health, Fort Dodge, Iowa.

than an hour, whereas others indicate a longer duration of up to 6 hours, particularly in cats.
OTHER COMMENTS

1. Interaction of butorphanol with pure agonists: Traditionally, it was thought that simultaneous or sequential administration of an agonist-antagonist such as butorphanol and a pure agonist such as oxymorphone or morphine would be counterproductive in that the agonist-antagonist might inhibit or even reverse the analgesic effects of the agonist. However, a recent study in cats, in which the colonic balloon model for visceral pain was used, suggests that combining butorphanol with oxymorphone (0.05 to 0.1 mg/kg of each) results in synergistic analgesia, minimal cardiopulmonary effects, and decreased excitement or dysphoria compared with oxymorphone alone.[1] Therefore a combination of an agonist-antagonist and a pure agonist may have advantages, particularly in species or individuals prone to opioid-induced dysphoria.

2. Partial antagonism of pure agonists: Another use for butorphanol and other agonist-antagonists is to partially antagonize the sedative or respiratory depressant effects of a pure μ agonist such as morphine or oxymorphone, without completely removing analgesia. This technique is particularly useful for reversal of excessive sedation and restoration of laryngeal reflexes so that a postoperative patient can be ex tubated in recovery. For this purpose, butorphanol, 0.1 mg/kg, administered intravenously, is generally effective.

Nalbuphine *

DESCRIPTION: *A κ agonist and partial μ antagonist, nalbuphine produces mild analgesia with little sedation, respiratory depression, or cardiovascular effect.*
OTHER COMMENTS

1. Cost: One of nalbuphine's main advantages is that it is inexpensive.
2. Nalbuphine is not a Drug Enforcement Agency (DEA)-scheduled substance because of its low abuse potential.

---

*Nalbuphine, Nalbuphine HCl Injection, Astra, Westborough, Massachusetts.

3. Partial antagonism of pure agonists: Nalbuphine, like butorphanol, may also be effective in partially antagonizing the
   sedative effects of a μ agonist, at a dosage of 0.1 to 0.5 mg/
   kg, administered intravenously.

Pentazocine*

DESCRIPTION: *Another κ agonist and μ antagonist similar to
butorphanol and nalbuphine, producing mild analgesia of uncertain
duration.*
OTHER COMMENTS: *Pentazocine appears to be less reliable than
butorphanol or nalbuphine as a partial antagonist for other opioids.*

Buprenorphine†

DESCRIPTION: *Buprenorphine is different from other agonist-
antagonists in that it is considered a partial agonist at μ receptors
and an antagonist at κ receptors.*
ANALGESIC EFFICACY: *Because it is only a partial agonist,
buprenorphine may not provide adequate analgesia for moderate to
severe pain, such as that following orthopedic or thoracotomy
procedures, and increasing dosages above those clinically
recommended may actually result in reduced analgesia.*
ONSET OF ACTION: *Buprenorphine has a slower onset of action than
many other opioids, with its peak effect delayed up to an hour after
IV administration.*
DURATION: *Although a purported advantage of buprenorphine is its
long duration of analgesia (up to 12 hours), its clinical analgesic
effect in animals often seems to wane by 6 hours.*
OTHER COMMENTS: *Once bound to μ receptors, buprenorphine is
difficult to displace, meaning that its effects may be difficult to
antagonize. Buprenorphine may be useful when administered orally
to cats, with a duration of 6 to 8 weeks.*
COST: *In addition, buprenorphine is considerably more expensive
than morphine.*

---

*Pentazocine, Talwin, Sanofi Winthrop, New York, New York.
†Buprenorphine, Buprenex Injectable, Reckitt & Colman Products, Rich-
mond, Virginia.

MECHANISM OF ACTION

- Inhibit pain transmission in the dorsal horn of the spinal cord
- Inhibit somatosensory afferents at supraspinal levels
- Activate descending inhibitory pathways
- Bind to receptors on the terminal axons of primary afferents within the substantia gelatinosa of the spinal cord, causing a decrease in the release of neurotransmitters such as substance P

EFFICACY/USE

Regional or Local Administration

Epidural

- Epidural administration of morphine is widely practiced in a variety of species, including dogs and cats.
- Morphine, 0.1 mg/kg, administered epidurally provides analgesia with fewer side effects than systemically administered morphine.
  1. Onset: Approximately 30 to 60 minutes.
  2. Duration: Approximately 18 hours.
- Preservative-free morphine is recommended, because preservatives may be neurotoxic.

Intraarticular

- Trauma or inflammation may activate opioid receptors on nociceptive nerve terminals and/or inflammatory cells (possibly μ 3 receptors).
- Morphine instilled into joint at the end of surgery reportedly provides up to 18 hours of analgesia.
- Application of a tourniquet proximal to the joint is recommended for 10 minutes after injection.
- Morphine may be combined with a local anesthetic such as bupivacaine.

Transdermal Administration

Fentanyl is available in a transdermal delivery system.*

---

*Duragesic, Janssen Pharmaceutical, Titusville, New Jersey.

DOSAGE: *2 to 4 µg/kg/hr*

1. Patch sizes = 25, 50, 75, or 100 µg/hr.
2. For very small animals, remove the backing from only a portion of the patch that represents an appropriate dose (i.e., for a 4-kg cat, use a 25 µg/hr patch with only half the backing removed → 12.5 µg/hr).

APPLICATION

1. Site: back of neck or shoulders, lateral thorax, metatarsus.
2. Clip hair; clean skin with water only.
3. Apply patch and hold firmly in place for at least 2 minutes.
4. Apply a bandage over the patch.

ONSET: *6 to 24 hours.*
DURATION: *72 to 104 hours.*

RELEVANT PHARMACOLOGY

Historical Classification

Opioid receptors were originally classified as sigma (σ), kappa (κ), mu (μ), and delta (δ).

Results of Opioid Agonist Occupying Opiate Receptor

Events that may occur when an opioid agonist occupies a particular opiate receptor, which result in inhibition of activation of neurons are:

- Depression of cyclic adenosine monophosphate formation
- Activation of potassium channels, resulting in membrane hyperpolarization
- Activation of G proteins
- Inhibition of opening of voltage-sensitive calcium channels
- Decreased release of neurotransmitters such as substance P

Location of Opiate Receptors

Traditionally, it was thought that opiate receptors were confined to the central nervous system. However, more recently, a peripheral, local action of opioids has also been demonstrated.

Brain (Predominantly μ Receptors)

- Mesencephalic periaqueductal gray
- Mesencephalic reticular formation

- Medulla
- Substantia nigra
- Ventral forebrain
- Amygdala

Spinal Cord (μ, κ, and δ Receptors)
- Dorsal horn laminae I-V
- Substantia gelatinosa

Peripheral Receptors
Opioids may have local actions under certain conditions of inflammation with hyperalgesia, suggesting that inflammatory cells that release cytokines and other nerve-sensitizing products may contain opiate receptors that can suppress these events.

SIDE EFFECTS/TOXICITY

Possible side effects of opioid administration are many and varied, although rarely problematic enough to prevent the use of opioids in pain management. One of the major advantages of opioids in pain management is their safety.

Sedation or Central Nervous System Depression
- Sedation commonly occurs after opioid administration in small animals, more so in dogs than in cats.
- Sedation is generally considered an advantage when an opioid is used as a preanesthetic, or in the immediate postoperative period when rest is desirable.
- Sedation may be undesirable if it interferes with return to normal behaviors such as eating and drinking.
- Options for preventing excessive sedation
  1. Reduce the dosage of opioid.
  2. Administer a low dose of an agonist-antagonist such as nalbuphine or butorphanol in conjunction with a pure agonist such as morphine.
  3. Administer a low dose of a pure antagonist such as nalmefene in conjunction with a pure agonist such as morphine.

Excitement or Dysphoria
- Excitement occurs in some, but not all, animals after opioid administration. There is a great deal of species and individual

variation, with cats and northern breeds of dogs (e.g., mala-
mutes, huskies) apparently more susceptible to dysphoria.
- The recommended dosages for most opioids in cats are about
  half those recommended for dogs to minimize the incidence of
  excitement. Use of lower-opioid dosages may minimize dysphoria in susceptible animals.
- If dysphoria or agitation occurs, administration of a tranquilizer
  such as acepromazine (0.01 to 0.03 mg/kg) or a sedative such as
  xylazine (0.1 to 0.3 mg/kg) or medetomidine (0.05 to 5 μg/kg)
  should help to calm the animal.
- Another option is to use an agonist-antagonist such as nalbuphine
  or butorphanol to antagonize the excitatory effects of a pure agonist such as morphine, without antagonizing analgesia. A study
  in cats demonstrated that 0.1 mg/kg each of oxymorphone and
  butorphanol provided synergistic analgesia without excitement.[1]
- It is important to determine whether an agitated animal is dysphoric or in pain, since the treatment for each situation may be
  different. (See Chapters 3 and 4 for more information on assessing pain and analgesia.)

Bradycardia

- Occurs as a result of opioid-induced medullary vagal stimulation.
- More likely to occur in an animal not in pain (e.g., when an opioid is given as a preanesthetic).
- Some animals may develop second-degree atrioventricular
  block.
- Prevention and treatment: Atropine (0.02 to 0.04 mg/kg) or glycopyrrolate (0.01 to 0.02 mg/kg), administered subcutaneously,
  intramuscularly, or intravenously, is generally effective at restoring heart rate to an acceptable level.

Other Cardiovascular Effects

- With the exception of meperidine, opioids generally cause little
  to no depression of myocardial contractility.
- Therefore as long as bradycardia is prevented, cardiac output
  and blood pressure should be minimally affected by opioid
  administration.

Respiratory Depression

- Results from an opioid-induced decrease in responsiveness of
  the brainstem respiratory center to $Paco_2$.

- In people, opioid-induced respiratory depression can be profound, but in animals, clinically useful analgesic dosages of opioids *alone* are unlikely to produce clinically significant respiratory depression.
- However, when opioids are used in high dosages to provide surgical analgesia (such as fentanyl infusions at 20 μg/kg/hr or higher) or when they are used in conjunction with other respiratory depressant drugs (such as thiopental, propofol, or the inhaled anesthetics), assisted or controlled ventilation may be required.

Panting

- May occur in some dogs after opioid administration, particularly after oxymorphone.
- Panting animals do not necessarily hyperventilate; in fact, they may hypoventilate and become hypercapnic.
- The cause of panting is resetting of the thermoregulatory center in the thalamus, which makes a normothermic dog "think" it is hot, causing it to pant to cool off.
- Panting can be annoying or inconvenient, for instance, during radiography when excessive motion is problematic.
- Panting can also interfere with rewarming a hypothermic animal, for instance, in the postoperative recovery period. However, hypothermia should not be a reason to withhold opioid analgesics from a patient during the postoperative period; rather, external warming devices such as circulating warm water blankets or heat lamps should be used to restore and maintain body temperature while analgesia is provided.

Cough Suppression or Depression of Laryngeal Reflexes

- Opioid-induced cough suppression can be desirable or undesirable, depending on circumstances.
- Many dogs can be intubated after receiving IV opioid and benzodiazepine, even though they remain conscious. This technique can be used to induce profound neuroleptanalgesia in critical patients, thus avoiding the use of more depressant anesthesia induction drugs.
- Depression of laryngeal reflexes might be desirable when a brachycephalic (or other airway-challenged) dog is recovering from anesthesia, since it will allow the animal to tolerate the endotracheal tube for a longer time, during which inhaled anesthetic will be eliminated.

- Some opioid-treated dogs have excessively prolonged recoveries from anesthesia, in part because of insensitivity to the endotracheal tube. In those cases, a small dose of an agonist-antagonist such as nalbuphine or butorphanol (0.1 mg/kg IV) or a very small dose of an antagonist such as naloxone (1 to 10 µg/kg IV) may restore laryngeal reflexes to the point that the dog can be extubated safely.

Histamine Release
- Can occur with administration of certain opioids, such as morphine and meperidine, particularly with IV administration.
- Sequelae of histamine release include vasodilation and hypotension.
- Morphine should be given cautiously and slowly by the IV route in low dosages. Morphine should generally not be given by the IV route to an animal during general anesthesia.
- It is best to avoid IV administration of meperidine.
- No significant histamine release occurs after administration of oxymorphone, hydromorphone, or fentanyl, so these opioids are considered safe for IV use.

Vomiting and Defecation
- Commonly follow administration of opioids, particularly when administered as preanesthetics to animals not in pain; less common when administered to animals in pain or those that have had surgery.
- Nausea and vomiting are caused by stimulation of the chemoreceptor trigger zone in medulla.
- Defecation may result from an initial increase in gastrointestinal tone.

Constipation
- With long-term opioid use, increased gastrointestinal sphincter tone and reduced peristalsis may lead to constipation.
- Not usually a clinical problem in short-term pain management.

Urinary Retention
- Caused by increased detrusor muscle tone and increased vesical sphincter tone.
- Especially common after epidural morphine administration.
- Bladder may need to be manually expressed or catheterized.

Effect on Biliary Smooth Muscle

- In people, morphine has been shown to cause constriction of the sphincter of Oddi, causing pain from increased pressure within the common bile duct.
- Other opioids such as meperidine, fentanyl, and pentazocine may similarly affect this sphincter, but nalbuphine and buprenorphine appear to have minimal effect. Thus certain opioids may be contraindicated in patients with pancreatitis or biliary disease.
- Dogs often have separate bile and pancreatic ducts, so use of opioids in dogs with pancreatitis may not be problematic.
- Most cats do have a common pancreatic and bile duct, so nalbuphine or buprenorphine may be the best choice for pain management in cats with pancreatitis.

SPECIAL ISSUES

Comprehensive Drug Abuse Prevention and Control Act (United States)

- Drugs are classified according to potential for abuse.
    1. Most opioid agonists have a high potential for abuse and are listed in Schedule II: morphine, hydromorphone, methadone, meperidine, and others.
    2. Butorphanol, an opioid agonist-antagonist with moderate abuse potential, is listed in Schedule IV.
- Regulations for prescribing controlled substances (in United States)
    1. Veterinarian must register with DEA (registration to be renewed annually).
    2. Veterinarian must keep inventory of controlled substances.
    3. Controlled substances must be ordered by using special forms.

Tolerance and Physical Dependence

- It has been shown that tolerance to the effects of opioids can develop rapidly.
- Nociceptive stimulation reportedly antagonizes or prevents development of tolerance to fentanyl; therefore tolerance is less likely to occur during pain management.
- Clinically, occurrence of tolerance or physical dependence in animals is anecdotal and apparently rare.

Hyperthermia

Cats may develop hyperthermia (103° to 105° F) several hours after the administration of μ-opioid agonists (morphine, oxymorphone, hydromorphone). They should be treated with antipyretics.

Antagonists

General comments: Opioid antagonists are often used to arouse animals that are excessively sedated or obtunded from opioid administration, for instance, when recovery from anesthesia is prolonged and the patient has not regained laryngeal/cough reflexes. It should be remembered that reversal of opioid effects, particularly in an animal that is potentially in pain, may result in intense acute pain with accompanying sympathetic stimulation that may be detrimental. Therefore opioid antagonists should be used conservatively and only with good reason in animals experiencing pain. If bradycardia is the main cause for concern, an anticholinergic such as atropine or glycopyrrolate should be used, instead of an opioid antagonist, to restore a normal heart rate without affecting patient comfort.

Naloxone*

DESCRIPTION: *Naloxone does not induce any effects when administered alone, but when administered to an animal that has previously been given an opioid agonist such as morphine, it effectively reverses the effects of the agonist, causing increased alertness, responsiveness, and coordination, as well as increased awareness of pain.*

DURATION: *The duration of naloxone is shorter than that of many opioid agonists; an IV injection of naloxone, 0.01 mg/kg, lasts 20 to 40 minutes, while 0.04 mg/kg, administered intramuscularly, lasts 40 to 70 minutes. Therefore animals should be watched for renarcotization or resedation after a dose of naloxone.*

OTHER COMMENTS

1. Excitement or anxiety may accompany naloxone reversal of the effects of an opioid agonist.
2. Although not common, cardiac dysrhythmias such as ventricular premature contractions can occur after naloxone reversal of an opioid's effects, particularly if conditions favor high levels of circulating catecholamines.

---

*Naloxone, P/M Naloxone HCl Injection, Mallinckrodt, St. Louis, Missouri.

3. In potentially painful situations (such as after surgery), the dose of naloxone should be greatly reduced and given in small increments, just to the point of arousal, to avoid precipitating a painful recovery. For this purpose, a total dosage of 0.001 to 0.01 mg/kg IV may be sufficient.

Nalmefene *

DESCRIPTION: *An opioid antagonist approximately four times as potent as naloxone.*

DURATION: *Nalmefene works as quickly as naloxone, but its duration of action is approximately 1 to 2 hours, about twice that of naloxone. Therefore nalmefene may be advantageous in preventing renarcotization when it is used to antagonize a long-acting opioid.*

OTHER COMMENTS: *Dosages for animals have not been well-established, but in people, may vary from 0.25 μg/kg to 30 μg/kg.*

Naltrexone†

DESCRIPTION: *Another pure opioid antagonist, about four times more potent than naloxone.*

DURATION: *About twice that of naloxone.*

OTHER COMMENTS: *Based on these findings, a dose of 0.0025 mg/kg IV should effectively antagonize a pure agonist for approximately 2 hours.*

REFERENCE

1. Briggs SL, Sneed K, Sawyer DC: Antinociceptive effects of oxymorphone-butorphanol-acepromazine combination in cats, *Vet Surg* 27:466-472, 1998.

SUGGESTED READINGS

Hansen Br Palh, *Semin Vet Med Surg Small Anim* 12(2):55-142, 1997.

Mathews KA: Management of pain, *Vet Clin North Am Small Anim Pract* 30(4):703-970, 2000.

Thurman JC, Tranquilli WJ, Benson GJ, editors: *Lumb & Jones' veterinary anesthesia,* ed 3, Baltimore, 1996, Williams & Wilkins.

---

*Nalmefene, Revex, Ohmeda (Baxter), Deerfield, Illinois.

†Naltrexone, Trexonil, Wildlife Pharmaceuticals, Fort Collins, Colorado.

10

Nonsteroidal Antiinflammatory Drugs

STEVEN BUDSBERG

Compounds that comprise the group known as nonsteroidal antiinflammatory drugs (NSAIDs) share therapeutic actions including analgesia and antiinflammatory and antipyretic capabilities. Although chemically related, these compounds vary widely in their structure, and their classification based on chemical structure still engenders some controversy.[1,2] For the sake of this review, we will focus on broad classifications such as the carboxylic and enolic acid groups. NSAIDs have a biochemically unifying action in the inhibition of the cyclooxygenase (COX) enzymes. Historically, NSAIDs are one of the most commonly used classes of drugs in humans.[3] The same statement is beginning to be made about NSAIDs in small animal clinical practice. There are several reasons for the dramatic increase in NSAID use in companion animals. First, there is now a better understanding for the need to manage acute and chronic pain in small animal medicine. Pain control, as evidenced by the current publication and others, is a very important mission for the practicing veterinarian. NSAIDs provide an effective means to accomplish this goal. Second, NSAIDs with improved safety and efficacy targeted for small animals (primarily the dog) are now available. For the most part, the current prescribed NSAIDs are very safe drugs, with only a small percentage of patients experiencing serious complications. However, these problems have achieved significant proportions based on the fact that so many patients are taking them each year; thus a small percentage becomes a very large number. Because these drugs are remarkably effective yet carry a significant risk potential, one must closely evaluate and monitor their use in each patient.

MECHANISM OF ACTION

Prostaglandin Inhibition

Review

Our understanding of the mechanisms of action of NSAIDs is a continually developing story that started in the early 1970s with the publication of two manuscripts that examined the ability of aspirin to inhibit prostaglandin production.[4,5] Eicosanoids, which include the compounds known as prostaglandins, are derived from arachidonic acid. The ability of NSAIDs to interfere with eicosanoid synthesis and the subsequent alteration of different physiologic systems explain the numerous effects seen in the body with NSAID administration.[6] A significant portion of the analgesic and antiinflammatory clinical effects seen with NSAIDs administration is related to the inhibition of the COX enzyme isoforms.

Cyclooxygenase Enzyme Isoforms

The last 10 years have seen the discovery, identification, and considerable elucidation of a group of COX enzymes. Currently, two isoforms have been well established. Discovery of the two distinct isoforms generated a hypothesis that their functions were mutually exclusive, with COX-1 involved in normal physiologic functions of various systems and COX-2 involved in pathologic processes. Increased knowledge about these enzymes has strongly suggested that this initial paradigm was an oversimplification.[7] COX-1 is now primarily considered the constitutive isoform of COX, and it is responsible for basal prostaglandin production for normal homeostasis in many tissues. It normally exists in many tissues of the body including the stomach, kidneys, platelets, and reproductive tract where it catalyzes the synthesis of prostaglandins involved in the daily "housekeeping" functions.[8] COX-1 is expressed at sites of inflammation, but this is likely a function of basal rather than induced expression.[9] COX-2 is usually thought of as the induced isoform and is found in sites of inflammation, yet it is expressed constitutively in the brain and kidneys in some species.[8] Cells that express COX-2 include endothelial cells, smooth muscle cells, chondrocytes, fibroblasts, monocytes, macrophages, and synovial cells.[9-11] Various cytokines and growth factors including interleukin (IL)-1α, IL-1β, tumor necrosis factor (TNF)-α, platelet-derived growth factor, epidermal growth factor, and TGF-β rapidly induce the formation of COX-2.[10]

Selective Cyclooxygenase Isoform Inhibition

The COX enzymes initiate a complex cascade that results in the conversion of polyunsaturated acids to prostaglandins and thromboxane.[12] Briefly, arachidonic acid is transformed into PGG_2 and then PGH_2 by COX. Further enzymatic conversion of PGH_2 leads to the production of functionally important prostaglandins (types D, E, F, and I) and thromboxane. In regard to pain, prostaglandins, primarily PGE_2, contribute to the inflammatory response by causing vasodilation and enhancing the effects of other cytokines and inflammatory mediators. The production of PGE_2 at various sites of inflammation appears to be mediated primarily by COX-2. Thus as an inflammatory event occurs within the tissue, COX-2 enzyme production is induced, followed by an increase in prostaglandin concentrations. Thus the preferential (selective) inhibition of certain prostaglandins primarily produced by COX-2 should allow for the therapeutic analgesic and antiinflammatory effects while greatly diminishing the unwanted side effects caused by COX-1 inhibition. However, complete COX-2 inhibition is detrimental to many normal physiologic functions including the healing of gastric ulcers. Thus it is important to accurately assess COX-2 selectivity, and current methods to make these assessments are not clear-cut. COX selectivity is a measure of the relative concentration of a drug required to inhibit each COX isoenzyme and is usually obtained by performing in vitro studies. The relative degree of isoform selectivity of a compound varies, depending on the assay used. Furthermore, the assessment of in vitro selectivity may not be informative of what happens in vivo at therapeutic serum concentrations. Recent ex vivo and limited in vivo data have become available, indicating the COX-2 selectivity or COX-1–sparing effects of certain compounds.[13-16] A recent study did provide a model that shows the physiologic effects of COX selectivity in target tissues in dogs with osteoarthritis.[13]

Site of Action

The previous discussion focuses on the peripheral (tissue injury site) actions of NSAIDs. There is mounting evidence that NSAIDs have antinociceptive effects at the level of the central nervous system (CNS). Recent studies have shown the production of antinociception with direct NSAID administration to both the supraspinal and spinal structures.[17] Although most of this inhibition is COX-mediated prostaglandin synthesis, several other modes of action may be involved. NSAIDs may have actions on excitable membranes, cellular metabolism, second messenger systems, or the expression of inflammatory mediators within the CNS.[18] These data, however, should not lead directly to the conclusion that spinal delivery of NSAIDs will be more effective than systemic delivery.[19] These data do provide insights into the potential value of developing centrally acting agents that alter receptor-mediated actions of prostanoids or enzyme inhibitors that can target specific sites in the prostaglandin cascade.

CLINICAL APPLICATIONS

Indications

NSAIDs can be used to relieve pain in a variety of patients. Efficacy of NSAIDs is comparable to that of opioids in many instances for treatment of musculoskeletal and visceral pain. However, for major pain such as fractures, data are not available to substantiate the same claim. NSAIDs can be used for cases of acute pain, either traumatic or surgically induced, as well as for chronic pain such as osteoarthritis (Tables 10-1 and 10-2). Please note that some of these drugs and dosages have not been approved in all countries (i.e., Food and Drug Administration [FDA] approval in the United States). Remember that efficacy and toxicity are often individualistic and individual monitoring is mandatory.

TABLE 10-1

Nonsteroidal Antiinflammatory Analgesic Dosing Regimen Per Body Weight

Drug	Perioperative NSAID Recommendations		
	Species/Dose	Route	Frequency
Ketoprofen	Dogs: 2.0 mg/kg	IV, SC, IM	Once (postoperative)
	Cats: 2.0 mg/kg	SC	
Meloxicam	Dogs: 0.2 mg/kg	IV, SC	Once on induction
	Cats: 0.2 mg/kg	SC	Once on induction
Carprofen	Dogs: 4.0 mg/kg	IV, SC, IM	Once on induction
	Cats: 4.0 mg/kg	SC	Once on induction

IV, Intravenously; *SC,* subcutaneously; *IM,* intramuscularly.

TABLE 10-2

Chronic Usage Recommendations for Nonsteroidal Antiinflammatory Drugs

Drug	Species	Initial Dose	Frequency	Subsequent Doses
Ketoprofen	Dogs and cats	2.0 mg/kg PO	q 24 hr	1.0 mg/kg PO*
Meloxicam	Dogs	0.2 mg/kg PO	q 24 hr	0.1 mg/kg PO
	Cats	≤0.2 mg/kg SC, PO	Once (initial dose)	Chronic dosing: ≤0.1 mg/kg PO for 2-3 days; then 0.025 mg/kg PO with a maximum dose of 0.1 mg per cat 2-3 times/wk
Carprofen	Dogs		q 12 hr	2.2 mg/kg PO
Etodolac	Dogs		q 24 hr	10-15 mg/kg PO
Tolfenamic acid	Cats and dogs		Once daily for 3 days on and 4 days off; repeat cycle	4 mg/kg SC, PO
Piroxicam	Dogs		q 24 hr for 2 treatments, then q 48 hr	0.3 mg/kg PO

PO, By mouth (per os); q, every; SC, subcutaneously.

*Recommended that dose and frequency be reduced after 3 to 5 days to avoid gastrointestinal and renal side effects.

Choosing and Monitoring Nonsteroidal Antiinflammatory Drug Use

- Use products with history of clinical experience and good safety profiles.
- Use only one NSAID at a time and ensure adequate dosing.
- Adapt therapy to suit patients' requirements. In patients with chronic pain, begin with the recommended dose, and if efficacious, attempt to reduce dose at regular intervals (e.g., weekly) until you have the lowest dose providing the maximum benefit.
- Review therapy frequently, and change to alternative NSAIDs if there is a poor response to therapy.
- Avoid NSAIDs in patients with known contraindications to their use.
- Observe for potential toxicity. Increased vigilance and monitoring are required for at-risk patients. If indicated, establish renal and hepatic status of the patient before NSAID administration.

Contraindications

The following recommendations are general guidelines and the type of NSAID (e.g., COX-2 selective) may alter these recommendations as more data become available.[19]

- Patients with renal or hepatic insufficiency or dysfunction.
- Patients with any clinical syndrome that creates a decrease in the circulating blood volume (e.g., shock, dehydration, hypotension, or ascites).
- Patients with any type of confirmed or suspected coagulopathies. (This may be less important with COX-2–selective drugs.)
- Patients with active gastrointestinal disease.
- Trauma patients with known or suspected significant active hemorrhage or blood loss.
- Pregnant patients or females attempting to become pregnant.
- Patients with significant pulmonary disease. (This may be less important with COX-2–selective drugs.)

Specific Compounds

Approved Compounds

Approved NSAIDs available to the veterinarian around the world are variable. The following list includes discussion of some of the more widely used products. It is very important for practitioners to remember that the clinical response to a particular drug is quite individualistic. Dogs may respond favorably to one product and not another, so if an NSAID is indicated in a case and the first product used does not achieve a positive clinical response, do not forsake NSAIDs, but try a different product.

Carprofen. Carprofen, a member of the arylpropionic acid class of NSAIDs, is a reversible inhibitor of cyclooxygenase and also demonstrates the ability to modify cell-mediated immune responses.[20,21] In vitro studies have shown COX-2 selectivity with carprofen in dogs.[14,22,23] It is widely approved in an oral formulation for chronic pain in dogs. It is also approved for single-dose perioperative administration in dogs and cats in Canada and Europe. Carprofen has been shown to improve limb function in clinical trials in dogs with naturally occurring osteoarthritis.[24,25] Carprofen is also effective in providing postoperative analgesia for both orthopedic and soft-tissue procedures.[26-30] Carprofen does not appear to affect platelet function or cause excessive bleeding during surgical procedures. Adverse effects associated with carprofen are very limited, with the majority being gastrointestinal.[24,25,31] The recent association of carprofen with liver dysfunction deserves special attention, but remember that the reported incidence of liver dysfunction is less than 0.06% of all dogs treated.[31,32]

Etodolac. Etodolac is a member of the pyranocarboxylic acid class with potent analgesic activity. Etodolac inhibits PGE_2 synthesis of macrophages and is effective in inhibiting PGE_2 biosynthesis by chondrocytes and synoviocytes.[33] Enterohepatic circulation in the dog maintains serum concentrations for extended periods. In vitro data suggest that etodolac is not COX-2 selective in dogs.[14,22,23] It is approved in the United States in an oral formulation. Clinically, it has been shown to improve rear limb function in dogs with chronic osteoarthritis.[34] Adverse events seem to be limited to the gastrointestinal tract.[35,36]

Ketoprofen. Ketoprofen is an arylpropionic acid, which is a potent inhibitor of COX.[37] Ketoprofen has no COX-2 selectivity in dogs. Because it inhibits both COX enzymes, ketoprofen is expected to have significant antithromboxane activity.[8,19] Data show that although ketoprofen effectively manages postoperative pain, it has a propensity for hemorrhage associated with perioperative administration.[26] Ketoprofen is approved for use in dogs and cats in oral and parenteral formulations in Europe and Canada. Unfortunately, the only data available to the clinician regarding clinical use of this product are in perioperative pain management.[19,26,38] Adverse events are excessive bleeding and gastrointestinal effects (primarily vomiting). Anecdotal reports suggest that vomiting commonly occurs in dogs when commercial over-the-counter products intended for human use are administered.

Meloxicam. Meloxicam is a member of the oxicam family. Meloxicam is a potent inhibitor of prostaglandin synthesis and exhibits antipyretic and analgesic properties.[39] In vivo and in vitro data reveal that meloxicam is COX-2 selective and thus has minimal antithromboxane activity in dogs.[13,19,39] It is approved for use in dogs in oral and parenteral formulations in Canada and Europe. Published objective efficacy data are limited to perioperative pain management and research models.[19,40-43] Adverse events with meloxicam are infrequent and primarily gastrointestinal. Although dosages for cats are available, no clinical trials proving clinical efficacy or safety are currently available with meloxicam.

Tolfenamic Acid. Tolfenamic acid is an anthranilic acid derivative and a member of the fenamates family. It is approved in both oral and parenteral formulations for dogs and cats in Canada and Europe. Little objective peer-reviewed data are available on tolfenamic acid.[42] Strict recommendations on limiting the use of this product are apparently related to its relatively narrow therapeutic range. Most common adverse events are gastrointestinal effects (diarrhea and vomiting) and perioperative bleeding.[19]

Deracoxib. Deracoxib is a COX-2–selective drug of the coxib class; it is similar to celecoxib and rofecoxib, which currently are marketed for human use. Although not yet on the market for use, deracoxib has been demonstrated to provide effective analgesia for acute postoperative pain involving cruciate ligament stabilization.[44,45] Deracoxib has also been demonstrated to provide effective relief of pain caused by osteoarthritis in a clinical trial in dogs.[46] In these studies, reported adverse effects were few and seemingly clinically insignificant. There was no difference with respect to adverse event development between dogs treated with deracoxib and dogs administered placebo. Although clinical experience with use of COX-2 selective drugs in humans suggests that fewer side effects occur with these agents than with nonselective NSAIDs, widespread clinical experience is required before a similar statement can be made with respect to COX-2–selective drug use in dogs.

Compounds Used Off-Label

Nonapproved NSAIDs that have been recommended for use off-label include aspirin, piroxicam, and a plethora of human products.

Be aware the vast majority of the human products have limited to no data for dogs or cats for either a correct efficacy or safety dosage range.

Aspirin. Aspirin is historically the most commonly used NSAID for a variety of problems in dogs and cats. It is relatively effective, inexpensive, and readily available. Aspirin is not COX-2 selective. However, with the introduction of more effective and safer products, aspirin use has declined. Adverse events are primarily gastrointestinal and are not uncommon. The frequency of gastrointestinal toxicity increases as the dose increases. Buffered aspirin has been demonstrated to cause less gastrointestinal irritation than plain aspirin when administered to dogs.[44] Aspirin also has antithromboxane effects and is used as an anticoagulant.

Piroxicam. Piroxicam is a member of the oxicam family. It is a potent antiinflammatory agent and analgesic. Data suggest that piroxicam is COX-2 selective in dogs.[14] Piroxicam has an elimination half-life of approximately 40 hours in the dog.[45] Piroxicam has been used as an antineoplastic agent to treat transitional cell neoplasia in dogs.[46] Based on clinical response and this long elimination half-life, once-daily or once-every-other-day dosing has been successfully used in the dog. Piroxicam has been administered at a dose of 0.3 mg/kg orally once daily for many months for the treatment of canine transitional cell neoplasia. Approximately 18% of patients demonstrated adverse gastrointestinal signs.[46] Gastroendoscopic evaluation of healthy dogs given piroxicam at a dose of 0.3 mg/kg orally once daily for 28 days failed to demonstrate a difference in gastroduodenal lesion development between treated and control dogs.[47] Additional data are needed before sweeping recommendations on use in pain management can be made.

POTENTIAL SIDE EFFECTS (Box 10-1)

Gastrointestinal

The most common problems associated with NSAID administration to dogs and cats involve the gastrointestinal tract. Some of the gastrointestinal toxicities associated with NSAID use are believed to be due to inhibition of endogenous prostaglandins. Signs may range from vomiting and diarrhea, including hematemesis and melena, to a silent ulcer that results in perforation. The true overall incidence of gastrointestinal toxicity in dogs and cats treated with NSAIDS is

---

BOX 10-1

Key Points to Minimize Adverse Reactions

---

1. Every effort should be made to prevent, rather than treat the adverse reactions associated with NSAID use. Use intermittent dosing schedules.
2. Chronic use may be necessary, and the goal should be to use the minimum amount of drugs to maintain the now improved patient function. NSAIDs may also be given on an as-needed basis to these improved patients, or to the less severely effected dogs initially.
3. Concurrent use of other NSAIDs or corticosteroids provides no additional therapeutic benefit but does increase the potential for adverse reactions.
4. As the patient ages or the addition of medications for nonrelated problems increases, so should the monitoring for potential problems.

---

unknown. Concurrent administration of other medications (especially other NSAIDs or corticosteroids), previous gastrointestinal bleeding, or the presence of other systemic diseases may contribute to adverse reactions.[31,48] The effect aging has on an individual patient's ability to metabolize NSAIDs is likely to be quite variable. However, given the potential toxicity of NSAIDs for these patients, it is appropriate to initially dose at the low end of the recommended range and to critically assess the response.[48]

Hepatic

Hepatotoxicosis caused by NSAIDs is generally considered to be idiosyncratic. Administration of carprofen has been associated with an idiosyncratic cytotoxic hepatocellular reaction.[37] Anorexia, vomiting, and icterus, along with increased hepatic enzyme levels, have been seen. The onset of signs was seen by 21 days in the majority of dogs. Most dogs recovered with cessation of treatment and supportive care.

Renal

Renal dysfunction may occur with NSAID administration as a consequence of prostaglandin inhibition. Renal prostaglandin synthesis is very low under normovolemic conditions. When normovolemia is challenged, prostaglandin synthesis is increased, and this is important for maintenance of renal perfusion.[48] NSAID use must be considered very carefully in hypovolemic animals. This is especially important to remember with the increasing use of NSAIDs for perioperative pain management.

Cartilage

NSAIDs are used frequently and often on a long-term basis in patients with osteoarthritis. Thus the effects on cartilage are of interest to the practitioner. Studies have demonstrated a variety of effects on proteoglycan synthesis when chondrocytes or cartilage explants are incubated with a NSAID in vitro. The most pronounced effects have been seen in chondrocytes from osteoarthritis joints, although a lesser effect on normal cartilage has been demonstrated. Aspirin is uniformly reported to cause inhibition of proteoglycan synthesis, although conflicting data exist for other NSAIDs, such as etodolac, which shows both potential negative and positive effects. In a final group including meloxicam, piroxicam, and carprofen, no effect, or even some increased synthesis of proteoglycan, has been noted.[49-55] The significance of these in vitro findings remains unclear. To the author's knowledge, no studies regarding the effect of long-term administration of an NSAID on progression of osteoarthritis in clinical canine patients have been performed.

FUTURE DEVELOPMENTS

The future uses of NSAIDs can be broken into two areas: types of available products and potential uses.

- In general, the near future will see an increase in the number of NSAIDs available for use. There is also a significant move toward compounds that are described as COX-2–specific products. In fact, one may see these products no longer listed as NSAIDs but simply classified as COX-2–selective products. Once these compounds show efficacy equivalent to that of current products, they will become attractive because of their probable lower adverse reaction profile.

- A second group of drugs that may start to enter the market will be products that target both the COX and lipooxygenase pathways, or solely the lipooxygenase pathway. There is growing evidence that alterations in LTB_4 and other mediators of the lipooxygenase pathway can alter clinical osteoarthritis.

- There are a variety of areas of research being pursued such as coupling NSAIDs to a nitric oxide (NO)-releasing moiety. These NO-NSAIDs inhibit both isoforms of COX with the same potency as the parent NSAID, but they have markedly decreased gastric toxicity.[56] Also, NO-NSAIDs inhibit NO synthase expression, which is unregulated during gastric injury and seems to improve healing of preexisting acutely induced ulcers. Other novel areas of research include the preassociation of NSAIDs with a zwitterionic phospholipid to prevent interactions between the NSAID and the mucosa.[56]
- More studies are examining the potential use of NSAIDs directly within the CNS and direct transdermal applications.
- The investigation of specific prostaglandin receptor antagonists is ongoing.

REFERENCES

1. Scarpinganto C: Nonsteroidal anti-inflammatory drugs: how do they damage gastroduodenal mucosa, *Dig Dis* 13(suppl 1):9-39, 1995.
2. Humber LG: On the classification of NSAIDs, *Drug News and Perspectives* 102-103, 1992.
3. Wolfe MM, Lichtenstein DR, Singh G: Gastrointestinal toxicity of nonsteroidal antiinflammatory drugs, *N Engl J Med* 340:1888-1898, 1999.
4. Vane JR: Inhibition of prostaglandin synthesis as a possible mechanism of action of aspirin like drugs, *Nature* 231:232-235, 1971.
5. Smith JB, Willis AL: Aspirin selectively inhibits prostaglandin production in human platelets, *Nature* 231:235-237, 1971.
6. Livingston A: Mechanism of action of nonsteroidal antiinflammatory drugs, *Vet Clin North Am Small Anim Pract* 30:773-781, 2000.
7. Patrignani P: Nonsteroidal antiinflammatory drugs, COX-2 and co lorectal cancer, *Toxicol Lett* 112-113:493-498, 2000.
8. Jones CJ, Budsberg SC: Physiologic characteristics and clinical importance of the cyclooxygenase isoforms in dogs and cats, *J Am Vet Med Assoc* 21:676-681, 2000.
9. Crofford LJ, Wilder RL, Ristimaki AP, et al: Cyclooxygenase-1 and -2 expression in rheumatoid synovial tissues: effects of interleukin-1β, phorbol ester, and corticosteroids, *J Clin Invest* 93:1095-1101, 1994.
10. Smith TJ: Cyclooxygenases as the principle targets for the action of NSAIDs, *Rheum Dis Clin North Am* 24:501-521, 1998.
11. Masferrer JL, Isakson PC, Seibert K: Cyclooxygenase-2 inhibitors: a new class of anti-inflammatory agents that spare the gastrointestinal tract, *Gastroenterol Clin North Am* 25:363-372, 1996.

12. Vane JR, Bakhle YS, Botting RM: Cyclooxygenases 1 and 2, *Annu Rev Pharmacol Toxicol* 38:97-120, 1998.

13. Jones CJ, Streppa HK, Budsberg SC: *In vivo* effect of a COX-2 selective and nonselective nonsteroidal anti-inflammatory drug (NSAID) on gastric mucosal and synovial fluid prostaglandin synthesis in dogs, *J Vet Intern Med* 15:273, 2001.

14. Streppa HK, Jones CJ, Budsberg SC: Differential biochemical inhibition of specific cyclooxygenases by various non-steroidal anti-inflammatory agents in canine whole blood, *Am J Vet Res* 63:91-94, 2002.

15. Cryer B, Feldman M: Cyclooxygenase-1 and cyclooxygenase-2 selectivity of widely used nonsteroidal anti-inflammatory drugs, *Am J Med* 104:413-421, 1998.

16. Brideau C, Kargaman S, Liu S, et al: A human whole blood assay for clinical evaluation of biochemical efficacy of cyclooxygenase inhibitors, *Inflamm Res* 45:68-74, 1996.

17. Vangeas H, Schaible HG: Prostaglandins and cyclooxygenases in the spinal cord, *Prog Neurobiol* 64:327-363, 2001.

18. Yakash TL, Dirig DM, Malmberg AB: Mechanism of action of nonsteroidal anti-inflammatory drugs, *Cancer Invest* 16:509-527, 1998.

19. Mathews KA: Nonsteroidal antiinflammatory analgesics, *Vet Clin North Am Small Anim Pract* 30:783-804, 2000.

20. Fox SM, Johnston SA: Use of carprofen for the treatment of pain and inflammation in dogs, *J Am Vet Med Assoc* 210:1493-1498, 1997.

21. McKellar QA, Pearson T, Gogan JA, et al: Pharmacokinetics, tolerance and serum thromboxane inhibition of carprofen in the dog, *J Small Anim Pract* 31:443-448, 1990.

22. Kay-Mugford P, Benn SJ, Lamarre J, et al: In vitro effects of nonsteroidal antiinflammatory drugs on cyclooxygenases activity in dogs, *Am J Vet Res* 61:802-810, 2000.

23. Ricketts AP, Lundy KM, Seibel SB: Evaluation of selective inhibition of canine cyclooxygenases 1 and 2 by carprofen and other nonsteroidal anti-inflammatory drugs, *Am J Vet Res* 59:1441-1446, 1998.

24. Vasseur PB, Johnson AL, Budsberg SC, et al: Randomized, controlled trial of the efficacy of carprofen, a nonsteroidal antiinflammatory drug, in the treatment of osteoarthritis in dogs, *J Am Vet Med Assoc* 206:807-811, 1995.

25. Holtsinger RH, Parker RB, Beale BS, et al: The therapeutic efficacy of carprofen in 209 clinical cases of canine degenerative joint disease, *Vet Comp Orthop Traumat* 5:140-144, 1992.

26. Grisneaux E, Pibarot P, Dupuis J, et al: Comparison of ketoprofen and carprofen administered prior to orthopedic surgery for control of postoperative pain in dogs, *J Am Vet Med Assoc* 215:1105-1110, 1999.

27. Balmer TV, Irvine D, Jones RS, et al: Comparison of carprofen and pethidine as postoperative analgesics in the cat, *J Small Anim Pract* 39:158-164, 1998.

28. Lascelles BDX, Cripps PJ, Jones A, et al: Efficacy and kinetics of carprofen, administered preoperatively or postoperatively, for the prevention of pain in dogs undergoing ovariohysterectomy, *Vet Surg* 27:568-582, 1998.

29. Nolan R, Reid J: Comparison of the postoperative analgesic and sedative effects of carprofen and papaveretum in the dog, *Vet Rec* 133:240-242, 1993.

30. Lascelles BDX, Butterworth SJ, Waterman AE: Postoperative analgesic and sedative effects of carprofen and pethidine in dogs, *Vet Rec* 134:187-191, 1994.

31. Hodge TM, Wahlstrom T: Three years (1997-1999) of U.S. clinical experience with Rimadyl (carprofen), *Technical Bulletin (Pfizer Animal Health)*, December 2000.

32. MacPhail CM, Lappin MR, Meyer DJ, et al: Hepatocellular toxicosis associated with administration of carprofen in 21 dogs, *J Am Vet Med Assoc* 212:1895-1901, 1998.

33. Neuman RG, Wilson BD, Barkley M, et al: Inhibition of prostaglandin biosynthesis by etodolac. I. Selective activities in arthritis, *Agents Actions* 21:160-166, 1987.

34. Budsberg SC, Johnston SA, Schwarz PD, et al: Evaluation of etodolac for the treatment of osteoarthritis of the hips in dogs: a prospective multicenter study, *J Am Vet Med Assoc* 214:1-5, 1999.

35. Sumi N, Uchimoto H, Fujimoto S, et al: Three-month oral toxicity of etodolac in dogs followed by one-month recovery test, *Oyo Yakuri/Pharmacometrics* 40:515-560, 1990.

36. Wrenn JM, Inhelder JL, Hemm RD, et al: One year chronic toxicity study of etodolac, a nonsteroidal anti-inflammatory agent, in the beagle dog, *Oyo Yakuri/Pharmacometrics* 40:599-646, 1990.

37. Sigurdsson GH, Youssef II: Amelioration of respiratory and circulatory changes in established endotoxic shock by ketoprofen, *Acta Anesthesiol Scand* 38:33-39, 1994.

38. Pibarot P, Dupuis J, Grisneaux E, et al: Comparison of ketoprofen, oxymorphone hydrochloride, and butorphanol in the treatment of postoperative pain in dogs, *J Am Vet Med Assoc* 211:438-444, 1997.

39. Engelhardt G, Bogel R, Schnitaka, et al: Meloxicam: influence on arachidonic acid metabolism, *Biochem Pharmacol* 51:21-38, 1996.

40. Van Bree H, Justus C, Quinke JF: Preliminary observations on the effects of Meloxicam in a new model for acute intra-articular inflammation in dogs, *Vet Res Commun* 18:217-224, 1994.

41. Mathews KA, Pettifer G, Foster R, et al: Safety and efficacy of preoperative administration of meloxicam, compared with that of ketoprofen and butorphanol in dogs undergoing abdominal surgery, *Am J Vet Res* 62:882-888, 2001.

42. Slingsby LS, Waterman-Pearson AE: Postoperative analgesia in the cat after ovariohysterectomy by use of carprofen, ketoprofen, meloxicam or tolfenamic acid, *J Small Anim Pract* 41:447-450, 2000.

43. Cross AR, Budsberg SC, Keefe TJ: Kinetic gait analysis assessment of meloxicam efficacy in a sodium urate-induced synovitis model in dogs, *Am J Vet Res* 58:626-631, 1997.

44. Lipowitz A, Boulay J, Klausner J: Serum salicylate concentrations and endoscopic evaluation of the gastric mucosa in dogs after oral administration of aspirin-containing products, *Am J Vet Res* 47:1586-1589, 1986.

45. Galbraith EA, McKellar QA: Pharmacokinetics and pharmacodynamics of piroxicam in dogs, *Vet Rec* 128:561-565, 1991.

46. Knapp DW, Richardson RC, Chan TC, et al: Piroxicam therapy in 34 dogs with transitional cell carcinoma of the urinary bladder, *J Vet Intern Med* 8:273-276, 1994.

47. Johnston SA: Personal communication, 1998.

48. Johnston SA, Budsberg SC: Nonsteroidal antiinflammatory drugs and corticosteroids for the management of canine osteoarthritis, *Vet Clin North Am* 27:841-862, 1997.

49. Rainsford KD, Ying C, Smith FC: Effects of meloxicam, compared with other NSAIDs, on cartilage proteoglycan metabolism, synovial prostaglandin E_2, and production of interleukins 1, 6 and 8, in human and porcine explants in organ culture, *J Pharm Pharmacol* 49:991-998, 1997.

50. Henrotin Y, Bassleer C, Reginster JY, et al: Effects of etodolac on human chondrocytes cultivated in three dimensional culture, *Clin Rheum* 8:36-42, 1989.

51. Redini F, Mauviel A, Loyau G, et al: Modulation of extracellular matrix metabolism in rabbit articular chondrocytes and human rheumatoid synovial cell by the non-steroidal antiinflammatory drug etodolac. II: Glycosaminoglycan synthesis, *Agents Actions* 31:358-367, 1990.

52. Benton HP, Vasseur PB, Broderick-Villa GA, et al: Effect of carprofen on sulfated glycosaminoglycan metabolism, protein synthesis, and prostaglandin release by cultured osteoarthritic canine chondrocytes, *Am J Vet Res* 58:286-292, 1997.

53. Ghosh P: Nonsteroidal antiinflammatory drugs and chondroprotection, *Drugs* 46:834-846, 1993.

54. Wilbrink B, Van derVeen MJ, Huber J, et al: In vitro influence of ketoprofen on the proteoglycan metabolism of human normal and osteoarthritis cartilage, *Agents Actions* 32:154-159, 1991.

55. Collier S, Ghosh P: Comparison of the effects of nonsteroidal antiinflammatory drugs (NSAIDs) on proteoglycan synthesis by articular cartilage explant and chondrocyte monolayer cultures, *Biochem Pharmacol* 41:1375-1385, 1991.

56. Wolfe MM: Future trends in the development of safer nonsteroidal antiinflammatory drugs, *Am J Med* 105(5A):44S-52S, 1998.

11

α_2-Agonists

LEIGH LAMONT AND WILLIAM TRANQUILLI

Xylazine, though not recognized as such at the time of its introduction into clinical practice, has been the prototypical α_2-adrenergic agonist used in veterinary medicine. It was first synthesized in Germany in 1962 for use as an antihypertensive agent, but it was soon discovered that it had potent sedative effects in animals. Xylazine was initially used in cattle and other ruminants in Europe, and in the early 1970s reports of its use as an anesthetic or anesthetic adjuvant began to appear. It has been used extensively in numerous species, often in combination with ketamine, to produce rapid and reliable sedation with accompanying muscle relaxation and analgesia. Unfortunately, xylazine was labeled for use in dogs and cats as an anesthetic agent years before its sedative-analgesic actions were definitively linked to stimulation of central α_2-adrenoceptors in 1981.[1] This discovery has prompted extensive investigation and development of novel α_2-agonists to be used as adjuncts in analgesic and anesthetic protocols in both humans and animals. Though still a mainstay in equine and food animal practice, the use of xylazine in companion animals has slowly been supplanted by other newer α_2-agonists, such as medetomidine and romifidine.

Medetomidine is an equal mixture of two optical enantiomers, dexmedetomidine and levomedetomidine. Dexmedetomidine is a potent α_2-agonist and has generated considerable interest in human anesthesiology. Levomedetomidine is considered to be pharmacologically inactive, though it may be involved in drug interactions. Racemic medetomidine is approved for use as a sedative-analgesic agent for dogs by the Center for Veterinary Medicine of the Food and Drug Administration. Its lipophilicity facilitates rapid absorption after intramuscular administration, with peak plasma concentrations reached in approximately 0.5 hours.[2] Elimination of medetomidine from plasma is also relatively rapid, with reported half-lives varying between 0.96[3] and 1.28 hours.[2] It has an α_2/α_1 binding ratio of 1620, compared with ratios of 260, 220, and 160 for detomidine, clonidine, and xylazine, respectively.[4] Romifidine is an imino-imidazolidine derivative of clonidine and is the newest α_2-agonist to be used as a sedative-analgesic agent in dogs. It, too, is a potent and selective α_2-adrenoceptor agonist that seems to produce sedative and analgesic effects comparable to those achieved with medetomidine. It is not currently approved for use in dogs or cats in the United States.[5,6]

The recognition of the importance of adrenergic pathways in mediating nociception has changed the way α_2-agonists, such as medetomidine, are used clinically. Although it is no longer common practice to administer large doses of α_2-agonists as monoanesthetic agents, it is generally accepted that low doses, often in combination with other analgesic drugs such as opioids, are extremely useful when used as adjuncts in a balanced analgesic protocol.

PHARMACOLOGY AND MECHANISMS OF ANALGESIC ACTION

Molecular Pharmacology of α_2-Adrenoceptors

Historically, adrenergic receptor classification has been based on pharmacologic and biochemical criteria only, and little was known about the structure and function of these specialized membrane proteins on the molecular level. Recently, the development of increasingly sophisticated molecular biologic and electrophysiologic techniques has led to the discovery of several gene families that code for a variety of adrenergic receptors, providing new insight into the events mediating intracellular biochemical signaling.

All α_2-adrenoceptor proteins are similar in size, ranging from 415 to 480 amino acids in length.[7] Each protein contains seven transmembrane domains composed of stretches of lipophilic amino acids separated by segments of hydrophilic amino acids, creating an extracellular amino terminus and an intracellular carboxyl terminus, with three small extracellular loops and three intracellular loops. Three distinct human α_2-adrenoceptor subtype genes or complementary DNAs have been cloned and are designated α_2-C10, α_2-C4, and α_2-C2, according to the locations of the receptor genes on human chromosomes 10, 4, and 2.[8] In terms of the earlier pharmacologic nomenclature, α_{2A} corresponds to α_2-C10, α_{2B} to α_2-C2, and α_{2C} to the α_2-C4 designation.[8] Related α_2-adrenoceptor subtypes have been cloned in a variety of other species, including rat, mouse, pig, opossum, and fish; and partial cDNA sequences from bovine and avian α_{2A}-receptors have also been identified. A fourth α_2-adrenoceptor subtype (α_{2D}) has been proposed in the rat; however, recent studies have indicated that this receptor is actually a species homologue of the rat α_{2A} subtype.[8] All three α_2 subtype genes apparently share a common evolutionary origin, despite only 50% protein homology at the amino acid level. However, several key structural and functional domains appear to be well conserved.

Numerous experimental limitations have precluded clarifying the role of each α_2-adrenoceptor subtype in catecholamine-mediated physiologic processes in both the periphery and the central nervous system (CNS). Most of the currently available α_2-agonists bind with similar affinity to all three receptor subtypes, although some compounds (such as prazosin and chlorpromazine) can discriminate to varying degrees in ligand-binding assays. The lack of subtype-specific agonists and antagonists has limited the utility of classic pharmacologic approaches, and even in cases in which subtype selectivity has been noted in vitro, questions surrounding the in vivo bioavailability of the agents have confounded interpretation of observed clinical effects.[9] Furthermore, α_2-adrenoceptor subtype expression and function appear to be species specific, resulting in varied physiologic effects and pharmacologic activity profiles and making extrapolation of data among species unwise.[10] Despite these difficulties, it is clear that the possibility of identifying a single receptor subtype that mediates a desired analgesic effect without producing any undesirable cardiorespiratory alterations may someday become a reality.

With techniques such as in situ hybridization and reverse-transcription polymerase chain reaction, the messenger RNA transcription patterns of these receptor subtypes can be elucidated. Furthermore, recombinant DNA methodology has made it possible to address the biologic role of individual α_2-adrenoceptor subtypes by creating genetically modified reagents with either dysfunctional ("transgenic") or deficient ("knockout") subtypes, eliminating the need for subtype-selective agonists or antagonists. Identification of the genome protein sequence has also made it possible to produce antibodies directed specifically against the cognate proteins, which facilitates immunologic investigations, such as qualitative immunohistochemistry.[11]

Studies in rats and mice have shown that the α_{2A} subtype is the predominant receptor in the brain and that it is widely distributed. In the rat spinal cord, both α_{2A} and α_{2C} subtypes have been identified, with α_{2A} being widely distributed, whereas α_{2C} is restricted mainly to cells of the dorsal root ganglia.[11] In contrast, in human spinal cord preparations, α_{2A} and α_{2B} subtypes predominate, with the α_{2C} subtype only sparsely represented.[11]

Functionally, based on studies in knockout mice, there seems to be agreement that the α_{2A} subtype mediates clinically relevant analgesic, sedative-hypnotic, and anesthetic-sparing responses in this species.[9,11,12] It is interesting that a single α_2-adrenoceptor subtype mediates both the analgesic and sedative clinical effects, because the proposed sites of action involved differ significantly. The α_{2A} subtype, not surprisingly, also appears to be responsible for the hypotensive and bradycardic actions associated with α_2-agonist administration. The α_{2B} subtype appears to have a dominant role in eliciting the immediate surge in systemic vascular resistance seen after administration of α_2-agonists, though the α_{2A} subtype may make a lesser contribution to peripheral vasoconstriction in certain vascular compartments.[13] The hypothermic effects and modulation of dopaminergic activity are attributed to the α_{2C} subtype.[11]

Several of the currently available α_2-agonists, such as clonidine and romifidine, contain an imidazole moiety that is able to bind to and activate a second class of nonnoradrenergic receptors known as *imidazoline receptors*.[14] Imidazoline receptors are involved in the central control of vasomotor tone and are located primarily in the nucleus reticularis lateralis of the ventrolateral region of the medulla.[14] Thus the central hypotensive effects observed after administration of α_2-agonists possessing imidazoline activity are a result of activation of two completely distinct receptor systems, α_{2A}-adrenoceptors and imidazoline receptors.

Signal Transduction Mechanisms of α_2-Adrenoceptors

G Proteins

All α_2-adrenoceptors belong to a class of excitable transmembrane proteins involved in mediating cell communication and activity. They interact selectively with extracellular compounds to initiate a cascade of biochemical changes that ultimately lead to a physiologic effect. In order to act as an interface between the extracellular environment and the intracellular space, transmembrane receptors require a mechanism by which they can notify the cell of receptor occupancy by a ligand. This process is frequently referred to as *signal transduction* and often involves a group of proteins known as guanine nucleotide binding proteins, or G proteins.

α_2-Adrenoceptors are members of the larger G protein–coupled receptor superfamily, which also includes dopaminergic, cholinergic, and serotonergic receptor systems. G proteins effectively link cell membrane receptors to intracellular effector mechanisms, amplify the signal, and transduce external chemical stimuli into cellular responses. In general, binding of a specific ligand (such as a neurotransmitter, endogenous hormone, or exogenous drug molecule) induces a conformational change in the receptor, enabling it to activate specific types of G proteins.[8] Such receptor-activated G proteins may either modulate the synthesis or availability of intracellular second messenger molecules or directly alter the activity of transmembrane ion channels.[8]

Mammalian G proteins are composed of three polypeptide subunits, α, β, and γ. To date, at least 20 different G protein α-subunits have been discovered, and each is capable of modulating the activity of specific effector pathways.[15] The coupling of α_2-adrenoceptors to various isoforms of the pertussis toxin–sensitive inhibitory G proteins, G_i and G_o, has been extensively characterized, but recent evidence indicates that other G proteins may also interact with α_2-adrenoceptors, including the stimulatory G protein, G_s.[8]

Effector Mechanisms

Adenylate Cyclase. Perhaps the most thoroughly documented α_2-adrenoceptor effector mechanism is the inhibition of adenylate cyclase activity. This response is mediated by α_2-activation of G_i, which inhibits enzyme activity and results in decreased accumulation of cyclic adenosine monophosphate (cAMP) within the cell.[16] The decreased availability of intracellular cAMP attenuates the stimulation of cAMP-dependent protein kinase, and hence, the phosphorylation of target regulatory proteins. However, it has been recognized that many of the physiologic processes attributed to α_2-adrenoceptor activation, including analgesia, cannot be explained solely or at all by decreased intracellular cAMP levels. Indeed, spinal antinociception seems to be dissociated from effects on cAMP, since it can be reproduced in systems in which elevated cAMP concentrations are maintained throughout.[8] Consequently, alternative mechanisms must exist to explain the diversity of events mediated by α_2-adrenoceptor activation.

Modulation of Ion Channel Activity. A second key effector mechanism involves the modulation of ion channel activity. α_2-Adrenoceptor activation of G-protein–gated potassium channels results in membrane hyperpolarization, causing a decrease in the firing rate of excitable cells in the CNS.[8] Evidence suggests that α_2-adrenoceptors are coupled to these potassium channels by the inhibitory G protein, Gi_3, although other pertussis toxin–sensitive G protein species cannot be excluded at this time. In many systems, this increased potassium conductance leading to hyperpolarization appears to be a calcium-dependent process, though the role of calcium availability in this setting remains to be clarified. Furthermore, it has also been proposed that potassium channel–mediated hyperpolarization may in fact occur secondary to inhibition of adenylate cyclase activity, perhaps arising from a cAMP-dependent change in the phosphorylation status of the ion channel.[8]

Potassium channels are not the only ion channels coupled to α_2-adrenoceptors via G proteins. Inhibition of calcium influx through N-type voltage-gated calcium channels presumably reduces fusion of synaptic vesicles with the postsynaptic membrane, thereby reducing neurotransmitter release after presynaptic α_2-adrenoceptor stimulation.[7] Although α_2-adrenoceptor–mediated inhibition of calcium conductance is modulated primarily by G_o-type G proteins, indirect calcium channel modulation is also possible through cAMP and protein kinase A.[8]

Other Biochemical Second Messengers. There are a number of other suggested G protein–dependent second messenger mechanisms linked with α_2-adrenoceptor activation. For example, acceleration of sodium/hydrogen exchange by α_2-adrenoceptor agonists, together with increased intracellular availability of calcium, is postulated to cause stimulation of phospholipase A_2 activity and arachidonic acid mobilization that increases formation of thromboxane A and other bioactive cyclooxygenase metabolites.[8] Other potential effector mechanisms include stimulation of phosphoinositol-mediated mobilization of intracellular calcium by phospholipase C via pertussis toxin–sensitive G proteins and calcium-stimulated activation of a calcium/calmodulin–sensitive form of adenylate cyclase. The biologic significance of these biochemical second messenger systems remains to be determined.

Neurophysiology of α_2-Adrenoceptor-Mediated Antinociception

Elucidating the neurophysiologic basis of α_2-adrenoceptor–mediated analgesia has proven to be a challenging task for a number of reasons. First, α_2-adrenoceptors within the CNS are not confined solely to noradrenergic neurons (so-called autoreceptors) but are also located on nonnoradrenergic neurons (called *heteroceptors*) in the dorsal horn of the spinal cord.[17,18] Both populations of receptors appear to be involved in α_2-mediated antinociception. In addition, there is evidence to suggest that both presynaptic and postsynaptic sites of action may contribute to analgesia and that this effect may be produced either directly, through stimulation at the level of the spinal cord, or indirectly, through activation of descending adrenergic nociceptive pathways.

Spinal Antinociception

Dense populations of α_2-adrenoceptors are concentrated in the dorsal horn of the mammalian spinal cord, located both presynaptically and postsynaptically on non-noradrenergic nociceptive neurons. Activation of these heteroceptors by norepinephrine or an exogenous α_2-agonist may produce direct spinally mediated analgesia by one of two potential mechanisms.[19] The first involves presynaptic α_2-adrenoceptors found on primary afferent C fibers terminating in the superficial laminae of the dorsal horn. When activated, G_o proteins mediate a decrease in calcium influx (as outlined in the preceding section), leading to decreased release of neurotransmitters and/or neuropeptides, including glutamate, vasoactive intestinal peptide, calcitonin gene-related peptide, substance P, and neurotensin. The net result of this presynaptic α_2 stimulation is spinal antinociception. In addition, α_2-heteroceptors are also located postsynaptically on wide-dynamic-range projection neurons targeted by primary afferent fibers in the dorsal horn. Ligand binding at these receptors produces neuronal hyperpolarization via G_i protein–coupled potassium channels (see previous section), thereby dampening ascending nociceptive transmission and producing postsynaptically mediated spinal analgesia.

Supraspinal Antinociception. It is generally accepted that the analgesic effects attributed to α_2-agonist administration are a result of direct activation of α_2-adrenoceptors located at the level of the spinal cord as discussed previously, while the sedative-hypnotic effects are mediated by activation of supraspinal α_2-autoreceptors located in the brainstem. However, there is now evidence to suggest that these supraspinal structures may also contribute indirectly to spinally mediated α_2-adrenoceptor–mediated antinociception.

Relatively high densities of α_2-agonist binding sites are concentrated in the mammalian brainstem. The catecholaminergic nuclei of the pons, designated *A5, A6* (also called the *locus ceruleus*), and *A7,* are the major origins of noradrenergic innervation of the spinal cord.[20,21] Of these, the locus ceruleus (LC) is the most important, with noradrenergic neurons originating here descending to all segments of the spinal cord and also modulating noradrenergic input from higher structures such as the periaqueductal gray matter of the midbrain. It has been proposed that in addition to the hypnotic effects observed after α_2-agonist binding in cell bodies of LC neurons, these nuclei may modulate descending noradrenergic pathways and augment spinal antinociception.

Based on a growing body of evidence, it is speculated that activation of α_2-autoreceptors, either by norepinephrine or an exogenous α_2-agonist located in the LC, results in neuronal inhibition and a decreased release of norepinephrine from the LC. This dampening of LC activity *dis*inhibits activity in the cell bodies of A5 and A7 nuclei, resulting in increased release of norepinephrine from their terminals in the dorsal horn of the spinal cord, which in turn activates presynaptic and postsynaptic α_2-heteroceptors to produce antinociception.[20] This hypothesis offers an explanation for the apparent paradox that supraspinal noradrenergic manipulation, characterized by diminished norepinephrine release, can somehow induce spinal release of norepinephrine and that the ensuing antinociceptive effect can be precisely mimicked by spinal delivery of α_2-adrenoceptor agonists. Furthermore, analgesia produced by the injection of α_2-agonists directly into the LC can be blocked by spinal administration of specific α_2-antagonists. Even higher supraspinal structures may play a role, adding another tier to the noradrenergic nociceptive pathway. The periaqueductal gray matter of the midbrain extends noradrenergic innervation to the LC and thus, when activated, may lead to α_2-mediated decreases in LC norepinephrine release, which indirectly feeds back on spinal α_2-adrenoceptors to produce antinociception.[17]

Clinical Use as Analgesic Adjuvants

Systemic Use

Despite the fact that α_2-agonists have been used extensively in veterinary clinical practice for over 30 years, the past decade has seen a new appreciation of the unique spectrum of anesthetic and analgesic properties of this novel class of compounds. These agents are not general anesthetics or even first-line analgesic agents but rather, in the opinion of the authors, should be classified as anesthetic and analgesic adjuncts. They are extremely effective when coadministered with other agents, such as opioids or dissociatives, in a balanced analgesic or anesthetic protocol. At low dosages, both the sedative and analgesic effects of the α_2-agonists are dose-dependent. At higher dosages, however, a maximal response is attained and further increases in dose serve only to prolong the duration of sedation without providing more intense analgesia.[22] In general, the sedative effect lasts significantly longer than the analgesic effect, so adequate analgesia cannot be inferred on the basis of clinical signs of sedation alone. α_2-Agonists contribute to effective analgesia in a variety of pain syndromes, including pain of musculoskeletal, visceral, and neuropathic origin. In addition, because α_2-agonists and opioids exert many of their analgesic effects through similar modulatory pathways within the CNS, combination therapy with these two classes has the potential to produce analgesic synergism. Therefore it is common practice to coadminister medetomidine or xylazine with one of a variety of opioids such as butorphanol, buprenorphine, morphine, oxymorphone, hydromorphone, or fentanyl to enhance analgesia and prolong its duration.

Considerations for Patient Selection

Regardless of the particular combination chosen, patient evaluation and selection is critical when administration of an α_2-agonist is considered. Even at the low doses currently advocated, α_2-agonists still induce immediate alterations in cardiopulmonary function, and consequently, their use should be restricted to young to middle-aged animals without significant systemic disease. Specific contraindications include patients that will be adversely affected by an increase in cardiac afterload or a decrease in cardiac output (e.g., mitral or tricuspid regurgitation or dilated cardiomyopathy); patients with cardiac arrhythmias or conduction disturbances (e.g., premature ventricular contractions or atrioventricular block); patients with pre-existing hypertension or with an increased potential for arterial hemorrhage (e.g., traumatic arterial laceration); and patients for whom vomiting could have serious detrimental effects (e.g., upper gastrointestinal obstruction or corneal descemetocele). α_2-Agonists may be contraindicated in some geriatric animals because of the diminished cardiovascular reserve capacity in this group of patients, and other alternative analgesic adjuncts should probably be considered first in this population.

α_2-Agonists can be used systemically in a number of ways as analgesic adjuvants in clinical practice. First, they can be used as sedative-analgesic agents for diagnostic or minor surgical procedures of short duration; second, they can be used as preanesthetic agents before induction of general anesthesia and transfer to an inhalation agent; and third, they can be used as anxiolytic-analgesic agents administered in very low dosages as constant-rate infusions.

α_2-Agonists as Sedative-Analgesic Agents. The sedative-analgesic effects of the α_2-agonists facilitate completion of a variety of short, noninvasive procedures including radiographs, sonograms, minor laceration repair, wound debridement, bandage placement, ear canal examination and cleaning, skin biopsy, and oral examination. In general, the addition of an opioid will necessitate a lower dose of α_2-agonist and result in better, longer-lasting analgesia. For procedures associated with minimal discomfort, xylazine or medetomidine (Table 11-1) can be combined with butorphanol or buprenorphine; and for potentially painful procedures, addition of morphine, oxymorphone, or hydromorphone is recommended. The intramuscular route of administration is used most commonly, with the two drugs mixed together in one syringe and injected 20 minutes before initiation of the procedure. If the intravenous route of administration is chosen, the dose of α_2-agonist can be reduced to approximately one half to one third of the intramuscular dose. The onset of action occurs within minutes of intravenous injection, and a smoother effect is often achieved if the opioid is administered after the patient begins to exhibit signs of sedation. The duration of analgesic action with α_2-agonists is relatively short at the dosages recommended in Table 11-1, ranging from 30 to 90 minutes, depending on the agent and the route of administration. The addition of an opi-

TABLE 11-1

Recommended Dosages of α_2-Agonists as Analgesic Adjuncts

	Systemic	Epidural	Perineural/ Intraarticular
Medetomidine	Dog: 5-10 µg/kg IM, SC* Dog: 1-4 µg/kg IV bolus* Cat: 10-20 µg/kg IM, SC* Cat: 2-6 µg/kg IV bolus*	Dog and cat: 1-5 µg/kg	Dog and cat: 2-5 µg/kg
Romifidine	Dog: 10-20 µg/kg IM, SC* Cat: 20-40 µg/kg IM, IV*		
Xylazine	Dog: 0.2-0.5 mg/kg IM, SC* Dog: 0.1-0.2 mg/kg IV* Cat: 0.2-0.5 mg/kg IM, SC* Cat: 0.1-0.3 mg/kg IV*		
Atropine	0.04 mg/kg IM, SC 0.02 mg/kg IV		
Glycopyrrolate	0.01 mg/kg IM, SC 0.005 mg/kg IV		

IM, Intramuscular; *SC,* subcutaneous; *IV,* intravenous; *CRI,* constant-rate infusion.
*May combine with an anticholinergic in exercise-tolerant patients free from heart disease.

oid will prolong this effect for anywhere from 1 to 4 hours, depending on the opioid chosen, the dose, and the route of administration.

The use of anticholinergics in conjunction with α_2-agonists remains controversial. The immediate increase in systemic vascular resistance caused by peripheral α_2-adrenoceptor stimulation causes a baroreceptor-mediated increase in vagal tone, which may produce severe bradycardia. Although anticholinergic administration will counteract this increase in vagal tone and drive the heart rate up, it also increases myocardial work and oxygen consumption in the face of the increased cardiac afterload. For short nonpainful procedures, it may be optimal to monitor heart rate closely throughout the procedure and, if necessary, reverse the effects of the α_2-agonist with the specific reversal agent, atipamezole. Alternatively, atropine or glycopyrrolate may be administered preemptively or added to the α_2-agonist–opioid combination at the time of injection. Some advocate the administration of the anticholinergic intramuscularly 15 minutes *before* administration of the α_2-agonist–opioid combination. This is based on the rationale that the initial reflex tachycardia often seen after atropine administration will be waning by the time the α_2-agonist–induced hypertensive phase occurs, which would, in theory, put less strain on the myocardium. In any case, these considerations underline the importance of ensuring normal cardiovascular function in patients before proceeding with α_2-agonist administration and attentive monitoring of heart rate and rhythm throughout the duration of effect.

α_2-*Agonists in the Preanesthetic Period.* α_2-Agonists produce consistently reliable analgesia, sedation, and muscle relaxation, making them attractive candidates for incorporation into a balanced anesthetic protocol. Addition of an α_2-agonist in the preanesthetic period will markedly reduce the required dose of induction agents, such as thiopental, propofol, and ketamine, and will also have a significant minimum alveolar concentration (MAC)–sparing effect after transfer to an inhalation agent.[23] Typically, xylazine or medetomidine is combined with butorphanol or buprenorphine and administered before surgical procedures associated with mild-to-moderate pain; whereas administration of morphine, oxymorphone, hydromorphone, or fentanyl is recommended before major surgeries associated with moderate-to-severe pain. Dosing guidelines and routes of administration are the same as discussed previously and are outlined in Table 11-1. Although concurrent anticholinergic administration in this setting is not mandatory, it is recommended for several reasons. First, when α_2-agonists are used during the preanesthetic period in conjunction with potent induction and maintenance anesthetic agents, the potential for a severe vagotonic response resulting in profound bradycardia and cardiovascular depression is compounded. Furthermore, many of these agents, most notably isoflurane, produce significant vasodilation, which effectively counteracts the hypertensive response caused by peripheral α_2-adrenoceptor stimulation and probably attenuates the immediate increase in cardiac afterload. In our experience, concurrent administration of atropine or glycopyrrolate with an α_2-agonist–opioid combination in the preanesthetic period has not been associated with excessive tachycardia at the time of induction or with prolonged systemic hypertension after transfer to inhalation anesthesia. The transient alterations in cardiopulmonary function induced by α_2-agonists are very well tolerated in young to middle-aged animals free of significant systemic disease; however, monitoring throughout the perianesthetic period is essential. In animals undergoing surgery, routine postoperative reversal of the α_2-agonist is not recommended, because this will also reverse any remaining analgesic effects. In most cases, recovery from anesthesia is calm and smooth and is rarely delayed as a result of residual α_2-agonist–mediated sedation. Additional opioids may be administered during the recovery period to ensure adequate postoperative analgesia.

α_2-Agonists as Constant-Rate Infusions. A third use for α_2-agonists involves intravenous administration of extremely low doses as a constant-rate infusion to provide sedation, anxiolysis, and analgesia. The α_2-agonist, dexmedetomidine, has recently been labeled for this purpose in human patients in the intensive care setting because the drug's relatively short half-life makes it suitable for administration as a continuous infusion. A growing body of evidence implicates the classic neuroendocrine stress response as a major factor in increasing morbidity and prolonging the clinical course in patients who have experienced trauma or undergone surgery.[24] Presumably, sedation and anxiolysis may improve outcome by reducing this stress response, which is often exacerbated by routine intensive care unit interventions, and by modulating the posttraumatic hormonal milieu. The additional benefit of supplemental analgesia makes the α_2-agonists attractive alternatives to other sedatives commonly used for these patients. Studies involving dexmedetomidine infusions in humans have demonstrated significant reductions in benzodiazepine and opioid requirements in intubated, mechanically ventilated patients without inducing serious impairment of cardiopulmonary parameters, most notably, respiratory function.[24,25] In addition, α_2-agonists also influence hormonal patterns to counteract protein catabolism and high nitrogen losses, which are characteristic sequelae of trauma and surgery. A significantly improved cumulative nitrogen balance has been documented in patients receiving α_2-agonist infusions after surgery, probably as a result of stimulation of growth hormone release.[26]

Unfortunately, to date, there have been no large-scale investigations examining the utility of medetomidine infusions in canine and feline patients in the intensive care unit, although we can assume that the deleterious effects associated with neurohormonal activation also affect clinical outcome negatively in these species. Dosing guidelines for continuous infusions of medetomidine have not been determined in dogs and cats. Because of the hemodynamic consequences associated with very low constant-rate infusion doses of medetomidine, cardiopulmonary monitoring is recommended. The unique combination of pharmacologic properties of α_2-agonists makes them candidates for use in this setting, and it would seem that future studies in veterinary patients are warranted.

Regional Use

Although systemic administration of α_2-agonists is effective, simple, and convenient, the anatomic distribution of α_2-adrenoceptors and our growing knowledge of the neurophysiology of adrenergic nociceptive pathways suggest that they may also be useful in a variety of regional anesthetic-analgesic techniques. Regardless of the technique chosen, the potential for systemic absorption of α_2-agonists still remains, and cardiopulmonary parameters should be monitored. Regional techniques targeting the CNS include epidural and intrathecal injection, while peripheral effects may be achieved with intraarticular or perineural administration.

Epidural/Intrathecal Administration of α_2-Agonists

A large body of evidence suggests that the spinal site of action is crucial in mediating the analgesic effect of α_2-agonists. Consequently, the epidural and intrathecal routes of administration have been investigated in an effort to specifically target the antinociceptive response while minimizing peripheral hemodynamic consequences. Several key observations support this reasoning: first, lumbar epidural injection of α_2-agonists in both humans and animals results in more intense analgesia in the caudal, dependent extremity, indicating that antinociception predominates at the skin dermatomes innervated by the cord segments near the site of spinal administration[27]; second, the correlation between blood α₂-agonist concentration and analgesia is relatively poor, while the correlation between the cerebrospinal fluid (CSF) concentration and analgesia is excellent, implicating a spinal site of action[28]; and third, the relatively brief duration of analgesia from an epidural bolus of α₂-agonist is consistent with the rapid elimination of these drugs from the CSF.[27,28]

In addition to the mechanisms underlying spinal analgesia discussed in Section II, regional neuraxial administration of α₂-agonists appears to produce analgesia, at least in part, by stimulation of cholinergic interneurons in the spinal cord.[28,29] Studies in animals have shown that epidurally or intrathecally applied α₂-agonists increase acetylcholine concentrations in spinal cord dorsal horn preparations and in lumbar CSF samples. Furthermore, epidural or intrathecal analgesia is enhanced by intrathecal injection of the cholinesterase inhibitor, neostigmine. This α₂-adrenergic–cholinergic interaction is apparently unique to the epidural and intrathecal routes of administration, since elevated acetylcholine levels in CSF have not been documented after systemic injection of α₂-agonists.[29,30]

Although intrathecal administration of analgesic agents is not routine in clinical veterinary medicine, the epidural route of administration is commonly used and is associated with fewer risks and adverse side effects compared with subarachnoid puncture. Incorporation of a low dose of an α₂-agonist into an epidural protocol will produce additive or even synergistic analgesic effects when combined with opioids and/or local anesthetics.[30a] Medetomidine may be combined with standard epidural doses of morphine, oxymorphone, buprenorphine, fentanyl, lidocaine, or bupivacaine and injected into the epidural space at the lumbosacral junction. As discussed previously, the lipophilic nature of medetomidine means that it is rapidly cleared from the CSF in the vicinity of the spinal injection site, thereby anatomically limiting the drug's action and resulting in a significant portion of the administered dose being absorbed systemically. Consequently, when the total dose administered approaches that which would otherwise be given systemically, the specificity of the regional analgesic effect may be lost. Similar observations have been made for highly lipid-soluble opioids, such as fentanyl, when compared with less soluble agents, such as morphine. Perhaps the best technique with which to optimize the regional spinal analgesic effects of medetomidine is a continuous infusion through an indwelling epidural catheter, where extremely low dosages can be administered directly to the desired segment of spinal cord while minimizing medetomidine plasma levels. Although epidural catheterization is probably not practical or justifiable in most patients, it may, in select cases, be the most effective means of managing severe pain, and in this setting, α_2-agonists may be valuable analgesic adjuncts.

Intraarticular Administration of α_2-Agonists

α_2-Adrenoceptors are not confined solely to the CNS but are also distributed throughout the peripheral nervous system, located on the terminals of primary afferent nociceptive fibers.[28] In addition to their central analgesic effects, α_2-agonists also appear able to produce some degree of antinociception peripherally by inhibition of norepinephrine release at nerve terminals. Decreases in neurotransmitter release modulate nociceptor activity and may help minimize peripheral sensitization arising from tissue injury.

Studies in human patients have demonstrated this peripheral analgesic effect by intraarticular administration of α_2-agonists to patients undergoing arthroscopic knee surgery. Intraarticular α_2-agonists produced significant analgesia when administered alone, and the effect is apparently unrelated to vascular uptake of the drug and redistribution to central sites.[31] Additive and synergistic analgesic effects have been documented for intraarticular combinations of α_2-agonists with both local anesthetics and opioids.[32] It has been suggested that peripherally mediated hypoalgesia is enhanced in conditions characterized by local tissue inflammation. Therefore veterinary patients undergoing routine arthrotomy may benefit from low dosages of medetomidine (see Table 11-1) combined with morphine, bupivacaine, or both injected into the joint at the end of surgery.

Perineural Administration of α_2-Agonists

Despite the fact that α_2-adrenoceptors are notably lacking on the axons of peripheral nerves, α_2-agonists enhance peripheral nerve block intensity and duration when added to local anesthetics administered perineurally. Three possible mechanisms accounting for this interaction have been proposed. First, α_2-agonists have been shown to block conduction in C fibers and, to a lesser degree, in Aδ fibers and increase potassium conductance in isolated neurons in vitro. This suggests a direct effect on neural transmission in the presence of high local concentrations, such as may occur after perineural injection. Second, α_2-agonists may cause local vasocon-striction in the clinical setting, thereby reducing vascular removal of local anesthetic surrounding neural structures and prolonging the duration of action. However, there is little evidence for this expla-nation, if clinically relevant concentrations of α_2-agonist are ad-ministered. Finally, it has become evident that both opioids and α_2-agonists can enhance the effects of perineural or spinal local anesthetics, regardless of whether they are administered regionally or systemically.[28] Although further studies are needed, it seems clear that the enhancement of peripheral nerve blockade produced by α_2-agonists is a complex, multifactorial phenomenon. In veterinary patients, medetomidine (see Table 11-1) may be combined with li-docaine or bupivacaine for brachial plexus and intercostal and den-tal nerve blocks to enhance nerve conduction blockade and improve analgesia.

SIDE EFFECTS OF α_2-AGONISTS

Sedation, Muscle Relaxation, and Anxiolysis

Compared with the other major classes of analgesic agents, α_2-agonists consistently produce significant sedative effects in dogs and cats when administered at clinically relevant dosages. The LC is the most important catecholaminergic nucleus of the mammalian brain-stem and is a major center for control of vigilance and arousal. Acti-vation of α_2-autoreceptors produces tonic inhibition of LC adrenergic neurons, characterized by a decreased release of norepinephrine re-sulting in sedation. The sedative-hypnotic effects are largely dose-dependent; however, at higher dosages a ceiling effect is attained and further increases in dose will simply prolong the duration of sedation.[33] The muscle-relaxant properties of α_2-agonists are well recognized and often exploited in veterinary medicine. This effect is mediated through inhibition of neuronal transmission at the level of the spinal cord. Mul-tiple studies have demonstrated the efficacy of α_2-agonists as anxi-olytics both perioperatively and during opiate and nicotine withdrawal. In both animals and humans, the α_2-agonists appear to be able to re-duce stress and anxiety independent of their sedative effects.[33]

Cardiovascular Effects

On intravenous injection, α_2-agonists bind peripheral postsynaptic α_2-adrenoceptors, which results in smooth muscle contraction and vasoconstriction. This increase in systemic vascular resistance produces a short-lived hypertensive phase accompanied by a compensatory baroreceptor-mediated reflex bradycardia.[33] The magnitude of the initial hypertension may be less after intramuscular administration, probably reflecting reduced peak plasma levels of the drug. Bradyarrhythmias may be encountered during this period as a result of increased vagal tone, and it is not uncommon for heart rates to decrease by as much as 50%.[33] Sinus arrhythmia, sinoatrial block, and first-degree and second-degree atrioventricular block are frequently seen, whereas third-degree atrioventricular block and sinoatrial arrest occur more rarely. After the transient peripherally mediated effects start to wane, central α_2-adrenoceptor effects will predominate. Decreased sympathetic tone results in reduced blood pressure and diminished cardiac output. It is not uncommon for blood pressure to fall by one quarter to one third and for cardiac output to decrease by one third to one half of baseline value.[33] These effects are observed consistently in almost all species and underline the importance of ensuring normal myocardial function and cardiovascular reserve capacity in patients before administration of an α_2-agonist.

The immediate alterations in cardiovascular function may be modified when α_2-agonists are coadministered with other agents, such as the dissociative, ketamine. Xylazine- or medetomidine-induced decreases in heart rate and cardiac output are attenuated to some degree by ketamine's sympathomimetic action, which also results in increased blood pressure, systemic vascular resistance, and myocardial oxygen consumption. The routine use of anticholinergics in conjunction with α_2-agonists remains controversial. The decision to administer atropine or glycopyrrolate probably depends on a number of factors including the species, the type and duration of procedure, and the concurrent use of other sedative or anesthetic agents. Regardless of whether an anticholinergic is incorporated into the protocol, monitoring of heart rate and rhythm is essential.

Concerns over the cardiodepressant and arrhythmogenic effects of the α_2-agonists have prevented some veterinarians from embracing these agents for use in everyday clinical practice. An understanding of the hemodynamic consequences associated with their use will guide patient selection and encourage monitoring of cardiopulmonary parameters, which will allow the practitioner to take full advantage of the unique spectrum of pharmacologic properties offered by this class of drugs.

Respiratory Effects

Although the respiratory rate decreases with the administration of both xylazine and medetomidine, at clinically recommended dosages, arterial pH, PaO_2, and $PaCO_2$ are not significantly altered. The decreased respiration rate is accompanied by an increased tidal volume, which effectively maintains alveolar ventilation.[33] However, at higher dosages, especially in combination with other CNS depressants, minute ventilation may be compromised, and decreases in venous PO_2 and oxygen content have been noted. This venous desaturation is presumably related to increased tissue oxygen extraction associated with decreased cardiac output.

Gastrointestinal Effects

α_2-Agonists can cause vomiting in both dogs and cats, although cats seem much more sensitive to the emetic effects of these drugs. Up to 20% of dogs and up to 90% of cats will vomit after medetomidine administration, apparently as a result of central stimulation of α_2-adrenoceptors.[34] Emesis is most often seen after subcutaneous and, to a lesser extent, intramuscular administration. Xylazine decreases esophageal sphincter pressure in dogs and may increase the likelihood of gastric reflux. In addition, acute abdominal distension has been reported in large-breed dogs after xylazine administration, which may be a result of drug-induced parasympatholytic activity promoting gastrointestinal atony and gas accumulation.[33]

Renal Effects

Increased urine output after administration of xylazine and medetomidine has been reported in both cats and dogs. Decreased urethral closure pressure has also been noted in both male and female dogs, although normal micturition reflexes are maintained. This effect is coupled to a reduction in electromyographic activity of the urethral sphincter.[29] Detrusor function appears unaffected.

Hormonal Effects

Transient hypoinsulinemia and hyperglycemia have been observed in dogs administered α_2-agonists. The magnitude and duration of these actions appear to be dose-dependent. Hyperglycemia is a result of inhibition of insulin secretion and is mediated by α_2-adrenoceptors located in pancreatic beta cells. Other hormonal changes include transient alterations in growth hormone, testosterone, prolactin, antidiuretic hormone, and follicle-stimulating hormone levels.

Miscellaneous Effects

Increased myometrial tone and intrauterine pressure have been noted in several species after xylazine administration. Mydriasis is also commonly observed, and this effect may be caused by central inhibition of parasympathetic innervation to the iris or direct sympathetic stimulation of α_2-receptors located in both the iris and the CNS. Decreased intraocular pressure has been reported in some species after systemic administration of xylazine and is a result of dampened sympathetic activity and decreased aqueous flow.

REFERENCES

1. Hsu WH: Xylazine induced depression and its antagonism by alpha-adrenergic blocking agents, *J Pharmacol Exp Ther* 218:188-192, 1981.
2. Salonen JS: Pharmacokinetics of medetomidine, *Acta Vet Scand* (suppl) 85:49-54, 1989.
3. Kuusela E, Raekallio M, Anttila M, et al: Clinical effects and pharmacokinetics of medetomidine and its enantiomers in dogs, *J Vet Pharmacol Ther* 23(1):15-20, 2000.
4. Virtanen R: Pharmacologic profiles of medetomidine and its antagonist, atipamezole, *Acta Vet Scand* (suppl) 85:29-37, 1989.
5. England GCW, Flack TE, Hollingworth E, et al: Sedative effects of romifidine in the dog, *J Small Anim Pract* 37:19-25, 1996.
6. Lemke KA: Sedative effects in intramuscular administration of a low dose of romifidine in dogs, *Am J Vet Res* 60(2):162-168, 1999.
7. Daunt DA, Maze M: α_2-Adrenergic agonist receptors, sites and mechanisms of action. In Short CE, Van Poznak A, editors: *Animal pain,* New York, 1992, Churchill Livingstone.
8. Aanta R, Marjamaki A, Scheinin M: Molecular pharmacology of α_2-adrenoceptor subtypes, *Ann Med* 27:439-449, 1995.
9. Lakhlani PP, MacMillan LB, Guo TZ, et al: Substitution of a mutant α_{2A}-adrenergic receptor via "hit and run" gene targeting reveals the role of this subtype in sedative, analgesic, and anesthetic-sparing responses *in vivo, Proc Natl Acad Sci USA* 94:9950-9955, 1997.
10. Ongioco RRS, Richardson CD, Rudner XL, et al: α_2-Adrenergic receptors in human dorsal root ganglia, *Anesthesiology* 92:968-976, 2000.
11. Maze M, Fujinaga M: α_2-Adrenoceptors in pain modulation: which subtype should be targeted to produce analgesia? *Anesthesiology* 92:934-936, 2000.

12. MacMillan LB, Lakhlani PP, Hein L, et al: In vivo mutation of the α_{2A}-adrenergic receptor by homologous recombination reveals the role of this subtype in multiple physiologic processes, *Adv Pharmacol* 42:493-496, 1998.

13. MacMillan LB, Hein L, Smith MS, et al: Central hypotensive effects of the α_{2A}-adrenergic receptor subtype, *Science* 273(5276):801-803, 1996.

14. Bousquet P: Imidazoline receptors: from basic concepts to recent developments, *J Cardiovasc Pharmacol* 26(suppl 2):S1-S6, 1995.

15. Hayashi Y, Maze M: Alpha$_2$-adrenoceptor agonists and anaesthesia, *Br J Anaesth* 71:108-118, 1993.

16. Schwinn DA: Adrenoceptors as models for G protein-coupled receptors: structure, function and regulation, *Br J Anaesth* 71:77-85, 1993.

17. Budai D, Harasawa I, Fields HL: Midbrain periaqueductal gray (PAG) inhibits nociceptive inputs to sacral dorsal horn nociceptive neurons through α_2-adrenergic receptors, *J Neurophysiol* 80(5):2244-2254, 1998.

18. Millan MJ, Bervoets K, Rivet JM, et al: Multiple alpha$_2$-adrenergic receptor subtypes. II. Evidence for a role of rat alpha$_{2A}$-adrenergic receptors in control of nociception, motor behavior and hippocampal synthesis of noradrenaline, *J Pharmacol Exp Ther* 270(3):958-972, 1994.

19. Buerkle H, Yaksh TL: Pharmacologic evidence for different alpha$_2$-adrenergic receptor sites mediating analgesia and sedation in the rat, *Br J Anaesth* 81:208-215, 1998.

20. Guo T, Jiang J, Butterman AE, et al: Dexmedetomidine injection into the locus ceruleus produces antinociception, *Anesthesiology* 84(4):873-881, 1996.

21. Peng YB, Lin Q, Willis WD: Involvement of alpha$_2$-adrenoceptors in the periaqueductal gray-induced inhibition of dorsal horn cell activity in rats, *J Pharmacol Exp Ther* 278(1):125-135, 1996.

22. Tranquilli WJ, Maze M: Clinical pharmacology and use of α_2-agonists in veterinary anesthesia, *Anaesthetic Pharmacology Review* 1(3):297-309, 1993.

23. Tranquilli WJ, Benson GJ: Advantages and guidelines for using alpha$_2$ agonists as anesthetic adjuncts, *Vet Clin North Am Small Anim Pract* 22(2):289-292, 1992.

24. Venn RM, Bradshaw CJ, Spencer R, et al: Preliminary UK experience of dexmedetomidine, a novel agent for postoperative sedation in the intensive care unit, *Anaesthesia* 54(12):1136-1142, 1999.

25. Hall JE, Uhrich TD, Barney JA, et al: Sedative, amnestic and analgesic properties of small-dose dexmedetomidine infusions, *Anesth Analg* 90(3):699-705, 2000.

26. Mertes N, Goeters C, Kuhmann M, et al: Postoperative alpha$_2$-adrenergic stimulation attenuates protein catabolism, *Anesth Analg* 82(2):258-263, 1996.

27. Sabbe MB, Penning JP, Ozaki GT, et al: Spinal and systemic action of the α_2-receptor agonist dexmedetomidine in dogs: antinociception and carbon dioxide response, *Anesthesiology* 80(5);1057-1061, 1994.

28. Eisenach J, De Kock M, Klimscha W: α_2-Adrenergic agonists for regional anesthesia: a clinical review of clonidine (1984-1995), *Anesthesiology* 85:655-674, 1996.

29. De Kock M, Eisenach J: Analgesic doses of intrathecal but not intravenous clonidine increase acetylcholine in cerebrospinal fluid in humans, *Anesth Analg* 84:800-803, 1997.

30. Eisenach JC, Hood DD, Curry R: Intrathecal, but not intravenous, clonidine reduces experimental thermal or capsaicin-induced pain and hyperalgesia in normal volunteers, *Anesth Analg* 87(3):591-596, 1998.

30a. Branson KR, Ko J, Tranquilli WJ, et al: Duration of analgesia induced by epidurally administered morphine and medetomidine in the dog, *J Vet Pharmacol Ther* 16:369-372, 1993.

31. Gentili M, Juhel A, Bonnet F: Peripheral analgesic effect of intra-articular clonidine, *Pain* 64(3):593-596, 1996.

32. Joshi W, Reuben SS, Kilaru PR, et al: Postoperative analgesia for outpatient arthroscopic knee surgery with intraarticular clonidine and/or morphine, *Anesth Analg* 90(5):1102-1106, 2000.

33. Thurman JC, Tranquilli WJ, Benson GJ: Preanesthetics and anesthetic adjuncts. In Thurman JC, Tranquilli WJ, Benson GJ, editors: *Lumb & Jones' veterinary anesthesia,* ed 3, Baltimore, 1996, Williams & Wilkins.

34. Vainio O: Introduction to the clinical pharmacology of medetomidine, *Acta Vet Scand Suppl* 85:85-88, 1989.

12

Local Anesthetics

KHURSHEED R. MAMA

- Local anesthetics reversibly block transmission of nerve endings or fibers.
- Autonomic nervous system blockade, anesthesia (analgesia), and/or muscle paralysis may result.
- A basic understanding of nerve physiology and drug pharmacology will facilitate the appropriate clinical use of local anesthetics.

PERIPHERAL NERVE ANATOMY

Nerve Fiber Classification
- Size and myelination
- Specific associated functions

Peripheral Nerves
- Individual nerve fibers or axons grouped together as fascicles within an outer sheath.
- Peripheral nerves may be myelinated or nonmyelinated. Schwann cells form multiple myelin layers around each axon of myelinated nerves and only a single membrane layer around nonmyelinated axonal fibers.
- In nonmyelinated nerves, ion channels supporting propagation of the action potential are distributed all along the axon. In myelinated nerves, these ion channels are concentrated at the nodes of Ranvier, which are periodic interruptions in the myelin sheath.

PHYSIOLOGY OF NERVE CONDUCTION

Action Potentials

Nerve signals are conducted by action potentials, which are rapid changes in the electrical gradients across the nerve membrane.[1]

- Depolarization is due to the rapid inward passage of sodium ions from the extracellular to the intracellular space via sodium channels in the nerve membrane.
- Repolarization results from the outward flow of potassium ions and resets the nerve membrane potential to resting conditions.
- The action potential moves along the unmyelinated nerve fiber (conduction of the impulse) until it reaches the fiber's end. In myelinated nerves, the impulse jumps from one node of Ranvier to the next (saltatory conduction).

Site of Local Anesthetic Action

- Local anesthetics inhibit the generation and propagation (conduction) of nerve impulses by blockage of sodium channels in the nerve membrane.
- The most prominent hypothesis is that the anesthetic enters the lipoprotein membrane and binds to a receptor site in the sodium channel to impede or prevent sodium ion movement. Sodium-generated currents are reduced because the drug inhibits channel conformational changes and thus drug bound channels fail to open. This slows the rate of depolarization of the membrane, preventing attainment of the membrane's threshold potential.
- To a lesser extent, movement through the channel is prevented because of the bound drug's physical blockade of the ion-conducting pore. A sodium channel that is inhibited by a local anesthetic is functionally similar to an inactivated channel. If the sodium movement is blocked over a critical length of the nerve, propagation across the blocked area is not possible.[2,3]

Differential Nerve Block

- Because of size and presence or absence of myelination, nerve fibers differ substantially in their susceptibility to local anesthetic blockade. Myelinated fibers are blocked before unmyelinated fibers of the same diameter. Smaller fibers with higher firing rates and less distance over which such fibers can passively propagate an impulse (type B and C fibers) are blocked before larger (type A) fibers.

BOX 12-1
Priority of Local Anesthetic Blockade

1. Pain
2. Warmth
3. Touch

4. Deep pressure
5. Motor function

- Although individual variation occurs, the disappearance of nervous function in response to local anesthetic blockade, in order of first to last, is generally: pain, warmth, touch, deep pressure, and finally motor function. Such variation in neural sensitivity to local anesthetics has made it possible to clinically block sensory transmission in patients without accompanying motor paralysis (differential nerve block) (Box 12-1).
- Exceptions to this general rule include large peripheral nerve trunks where motor nerves are more circumferentially located and hence exposed to the local anesthetic agent first, allowing for motor blockade to occur before sensory blockade. It is also important to remember that in general the mantle of the peripheral nerve trunk contains sensory innervation to the proximal aspect of an extremity while the core contains distal sensory innervation. Thus anesthesia will develop proximally before distal areas become desensitized.

PHARMACOLOGY

Chemical Structure

- The typical local anesthetic molecule consists of an unsaturated aromatic group linked by an intermediate chain to a tertiary amine end.
- The clinically important local anesthetics are divided into two distinct chemical groups based on their intermediate chain.
- Aminoamides (e.g., lidocaine, bupivacaine) have an amide link between the aromatic and amine ends, and aminoesters (e.g., procaine, benzocaine) have an ester link.
- These linkages, in large part, determine drug disposition within the body. Drug actions are also influenced by chemical substitutions

at either the aromatic or amine end of the basic molecule and are discussed in the following section (Table 12-1).

Structure-Activity Relationships
Lipophilic-Hydrophilic Balance
The aromatic portion of a local anesthetic is considered relatively lipophilic. Alkyl substitution at either the aromatic region or amine end of the basic local anesthetic molecule also imparts lipophilic characteristics to the molecule that in turn affects the tendency of a compound to associate with membrane lipids. A longer duration of action and increased anesthetic potency are correlated with increased lipid solubility.

Hydrogen Ion Concentration
Local anesthetics are weak bases with negative logarithm of the acid ionization constant (pK_a) values in the range of 8 to 9. Thus the predominant form of the compound in solution at physiologic pH is the ionized or cationic form. Although this form is important for local anesthetic activity at the receptor site, it is the uncharged base that is important for rapid penetration and diffusion through biologic membranes. Thus the amount of drug in the base form at physiologic pH strongly influences the onset of drug action and the drug's potency.

TABLE 12-1
Physicochemical Properties of Selected Local Anesthetic Agents

Drug	pK_a	Protein Binding (%)	Lipid Solubility
Esters			
Procaine	8.9	6	0.6
Tetracaine	8.5	76	80
Amides			
Lidocaine	7.8	70	2.9
Mepivacaine	7.6	77	1
Bupivacaine	8.1	95	28
Ropivacaine	8.1	94	Less than bupivacaine

Protein Binding

The tertiary amine is considered relatively hydrophilic and bears some positive charge in the physiologic pH range. The degree of ionization has been positively correlated to protein binding, and in general, the greater the protein binding, the longer the duration of action.

Chirality

Many newer local anesthetics are asymmetric compounds that exhibit two distinct spatial arrangements (mirror images), despite having the same physicochemical properties. Pharmacodynamic and pharmacokinetic actions vary as a result of these differences in structure.

Drug Disposition

Local anesthetic agents are usually injected into a localized area of the body to block specific nerves or areas. The absorption of drug from the injection site, distribution within the body, and excretion from the body are of primary importance in determining the systemic disposition of the drug and potential for side effects.

Absorption

The rate of systemic absorption of local anesthetic agents is inversely related to the duration of effect at the site of action. In addition to drug physicochemical and pharmacologic properties, drug dose, site of injection, and use of a vasoconstrictor influence drug absorption.

- The effect on systemic absorption of a change in either volume or concentration (at a constant dose) of local anesthetic is variable and generally not significant, but if the overall dose is increased, a higher systemic peak drug concentration is likely
- The site of injection also significantly influences the peak drug concentrations in the blood. Local anesthetic deposited in a highly vascular area will be absorbed more rapidly and result in higher blood levels of drug than if injected into tissue with less blood flow. Epinephrine (a vasoconstrictor) tends to reduce systemic absorption by reducing local blood flow. This effect may vary somewhat depending on the nature of the local anesthetic (i.e., concurrent use of a vasoconstrictor such as epinephrine reduces the peak blood levels of the shorter-acting drugs but has a

less pronounced effect on the more lipophilic and longer-acting agents).

Distribution

- Because of rapid breakdown by plasma pseudocholinesterase and the resulting short plasma half-life, distribution of ester anesthetics in body tissue is limited.
- Conversely, amide local anesthetic agents are widely distributed in the body after an intravenous bolus injection; a two- or three-compartment model usually describes their pharmacokinetic properties.
- Distribution of an amide-type local anesthetic, in particular, may be further influenced by anatomic and pathophysiologic factors.
  1. Hypercapnia and resulting acidosis in the central nervous system (CNS) will likely increase regional blood flow, and as a result, increase local anesthetic concentrations in the brain and increase the risk of toxicity.
  2. Conversely, drug reaching the systemic circulation may be reduced in some circumstances, because the lungs are capable of extracting at least some amide local anesthetics.[4] Protein binding may influence the free drug available for both activity and clearance by the liver and is inversely related to toxic plasma concentrations.

Biotransformation and Excretion

A major difference between the amino amides and amino esters is the pattern of metabolism. This has implications for both clinical usefulness and observed toxicity for the two classes of compounds.

- The principal metabolic pathway of local anesthetics with ester linkages is enzymatic hydrolysis in the plasma by nonspecific pseudocholinesterases. The rate of plasma hydrolysis varies (chloroprocaine > procaine > tetracaine) and is inversely related to toxicity.
  1. Pregnancy reduces plasma cholinesterase activity and might prolong the clearance of the ester anesthetics and increase the potential for toxicity.
  2. Because of the lack of significant pseudocholinesterase activity in the cerebrospinal fluid, subarachnoid administration of ester anesthetics will result in a clinical effect until the drug is systemically absorbed.

3. Products of hydrolysis can be directly excreted by the kidneys, but more commonly, they undergo metabolic transformation.
4. Para-aminobenzoic acid (PABA) is a breakdown product of the esters responsible for allergic reactions in some human patients.
5. Cocaine is an atypical ester in that it undergoes significant hepatic metabolism and urinary excretion.

- Amide local anesthetics are metabolized primarily in the liver. The order of clearance of amides is prilocaine (most rapid) > etidocaine > lidocaine > mepivacaine/ropivacaine > bupivacaine (least rapid).
  1. A common pathway in biotransformation of amide local anesthetics is dealkylation of the parent compound to an intermediate compound. This occurs primarily in the hepatic microsomes.
  2. Generally, this intermediate compound is hydrolyzed and excreted in the urine, but further conjugation (e.g., with glucuronide) before excretion is sometimes necessary. Toxicity could occur in species (e.g., cat) that have a limited ability to perform this step.
  3. Metabolism of certain compounds may also directly result in toxicity, as in the case of prilocaine, which is metabolized to ortho-toluidine, a compound capable of oxidizing hemoglobin to methemoglobin.
  4. Changes in hepatic or renal function or blood flow (as may be induced with hypotension during regional or general anesthesia and in certain disease states) will prolong the clearance of the local anesthetic drugs from the body and may increase the potential for side effects.

FACTORS INFLUENCING ANESTHETIC ACTIVITY

In addition to the chemical structure and physicochemical properties of local anesthetics that influence anesthetic potency, differential sensitivity, and onset and duration of anesthetic action, a number of other drug and patient factors are worthy of consideration. These include dose, site of injection, addition of hyaluronidase or vasoconstrictors to the injectate, carbonation and pH adjustment, influence of varying baricity, mixture of local anesthetics, and the influence of physiologic states such as pregnancy.

Dose of Anesthetic Agent

A more rapid anesthetic onset is facilitated by use of a greater volume of anesthetic or a more concentrated solution because this increases the number of agent molecules in the region of the nerve. When a local anesthetic is injected in the epidural or intrathecal space, increased volume of the solution will also influence the cranial spread of the agent.

Site of Injection

The shortest duration of action is usually seen after intrathecal administration, and the longest duration, after peripheral nerve blocks (e.g., brachial plexus, sciatic). This is generally independent of the agent used.

Use of Hyaluronidase

Addition of the mucolytic enzyme hyaluronidase is thought to enhance the diffusion of local anesthetic agents to the site of action (e.g., peripheral nerve). However, it may also enhance systemic absorption (and thus toxicity) and is currently not believed to be cost-effective.

Use of Vasoconstrictors

In vivo, the duration of action is influenced not only by the drug's intrinsic action on nerves but also by its action on local blood vessels. At low concentrations, local anesthetics tend to cause vasoconstriction, whereas in clinical doses, vasodilation is usually present. Thus the duration of block may be shorter in vivo than that determined in vitro. Addition of a vasoconstrictor to the local anesthetic solution decreases local perfusion, delays the rate of vascular absorption of local anesthetic, and therefore prolongs anesthetic action. Epinephrine (5 μg/ml or 1:200,000) is the agent most commonly added to the local anesthetic. Phenylephrine and norepinephrine have no substantial clinical advantage over epinephrine. Lack of clinical benefit from the addition of epinephrine may be related to the low pH of the epinephrine preparation; this potentially decreases available free base for diffusion, thus delaying the onset of the local anesthetic block (Box 12-2).

Carbonation and pH Adjustment

In the isolated nerve preparation, addition of bicarbonate to the local anesthetic solution results in a more rapid onset of nerve blockade

---

BOX 12-2
Effect of Addition of Epinephrine

Addition of epinephrine to lidocaine and bupivacaine delays local anesthetic absorption and prolongs anesthetic action.

---

and at a reduced anesthetic concentration. This is likely due to an increase in the amount of drug in the uncharged base form. Controversy exists concerning the merits of this practice under clinical conditions.

Baricity

Varying the baricity of local anesthetic solutions may influence the spread within the spinal cord. Hypobaric solutions (i.e., those with a specific gravity less than that of cerebrospinal fluid [CSF]) will tend to migrate to nondependent areas, whereas hyperbaric solutions (i.e., those with a specific gravity greater than that of CSF) will migrate from the site of injection to dependent areas.

Mixtures of Local Anesthetics

Although the clinical practice of mixing local anesthetics to enhance onset and prolong the duration of neural blockade is sometimes useful, it is not universally effective. Potentially beneficial effects are likely negated by drug interactions. For example, in isolated nerve studies, it has been suggested that when chloroprocaine (short onset and duration) and bupivacaine (long onset and duration) are mixed, metabolites of chloroprocaine may inhibit the binding of bupivacaine to receptor sites. Thus at present, mixing of local anesthetics remains controversial.

Pregnancy

Duration of the ester local anesthetics may be prolonged in pregnant patients because plasma cholinesterase activity is reduced. The spread and depth of an epidural or spinal local anesthetic is also reported to be greater in pregnant patients. Mechanical factors (smaller epidural space) and hormonal changes (elevations in progesterone levels) associated with pregnancy have been implicated. It is therefore generally recommended that the dose of spinal or epidural local anesthetics be reduced during pregnancy.

TOXICITY

When administered at an appropriate dose, local anesthetic agents are relatively free of harmful side effects. Most potentially harmful reactions occur after accidental intravenous (IV) administration or following vascular absorption of large amounts of anesthetic after regional administration.

Systemic Toxicity

Central Nervous System

- Low systemic doses of local anesthetic administered to awake, unmedicated humans are reported to cause numbness of the tongue and oral cavity. Low systemic doses will also likely contribute to reduced anesthetic requirement during general anesthesia.[5-7] As the plasma concentration of the drug increases, local anesthetics produce a predictable pattern of CNS excitement and then depression that may be accompanied by apnea and cardiovascular collapse.

- Plasma concentrations producing the various phases of overdose are drug-related (and perhaps species-related). For example, in cats, procaine is least potent in terms of CNS effects (convulsions at about 35 mg/kg), and bupivacaine is one of the most potent (convulsions beginning at about 5 mg/kg).[8] In dogs, the relative CNS toxicity of bupivacaine, etidocaine, and lidocaine is 4:2:1.[9]

Cardiovascular System

Local anesthetics can produce direct effects on both the heart and peripheral vascular smooth muscle and indirect effects through influence on autonomic nervous activity.

- Direct effects on the heart may be both electrophysiologic and mechanical. Both effects on the heart result in a decrease in cardiac output. Bupivacaine and etidocaine may produce severe cardiac dysrhythmias, including ventricular fibrillation[10,11] (Box 12-3).

BOX 12-3

Caution with Injections

Always aspirate before injection. Bupivacaine can cause cardiac dysrhythmias and ventricular fibrillation if injected intravenously.

- The effect of local anesthetics on peripheral vascular smooth muscle may be biphasic. When low concentrations are used, constriction may occur, especially in the pulmonary circulation, resulting in increases in pulmonary artery resistance and hypertension.[3] The more usual clinical response, especially with increasing concentrations, is relaxation resulting in vasodilation.
- Both the vasodilation and the decrease in cardiac output result in arterial hypotension. When an anesthetic is administered via the epidural or intrathecal route, cardiovascular collapse may be further exacerbated by sympathetic nervous system blockade as the agent spreads cranially.

Local Toxicity

Neural Toxicity

Although local anesthetics are rarely neurotoxic at clinically administered concentrations, irreversible conduction blockade in isolated nerves has been reported.[3] Prolonged sensory and motor deficits reported after epidural or subarachnoid administration of chloroprocaine are now believed to be related to the antioxidant sodium bisulfite and not the parent drug itself.

Skeletal Muscle Toxicity

When properly used, local anesthetics rarely produce localized tissue damage. However, some reports indicate that even when clinical doses are used for local infiltration, skeletal muscle damage may be associated with the longer-acting agents.[12,13]

Other Effects

Methemoglobinemia

Methemoglobinemia has been reported to develop after exposure to a number of local anesthetics, most notably prilocaine.[14,15] Breakdown products (e.g., o-toluidine) from the metabolism of the local anesthetic are likely responsible.

Allergies

Although allergic-type reactions to the amide local anesthetics are rare, it is possible for the aminoester local anesthetics such as procaine to cause hypersensitivity or anaphylactic responses. PABA, a product of ester metabolism, is most commonly implicated. Preservatives (e.g., methylparaben) contained in local anesthetic solutions may also result in allergic reactions.

Addiction

Although cocaine is rarely used in veterinary medicine, abuse both directly (e.g., by human beings with access to the compound) and indirectly (e.g., administration to horses as a stimulant before a race) are possibilities.

CLINICAL APPLICATION OF LOCAL ANESTHETICS

Local anesthetics are most often used to produce regional anesthesia and analgesia (Table 12-2). *Regional anesthesia* is a term loosely used to refer to a variety of applications of local anesthetics for anesthetic purposes. The term implies that a region of the body is affected as opposed to the entire body as with general anesthesia. The region affected may be very limited or broad in scope. In terms of organization, regional anesthesia includes the subcategories listed below. These are discussed in depth in Chapter 15.

- Topical anesthesia
- Local infiltration

TABLE 12-2

Clinical Attributes of Selected Local Anesthetic Agents

Drug	Onset	Duration (min)	Main Clinical Uses
Esters			
Procaine	Slow	45-60	Local and perineural infiltration
Tetracaine	Slow	60-180	Topical application
Amides			
Lidocaine	Rapid	60-120	Local and perineural infiltration, intravenous regional, epidural, and subarachnoid administration
Mepivacaine	Intermediate	90-180	Local and perineural infiltration
Bupivacaine	Intermediate	180-480	Local and perineural infiltration, epidural and subarachnoid administration
Ropivacaine	Intermediate	180-480	Local and perineural infiltration, epidural and subarachnoid administration

- Peripheral nerve block
- Intraarticular administration
- Intravenous block
- Epidural block
- Spinal (subarachnoid) block

Occasionally, local anesthetics may be used to supplement actions of intravenous and inhalation anesthetics or to prevent or treat cardiac dysrhythmias. In rare cases, lidocaine may be administered in low doses to suppress grand mal seizures and to prevent or treat increases in intracranial pressure.

LOCAL ANESTHETIC AGENTS

Amino-Ester Local Anesthetics

Procaine Hydrochloride

- Procaine hydrochloride is a weak organic base, with a pK_a of 8.9. It is nonirritant and promptly effective when injected subcutaneously. It provides a relatively brief period of anesthesia (45 to 60 minutes), which may be prolonged by addition of a vasoconstrictor.
- The drug is rapidly hydrolyzed, primarily in blood plasma by nonspecific pseudocholinesterases. The plasma half-life is about 25 minutes.[16] The kidneys excrete procaine and PABA, a product of procaine degradation.
- Procaine is used in veterinary medicine for infiltration and nerve block. A concentration of 1% is used for small patients, and 2% is preferable for larger animals. Procaine is rarely used for surface anesthesia because it is not very effective with this route of administration.

Tetracaine Hydrochloride

Tetracaine is eight times as potent as procaine and has a pK_a of 8.5. Although the onset of drug action is slow, it is rapidly absorbed from mucosal surfaces to which it is applied. The duration of effect is intermediate (60 to 180 minutes).

- Because of rapid absorption and slower metabolism (than that for procaine) by plasma cholinesterases, there is an increase in the potential for systemic toxicity.
- Tetracaine is used to provide topical anesthesia of the eye, nose, and throat and for spinal anesthesia when both sensory and

motor blockade are desired. It is a component of the topical local anesthetic mixture cetacaine. Recently, both a patch application system and a gel preparation have been evaluated as percutaneous analgesia with favorable results.[17]

Benzocaine

- Benzocaine is structurally similar to procaine except that it lacks a terminal diethyl amino group. It is available as a dusting powder or as oil in an ointment for surface application.
- Benzocaine is relatively nonirritating to tissues, and after absorption, it is metabolized to PABA and acetyl PABA. It has been reported to cause methemoglobinemia in some species (e.g., sheep), which may limit its widespread use in clinical practice.
- It has been used to varying degrees in dentistry to provide anesthesia of the gums and buccal mucosa and for cutaneous analgesia. Its low solubility allows it to remain localized in wounds to provide long-term pain relief. Benzocaine is also a component (as is tetracaine) in a topical local anesthetic mixture known as *cetacaine*, which is commonly used as a spray to anesthetize the larynx before intubation.

Proparacaine Hydrochloride

- Proparacaine hydrochloride is about equal in potency to tetracaine. It is chemically distinct from procaine and exhibits little cross-sensitivity.
- Unlike some topical anesthetics, it produces little or no tissue irritation.[18] Because proparacaine induces little discomfort on instillation into the human eye, it is widely used as an ophthalmic anesthetic.

Amino-Amide Local Anesthetics
Lidocaine Hydrochloride

- Lidocaine is one of the most versatile and most widely used local anesthetics in veterinary medicine. The compound has a pK_a of 7.9 and is considered twice as potent as procaine. Its clinical use is associated with a rapid onset of action and short (60 to 120 minutes) duration of effect. It is available as a sterile aqueous solution in concentrations of 0.5% to 5% with or without epinephrine and in a gel preparation in concentrations of 2.5% to 5%.
- Lidocaine is relatively quickly absorbed from the gastrointestinal tract and after injection.[19] The kinetics and oral absorption

rate of lidocaine have been determined in the dog; 78% of the administered dose reaches the general circulation.[20] Emesis occurs regularly at 2.5 hours after administration.

- The rate of systemic absorption after parenteral administration is slowed, and the duration of action is prolonged when lidocaine is used with a vasoconstrictor. Lidocaine is metabolized in the liver by mixed-function oxidases at a rate nearly as rapid as that for procaine. The metabolites and 10% to 20% of the unchanged form are excreted in urine of the dog.

- Lidocaine is used for all forms of local anesthesia. The transdermal (Lidoderm patch) administration of lidocaine produces local tissue concentrations far below those capable of producing toxicity but high enough to produce clinically effective local analgesia for periods of up to 24 hours without complete sensory block. The patches have been used to provide analgesia for skin abrasions, lacerations, and severe local skin irritation and itching (hot spots). The patch is supplied as a 10 × 14 cm adhesive bandage that may be cut into smaller sizes with a scissors before removing the protective drug release liner. Care should be taken to avoid contact with the attendant's skin or eyes to prevent numbing of the fingers or irritation, respectively. In addition to its use as a local anesthetic, it is used intravenously as an antidysrhythmic agent and also as a supplement to general anesthesia (25-50 μg/kg/min). It decreases the requirement for inhalation and injectable anesthetics.[5-7,21]

Prilocaine Hydrochloride

Prilocaine hydrochloride has pharmacologic properties resembling those of lidocaine. However, it causes significantly less vasodilation and hence may be used without the addition of epinephrine to prolong the duration of effect. It is also reported to be the least toxic of the amide local anesthetics and thus best suited for intravenous anesthesia. Methemoglobinemia is a side effect of overdose and accounts for its declining use, especially for human patients.

Eutectic Mixture of Lidocaine and Prilocaine

- Eutectic mixture of lidocaine and prilocaine (EMLA), a 1:1 mixture of lidocaine and prilocaine, is available commercially for transcutaneous application. It has been shown that when the base forms of these two compounds are mixed, oil is formed at temperatures over 18° C.[22] This eutectic mixture is commercially available in a preparation containing arlacton as an emulsifier and carbapol as a thickening agent. Each gram (or milliliter) contains 25 mg of lidocaine and 25 mg of prilocaine. The reported bioavailability is 3% for lidocaine and 5% for prilocaine.[23] This may, however, vary with the site of application, skin pigmentation, and condition.

- The toxicity of EMLA is related primarily to the metabolism of prilocaine to *o*-toluidine, which can result in methemoglobinemia. Blanching or hyperemia may be noted in the area of application after removal of the occlusive bandage and is likely due to the relative vasoactivity of the two compounds.

- EMLA has been evaluated as a percutaneous analgesic before venipuncture in dogs, cats, rabbits, and rats.[24] Its efficacy after a 60-minute application was good in dogs, cats, and rabbits but questionable in study rats.

Mepivacaine Hydrochloride

- The pharmacologic properties of mepivacaine hydrochloride are similar to those of lidocaine. Although actual potency figures vary, it is about equal (or slightly less) in local anesthetic potency to lidocaine. It has a slightly longer duration (90 to 180 minutes) of action, likely due to less intrinsic vasodilator activity when compared with lidocaine.

- Although its use in clinical practice is similar to that of lidocaine, mepivacaine is not recommended for obstetrical anesthesia because its actions are markedly prolonged in the fetus. In the adult, the toxicity of mepivacaine is about 1.5 to 2 times that of procaine but slightly less than that of lidocaine.

Bupivacaine Hydrochloride

- Bupivacaine is a long-acting local anesthetic chemically related to mepivacaine and about four times more potent than lidocaine. The onset of action is slow to intermediate, and the duration of action ranges from 3 to 10 hours.

- It is most commonly used for regional and epidural nerve blocks and was the first local anesthetic agent to show significant separation of sensory and motor blockade, making it the drug of choice for obstetric anesthesia. CNS and cardiac toxicity result from lower doses and blood levels than those reported for lidocaine.

Ropivacaine Hydrochloride

- Ropivacaine, a new long-acting aminoamide local anesthetic, is structurally related to mepivacaine and bupivacaine but differs in that it is an *S*-isomer, whereas the latter agents are racemic mixtures. (Previous studies of isomers of local anesthetics suggested that the systemic toxicity of the *S*-isomer of various compounds may be less than that of racemic preparations.) The physiochemical properties of ropivacaine are similar to those of bupivacaine with the exception of its lipid solubility (ropivacaine is substantially less lipid soluble).[25] At low concentrations, ropivacaine has intrinsic vasoconstricting properties, whereas higher concentrations result in vasodilation.
- Ropivacaine is used in a manner similar to bupivacaine. Reports indicate that the motor block after epidural administration is less dense and of a shorter duration than for bupivacaine. This, along with ropivacaine's reduced cardiotoxic potential when compared with bupivacaine, offers advantages for clinical use when differential blockade is desired.[26,27] Ropivacaine also reportedly caused fewer CNS symptoms in human volunteers and was at least 25% less toxic than bupivacaine in regard to the dose tolerated.[28]

ACKNOWLEDGMENT

Portions of this chapter are reproduced with modification with permission from Mama KR, Steffey EP: Local anesthetics. In Richard AH, editor: *Veterinary pharmacology and therapeutics,* ed 8, Ames, 2001, Iowa State University Press.

REFERENCES

1. Guyton AC, Hall JE: *Textbook of medical physiology,* ed 9, Philadelphia, 1996, WB Saunders.
2. Butterworth JF, Strichartz GR: Molecular mechanisms of local anesthesia: a review, *Anesthesiology* 72:711-734, 1990.
3. Strichartz GR, Berde CB: Local anesthetics. In Miller RD, editor: *Anesthesia,* ed 4, New York, 1994, Churchill Livingstone.
4. Tucker GT: Pharmacokinetics of local anesthetics, *Br J Anaesth* 58:717-731, 1986.

5. Himes RS, Jr, DiFazio CA, Burmey RC: Effects of lidocaine on the anesthetic requirements of nitrous oxide and halothane, *Anaesthesiology* 47:437-440, 1977.

6. Himes RS, Jr, Munson ES, Embro WJ: Enflurane requirement and ventilatory response to carbon dioxide during lidocaine infusion in dogs, *Anesthesiology* 51:131-134, 1979.

7. Doherty TJ, Frazier DL: Effect of intravenous lidocaine on halothane minimum alveolar concentration in ponies, *Equine Vet J* 30:300-303, 1998.

8. Englesson S: The influence of acid-base changes on central nervous system toxicity of local anesthetic agents. I. An experimental study in cats, *Acta Anaesth Scand* 18:79-87, 1974.

9. Liu PL, Feldman HS, Giasi R, et al: Comparative CNS toxicity of lidocaine, etidocaine, bupivacaine and tetracaine in awake dogs following rapid IV administration, *Anesth Analg* 62:375-379, 1983.

10. Kotelko DM, Shnider SM, Dailey PA, et al: Bupivacaine-induced cardiac arrhythmias in sheep, *Anesthesiology* 60:10-19, 1984.

11. Bruelle P, Lefrant J-Y, de La Coussaye JE, et al: Comparative electrophysiologic and hemodynamic effects of several amide local anesthetic drugs in anesthetized dogs, *Anesth Analg* 82:648-656, 1996.

12. Basson MD, Carlson BM: Myotoxicity of single and repeated injections of mepivacaine (Carbocaine) in the rat, *Anesth Analg* 59:275-282, 1980.

13. Benoit PW, Belt WD: Destruction and regeneration of skeletal muscle after treatment with a local anesthetic, bupivacaine (Marcaine), *J Anat* 107:547, 1970.

14. Ferraro L, Zeichner SGG, Groeger JS: Cetacaine-induced acute methemoglobinemia, *Anesthesiology* 69:614-616, 1988.

15. Paddleford RR, Krahwinkel DJ, Fuhr JE, et al: *Experimentally induced methemoglobinemia in the dog following exposure to topical benzocaine HCl.* In Grandy J, Hildebrand S, McDonell W, et al, editors: Proceedings of the second International Congress of Veterinary Anesthesia, Santa Barbara, 1985, Veterinary Practice Publishing.

16. Tobin T, Blake JW, Tai CY, et al: Pharmacology of procaine in the horse: a preliminary report, *Am J Vet Res* 37:1107-1110, 1976.

17. McCafferty DF, Woolfson AD: New patch delivery system for percutaneous local anaesthesia, *Br J Anaesth* 71:370-374, 1993.

18. Ritchie JM, Greene NM: In Goodman AG, Goodman LS, Gilman A, editors: *The pharmacological basis of therapeutics,* ed 8, New York, 1990, Pergamon Press.

19. Keenaghan JB, Boyes RN: The tissue distribution, metabolism and excretion of lidocaine in rats, guinea pigs, dogs and man, *J Pharmacol Exp Ther* 180:454-463, 1972.

20. Boyes RN, Adams HJ, Duce BR: Oral absorption and deposition kinetics of lidocaine hydrochloride in dogs, *J Pharmacol Exp Ther* 174:1-8, 1970.

21. Kissin I, McGee T: Hypnotic effect of thiopental-lidocaine combination in the rat, *Anesthesiology* 57:311-313, 1982.

22. Brodin A, Nyqvist-Mayer A, Wadsten T, et al: Phase diagram and aqueous solubility of the lidocaine-prilocaine binary system, *J Pharm Sci* 73:481-484, 1984.

23. Klein J, Fernandes D, Gazarian M, et al: Simultaneous determination of lidocaine, prilocaine and the prilocaine metabolite *o*-toluidine in plasma by high-performance liquid chromatography, *J Chromatogr B Biomed Sci Appl* 655:83-88, 1994.

24. Flecknell PA, Liles JH, Williamson HA: The use of lidocaine-prilocaine local anesthetic cream for pain-free venepuncture in laboratory animals, *Lab Anim* 24:142-146, 1990.

25. Rosenberg PH, Heinonen E: Differential sensitivity of A and C nerve fibres to long-acting amide local anaesthetics, *Br J Anaesth* 55:163-167, 1983.

26. Feldman H, Arthur G, Covino B: Comparative systemic toxicity of convulsant and supraconvulsant doses of intravenous ropivacaine, bupivacaine, and lidocaine in the conscious dog, *Anesth Analg* 69:794-801, 1989.

27. Reiz S, Haggmark S, Johansson G, et al: Cardiotoxicity of ropivacaine: a new amide local anaesthetic agent, *Acta Anaesth Scand* 33:93-98, 1989.

28. Scott DB, Lee A, Fagan D, et al: Acute toxicity of ropivacaine compared with that of bupivacaine, *Anesth Analg* 69:563-569, 1989.

13

Glucocorticoids

MARY O. SMITH

PROTOTYPE[1,2]

- Cortisol is the major endogenous glucocorticoid in most mammals.
- Cortisol is synthesized from cholesterol in the adrenal gland (*zona fasciculata* and *zona reticularis*).
- It is released into the circulation under the influence of corticotropin, which is secreted by the pituitary gland.
- Corticotropin secretion is controlled by the hypothalamus through the action of corticotropin-releasing hormone (CRH).
- CRH is secreted in response to physiologic stress (see Chapter 3).
- Negative feedback control exists at both the pituitary and hypothalamic levels.
- Some studies suggest that there are diurnal variations in circulating cortisol levels in animals, whereas others do not support this.[3,4]
- Plasma cortisol is >90% protein-bound:
  - Most is bound to cortisol-binding protein synthesized by the liver.
  - A small amount is loosely bound to albumin.
  - Ten percent is free in plasma and physiologically active.
  - Increased release of cortisol from the adrenal glands produce higher levels of free cortisol in plasma and greater effects on target cells.
  - Circulating synthetic glucocorticoids are mostly bound to albumin.
  - Most cortisol (>80%) is metabolized within and excreted by the liver: reduction and conjugation to glucuronides and sulfates.
  - The half-life of circulating cortisol is approximately 90 minutes and is increased by stress, hypothyroidism, and hepatic disease.

EFFECTS

Glucocorticoid Receptors

- Effects of glucocorticoids are mediated by a variety of glucocorticoid receptors on target cells.
- Binding to the glucocorticoid receptor induces conformational changes in the receptor.
- The glucocorticoid-receptor complex is actively transported to the cell nucleus where it binds to glucocorticoid receptor elements, altering the regulation of gene transcription.
- The precise effect of the hormone within the target cell depends on the type of receptor to which it binds and the target gene for that receptor.
- There are a large number of different glucocorticoid receptors.
- Target gene expression varies among cell types.
- Both of these factors contribute to the wide diversity of action of glucocorticoids within target cells.
- Activation of glucocorticoid receptors alters protein synthesis within the cell.

Adverse Effects of Glucocorticoids

Many of the effects of glucocorticoids may be adverse when supraphysiologic doses are administered.
- Increased gluconeogenesis and glycogen synthesis.
- Increases in both lipolysis and lipogenesis produce a net increase in body fat.
- Catabolism of fat, muscle, skin, bone, lymphoid tissue, and connective tissue.

Antiinflammatory Effects

- Pain relief afforded by glucocorticoid administration is due to a reduction in inflammation.

MECHANISMS OF ACTION

- The main mechanism of the antiinflammatory effects of glucocorticoids is the inhibition of phospholipase A_2, the precursor of arachidonic acid.[5]
- Phospholipase A_2 inhibition decreases the production of prostaglandins and leukotrienes.

- Prostaglandins and leukotrienes lower the nociceptive threshold, increasing sensitivity to substances that cause pain, such as histamine and bradykinin.
- Glucocorticoids reduce levels of cyclooxygenase (COX) enzymes in inflammatory cells, further inhibiting the production of prostaglandins.[1]
- Glucocorticoids have marked effects on leukocyte activity and distribution.[1]
- Glucocorticoid administration induces neutrophilia and lymphopenia.
  - Neutrophils are recruited from the bone marrow into the systemic circulation.
  - Migration of neutrophils from the vascular system into tissues is decreased, thereby decreasing inflammation.
  - Lymphocytes and other circulating leukocytes are recruited into lymphoid tissues.
- Glucocorticoids inhibit the activity of lymphocytes and tissue macrophages.
- Basal levels of endogenous glucocorticoids appear to be critical for facilitating certain mechanisms of analgesia, such as those mediated by endogenous opioids.[6]

EFFICACY AND USE (Box 13-1)

- Glucocorticoids are most commonly administered by systemic routes, either oral or injectable.
- There are many indications for the use of this group of drugs, but only painful conditions will be discussed here.
- Dosages used for the alleviation of pain should be those that suppress inflammation and not those that are immunosuppressive.
- Shorter-acting drugs, such as prednisone, prednisolone, or methylprednisolone, are preferred for systemic administration.

BOX 13-1

Most glucocorticoid dosage regimens are empirical or have been extrapolated from use in humans.

These drugs carry a lower risk of toxic side effects compared with drugs with long half-lives and durations of action.

Intervertebral Disk Disease

- Prednisone 0.1 to 0.2 mg/kg, administered orally once or twice daily, has been used successfully in combination with strict cage rest to treat mild cases of intervertebral disk disease (pain only or pain and mild paresis).[7]
- Successful treatment of animals with severe clinical signs (paraplegia) has been reported, although surgery is preferred.[8]
- High-dose methylprednisolone sodium succinate treatment within 8 hours of spinal cord trauma (including acute disk extrusion), although controversial, is widely used in dogs and cats. The main rationale for this use is to reduce inflammation and improve neurologic function, but some analgesic benefits may also be derived. A single dose of 30 mg/kg by slow intravenous injection (over 2 to 5 minutes) should be followed by a constant infusion of 5.4 mg/kg/hr for 24 to 48 hours.[9,10]

Systemic Inflammatory Diseases

- A variety of systemic inflammatory diseases may cause pain. Examples include polymyositis, masticatory myositis, polyarthritis, meningitis, and systemic lupus erythematosus.
- Glucocorticoids are generally used at immunosuppressive doses (e.g., prednisone, 1.1 to 2.2 mg/kg twice daily) to treat these diseases.
- Alleviation of pain is secondary to the main goal of glucocorticoid therapy, which is to suppress the immune-mediated disorder that underlies these diseases.

Otitis Externa[11]

- Topical or systemic use of glucocorticoids is often indicated for the treatment of otitis externa to reduce inflammation and edema in the ear. A decrease in pain is another beneficial effect.
- A wide variety of otic preparations that contain glucocorticoids are available, including 0.1% dexamethasone, betamethasone, or triamcinolone and 1.0% to 2.5% hydrocortisone. These drugs are administered as sole constituents or in combination with other drugs such as antibiotics.

- Oral prednisone or prednisolone may be indicated when inflammation is severe, at an antiinflammatory dose of 0.1 to 0.5 mg/kg once or twice daily.

Intralesional Administration

Intraarticular Administration

- The major route for intralesional use of glucocorticoids is intraarticular.
- Conflicting data exist on the effects of glucocorticoids on joint cartilage. One study demonstrated minimal or even beneficial effects, whereas others have demonstrated evidence of cartilage damage.[12-15]
- Methylprednisolone (20 to 40 mg) and, particularly, triamcinolone (1 to 3 mg) are the preferred drugs for intraarticular administration.[16]

Perineural Injection

- Injection of glucocorticoids around spinal nerve roots or peripheral nerves has been shown to alleviate pain in people with nerve root disease or peripheral neuropathies.[17]
- This use has not been described in veterinary medicine to date.

Epidural Administration

- Epidural glucocorticoid administration often is used in humans as a conservative treatment for lumbar pain.
- The procedure is generally considered safe with minor temporary side effects such as headache.[18,19]
- Efficacy is most likely due to reduction in nerve root and meningeal inflammation.[20]
- A recent study showed that wound irrigation with 20 or 40 mg of triamcinolone substantially reduced postoperative pain in humans after lumbar spinal surgery.[21]
- Beneficial effects of epidural injection of betamethasone have been demonstrated in a rat model of lumbar nerve root disease.[22]
- No recommendations or dosages for epidural glucocorticoid have been developed for animals.
- Cervical epidural administration of a corticosteroid has a potential for severe deleterious effects if the drug is accidentally administered into the cervical spinal cord parenchyma.[23]

Other Uses

- Methylprednisolone has been shown to be effective in controlling cancer pain in humans when added to 0.5% bupivacaine and administered intrapleurally.[24]
- Glucocorticoids have been used to produce an analgesic-sparing effect in humans for the treatment of cancer pain or during spinal surgery.[25,26]

RELEVANT PHARMACOLOGY

- Synthetic steroids are synthesized from bovine cholic acid or from plant sapogenins.
- Metabolism and excretion of synthetic glucocorticoids occur primarily within the liver and are similar to metabolism and excretion of endogenous glucocorticoids.
- Synthetic glucocorticoids have stronger antiinflammatory effects than do endogenous glucocorticoids (Table 13-1).
- Synthetic glucocorticoids generally have longer half-lives than the naturally occurring forms (Table 13-1).
- Synthetic glucocorticoids have greater affinity for cellular glucocorticoid receptors than do endogenous glucocorticoids.

TABLE 13-1
Characteristics of Glucocorticoids Commonly Used in Veterinary Medicine

Glucocorticoid	Relative Antiinflammatory Effect	Duration of Action After IV or Oral Administration (hr)[31]	Routes of Administration
Hydrocortisone	1	<12	PO, IV, IM
Prednisone	4	12-36	PO, IV, IM, SQ
Prednisolone	5	12-36	PO, IV, IM, SQ
Methylprednisolone	5	12-36	PO, IV, IM, SQ
Triamcinolone	5	12-36 (-weeks)	PO, IM, SQ
Betamethasone	25-40	>48	PO, IM
Dexamethasone	30	>48	PO, IV, IM, SQ

PO, By mouth (per os); *IV,* intravenous injection; *IM,* intramuscular injection; *SQ,* subcutaneous injection.
Veterinary-approved products are not necessarily available.

SIDE EFFECTS AND TOXICITY

- Glucocorticoids have a high potential for diverse toxicities because of their effects on almost every tissue in the body.
- Toxicity is dose- and treatment duration–dependent.
- Patient-dependent variations in toxicity also exist.
- Toxicity may result not only from systemic use of glucocorticoids but also from localized use (e.g., ophthalmic, intraarticular, topical).
- Concurrent medications may potentiate toxicity (e.g., nonsteroidal antiinflammatory agents).
- Some side effects are managed fairly readily (e.g., polyphagia), whereas others may be life-threatening (e.g., gastric ulceration).
- Use of glucocorticoids may not slow progression of the primary disease for which they are being used and may mask the primary disease and development of intercurrent disease.[5]

Iatrogenic Hyperadrenocorticism (Cushing's Syndrome)

Administration of glucocorticoids for a medium-term or longer period (weeks to months) often results in clinical signs that mimic Cushing's syndrome, including polydipsia, polyuria, skin thinning, and hair loss.

Hypoadrenocorticism (Addison's Disease)

Prolonged use of exogenous glucocorticoids produces atrophy of the adrenal gland (*zona fasciculata* and *zona reticularis*), resulting in the decreased production of endogenous glucocorticoids. Sudden withdrawal of exogenous drugs may produce signs of adrenocortical insufficiency.

Neuropathy and Myopathy

Signs of both myopathy and neuropathy may develop, particularly with chronic glucocorticoid use. Generalized weakness and muscle atrophy are the major clinical signs.

Polyphagia

Increased appetite is a common side effect of glucocorticoid use and appears to be mediated by central nervous system (CNS) centers. Obesity can develop when administration is prolonged for more than a few days to weeks.

Effects on Electrolyte and Fluid Balance

Glucocorticoids play a key role in the maintenance of normal fluid balance and do have some mineralocorticoid activity. Glucocorticoids promote polydipsia and polyuria as a result of inhibition of antidiuretic hormone release. They also result in excretion of calcium and potassium, sodium and chloride retention, and increased extracellular fluid volume. In rare cases, hypokalemia or hypocalcemia may result from chronic administration.

Glaucoma and Cataracts

Chronic use of glucocorticoids in the eye can result in the development of glaucoma or cataracts.

Gastric Ulceration

Glucocorticoids promote acid secretion in the stomach and can result in life-threatening gastric and intestinal ulceration. Although experimental studies have suggested that steroid administration alone does not usually cause ulceration, other factors, such as stress, increased autonomic nervous system activity, or the concurrent administration of drugs such as nonsteroidal antiinflammatory drugs, may collaborate to cause ulceration.[27]

Delayed Wound Healing

Use of glucocorticoids can result in delayed wound healing.

Immunosuppression

Prolonged administration of high doses of glucocorticoids can result in immunosuppression and an increased susceptibility to infections in almost any organ system.

The antiinflammatory effects of glucocorticoids may mask the presence of infections until they are severe.

Glucocorticoids are contraindicated in the presence of infection, except when adequate measures (e.g., antibiotics) are used to control the infection.

Systemic fungal infections are a particular contraindication to glucocorticoid use.

Insulin Resistance

Glucocorticoids antagonize insulin, resulting in increased gluconeogenesis and often hyperglycemia.

An appetite increase secondary to prolonged glucocorticoid administration results in hyperinsulinism and may lead to diabetes mellitus.

Hepatopathy

Prolonged or high-dose glucocorticoid administration in dogs, but not cats, results in a steroid-induced production of an isoenzyme of alkaline phosphatase by the liver. High levels of this isoenzyme are found in serum of most dogs receiving glucocorticoids and can result in a significant hepatopathy in some animals, even resulting in hepatic failure.

Central Nervous System Effects

Glucocorticoids can cause changes in behavior, particularly restlessness and increased aggression.

Experimental studies in the rat suggest that glucocorticoids may lower the seizure threshold in the brain.[28]

Iatrogenic Bacterial and Fungal Infections

Glucocorticoids have diverse effects that combine to induce immunosuppression, making patients susceptible to opportunistic local or systemic infections.

Intralesional use of glucocorticoids may result in bacterial infections caused by contamination introduced during injection. This could become life-threatening after epidural injections that result in CNS infection.[29]

Other Side Effects and Toxicities

Increased intracranial pressure resulting in blindness caused by retinal and vitreal hemorrhages has been reported in one person after epidural steroid injection.[30]

CONCLUSIONS

- Glucocorticoids reduce pain by decreasing inflammation.
- Glucocorticoids have diverse and often deleterious effects on many tissues. Glucocorticoid administration can mask progression of the specific disease being treated and can also mask the development of new diseases (e.g., opportunistic infections).
- Although glucocorticoids may play a role in the control of pain in some patients, they should be used sparingly and with caution.

- The role of glucocorticoids for adjunctive analgesia and their use by novel routes (e.g., epidural administration) has not yet been thoroughly investigated in veterinary medicine.

REFERENCES

1. Goldfien A: Adrenoglucocorticoids and adrenocortical antagonists. In Katzung BG, editor: *Basic and clinical pharmacology,* Stamford, Conn, 1998, Appleton & Lange.
2. Ferguson D, Hoenig M: Glucocorticoids, mineralocorticoids, and steroid synthesis inhibitors. In Adam HR, editor: *Veterinary pharmacology and therapeutics,* ed 7, Ames, 1995, Iowa State University Press.
3. Kempainnen RJ: Principles of glucocorticoid therapy in nonendocrine disease. In Kirk RW, editor: *Current veterinary therapy IX,* Philadelphia, 1986, WB Saunders.
4. Feldman EC, Nelson RW: *Canine and feline endocrinology and reproduction,* Philadelphia, 1987, WB Saunders.
5. Johnston SA, Fox SM: Mechanisms of action of anti-inflammatory drugs used for the treatment of osteoarthritis, *J Am Vet Med Assoc* 210:1486-1492, 1997.
6. Sutton LC, Fleshner M, Mazzeo R, et al: A permissive role of corticosterone in an opioid form of stress-induced analgesia: blockade of opiate analgesia is not due to stress-induced hormone release, *Brain Res* 663:19-29, 1994.
7. Coates JR: Intervertebral disc disease, *Vet Clin North Am Small Anim Pract* 30:77-110, 2000.
8. Hoerlein BF: Further evaluation of the treatment of disc protrusion paraplegia in the dog, *J Am Vet Med Assoc* 129:495-502, 1956.
9. Bracken MB, Shephard MJ, Collins WF Jr, et al: A randomized controlled study of methylprednisolone or naloxone in the treatment of acute spinal cord injury, *N Engl J Med* 322:1045, 1990.
10. Siemering GB: High dose methylprednisolone sodium succinate: an adjunct to surgery for canine intervertebral disc herniation, *Vet Surg* 21:406, 1992.
11. Logas D: Appropriate use of glucocorticoids in otitis externa. In Bonagura JD, editor: *Kirk's current veterinary therapy: small animal practice,* ed 13, Philadelphia, 2000, WB Saunders.
12. Pelletier JP, Martel-Pelletier J: Protective effects of glucocorticoids on cartilage lesions and osteophyte formation in the Pond-Nuki model of osteoarthritis, *Arthritis Rheum* 32:181-193, 1989.
13. Chunckamrai S, Krook LP, Lust G, et al: Changes in articular cartilage after intra-lesional injections of methylprednisolone acetate in horses, *Am J Vet Res* 50:1733-1741, 1989.

14. Behrens F, Shepard N, Mitchell N: Alterations of rabbit articular carti-
    lage by intra-articular injections of glucocorticoids, *J Bone Joint Surg
    Am* 57:70-76, 1975.
15. Miller SL, Wertheimer SJ: A comparison of the efficacy of injectable
    dexamethasone sodium phosphate versus placebo in postoperative po-
    diatric analgesia, *J Foot Ankle Surg* 37:223-226,1998.
16. Caldwell JR: Intra-articular corticosteroids: guide to selection and indi-
    cations for use, *Drugs* 52:507-514, 1996.
17. Abram SE: Neural blockade for neuropathic pain, *Clin J Pain* 16:S56-
    S61, 2000.
18. Botwin KP, Gruber RD, Bouchlas CG, et al: Complications of fluoro-
    scopically guided transforaminal lumbar epidural injections, *Arch Phys
    Med Rehab* 81:1045-1050, 2000.
19. Reale C, Turkiewicz AM, Reale CA, et al: Epidural steroids as a phar-
    macological approach, *Clin Exp Rheumatol* 18:S65-S66, 2000.
20. Cannon DT, Aprill CN: Lumbosacral epidural steroid injections, *Arch
    Phys Med Rehab* 81:S87-S98, 2000.
21. Pobereskin LH, Sneyd JR: Does wound irrigation with triamcinolone
    reduce pain after surgery to the lumbar spine? *Br J Anaesth* 84:731-734,
    2000.
22. Hayashi N, Weinstein JN, Meller ST, et al: The effect of epidural injec-
    tion of betamethasone or bupivacaine in a rat model of lumbar radicu-
    lopathy, *Spine* 23:877-885, 1998.
23. Hodges SD, Castleberg RL, Miller T, et al: Cervical epidural steroid in-
    jection with intrinsic spinal cord damage: two case reports, *Spine*
    23:2137-2142, 1998.
24. Klein DS, Klein PW: Intermittent interpleural injection of bupivacaine
    and methylprednisolone for analgesia in metastatic thoracic neoplasm,
    Clin J Pain 7:232-236, 1991.
25. Twycross R: The risks and benefits of corticosteroids in advanced can-
    cer, *Drug Saf* 11:163-178, 1994.
26. Korman B, MacKay RJ: Steroids and postoperative analgesia, *Anaesth
    Intens Care* 13:395-398, 1985.
27. Hanson SM, Bostwick DR, Twedt DC, et al: Clinical evaluation of
    cimetidine, sucralfate, and misoprostol for prevention of gastrointestinal
    tract bleeding in dogs undergoing spinal surgery, *Am J Vet Res* 58:1320-
    1323, 1997.
28. Lee PH, Grimes L, Hong JS: Glucocorticoids potentiate kainic acid-
    induced seizures and wet dog shakes, *Brain Res* 480:322-325, 1989
29. Cooper AB, Sharpe MD: Bacterial meningitis and cauda equina syn-
    drome after epidural steroid injections, *Can J Anaesth* 43:471-474, 1996.
30. Victory RA, Hassett P, Morrison G: Transient blindness following
    epidural analgesia, *Anaesthesia* 46:940-941, 1991.
31. Plumb DC, editor: *Veterinary drug handbook,* ed 3, Ames, 1999, Iowa
    State University Press,

14

Other Drugs Used to Treat Pain

JAMES S. GAYNOR

This section outlines drugs that have demonstrated or perceived analgesic efficacy but are not in the mainstream of veterinary practice. Many of these drugs are commonly used in the management of human pain. Much of the evidence substantiating their use comes from laboratory animal research, clinical trials in humans, or anecdotal reports in humans and animals.

KETAMINE

Mechanism of Action

Ketamine has traditionally been considered a dissociative anesthetic. Recently it has been characterized as an N-methyl-D-aspartate (NMDA) receptor antagonist (Box 14-1).

Efficacy and Use

NMDA receptor stimulation has been associated with central nervous system sensitization. Blockade of the NMDA receptor results in the ability to provide analgesia with potentially lower doses of opioids and less dysphoria.[1-2]

- Microdoses of ketamine, much lower than those used for anesthesia or chemical restraint, are used as an adjunct to analgesia protocols.
- Initial dose of ketamine is 0.5 mg/kg intravenously (IV) before surgical stimulation.
- An infusion of 10 μg/kg/min is administered during the procedure until the end of stimulation.
- A lower infusion rate of 2 μg/kg/min is administered for the next 24 hours.

BOX 14-1

Novel Use of Ketamine

Microdose ketamine intraoperatively can decrease analgesia requirements postoperatively.

- Some studies have advocated an additional lower infusion rate of 1 μg/kg/min for the next 24 hours postoperatively.
- In the absence of an infusion pump, 0.6 ml (60 mg) of ketamine can be added to a 1 L bag of crystalloid solutions to be administered at 10 ml/kg/hr to achieve the intraoperative dosing rate of 10 μg/kg/min.
- For postoperative administration of ketamine at 2 μg/kg/min without a syringe pump, 0.6 ml (60 mg) of ketamine for every 20 kg of body weight can be added to a 1-L bag of crystalloid solutions to be administered at 2 ml/kg/hr, approximately the normal maintenance fluid rate for an awake patient.

Pharmacology

The pharmacology of microdose ketamine dosing has not been well established. Even with the low doses, ketamine does bind with NMDA receptors in dogs.[3]

Side Effects and Toxicity

The microdose ketamine appears to have little if any side effects. Anecdotal accounts exist of several patients developing tachycardia.

Special Issues

It is important to remember that microdose ketamine by itself produces minimal if any analgesia. It must be used in conjunction with an analgesic such as an opioid.

AMANTADINE

Amantadine was originally developed as an antiviral drug for use in humans. It has been shown to have efficacy for treatment of drug-

---

BOX 14-2

Use of Amantadine

Amantadine may help with allodynia and opioid tolerance in patients
with chronic pain.

---

induced extrapyramidal effects and for Parkinson's disease. Its use
for treating pain has recently been described (Box 14-2).

Mechanism of Action

As a drug used in control of pain, amantadine has antagonist effects
at the NMDA receptor.

Efficacy and Use

- In humans, amantadine has been used for neuropathic pain.[9-10]
- Amantadine is used for veterinary patients suffering from allodynia and opioid tolerance. Amantadine use in these patients allows lowering of the opioid dose and helps increase analgesia
  provided by opioids.
- The dose for dogs and cats is approximately 3 to 5 mg/kg PO
  once daily. Amantadine is available in 100 mg capsules and a
  10 mg/ml liquid.

Pharmacology

The pharmacology of amantadine in dogs and cats has not been well
established, although the pharmacology of rimantadine, a similar
drug, is known for dogs.[10] In humans, amantadine is well absorbed,
not metabolized, and excreted in the urine.

Side Effects and Toxicity

- The feline toxic dose is 30 mg/kg.[10]
- Behavioral effects in dogs and cats[10] begin at 15 mg/kg PO.

Special Issues

The duration of action of amantadine may be prolonged in patients
with renal insufficiency.

TRAMADOL

Mechanism of Action

Tramadol is a synthetic, centrally acting analgesic that is not related to opioids.[4]

- Tramadol binds to μ-opioid receptors.
  - The parent compound has weak binding affinity.
  - The metabolites have 200 times the binding affinity for the μ-receptor.
- Tramadol inhibits reuptake of norepinephrine and serotonin, thus acting somewhat like an α_2-agonist.
- The mixed mechanism of action helps explain why naloxone (an opioid antagonist) only partially reverses tramadol-induced analgesia.

Efficacy and Use

- Tramadol is useful for moderate-to-severe pain. It has analgesic potency similar to meperidine.[5]
- In humans it has been used to alleviate pain associated with osteo-arthritis, fibromyalgia, diabetic neuropathy, and neuropathic pain.
- Tramadol may also be useful in patients with allodynia.[6]
- Humans dosed with 50 to 200 mg orally (PO) postoperatively or for chronic pain seem to experience good analgesia.
- The appropriate dose for dogs is unclear but is probably about 2.5-10 mg/kg PO SID-BID.
- Tramadol can be administered to dogs and cats at 2 to 4 mg/kg IV.

Pharmacology

- Oral dosing of tramadol in dogs results in rapid absorption with approximately 75% bioavailability. Dosing with or without food seems to make no difference.
- The biotransformation of tramadol is qualitatively similar between dogs and humans. Dogs metabolize approximately 99% of tramadol, whereas humans metabolize about 30%. The balance of the drug appears to be excreted unchanged by the kidneys.[7]

Side Effects and Toxicity

- Tramadol may cause respiratory depression when combined with other anesthetics.

- Short-term administration of tramadol may cause some nausea and vomiting.
- Long-term administration may cause constipation or diarrhea

Special Issues

Tramadol is less likely to induce tolerance in animals and humans compared with morphine. This is related to its nonopioid mechanism of action.[8]

GABAPENTIN

Gabapentin is a structural analog of gamma-aminobutyric acid (GABA).[11] It was originally introduced as an antiepileptic drug.

Mechanism of Action

The mechanism of action of gabapentin is unclear and elusive.
- Although gabapentin is related to GABA, it does not appear to have any analgesic effect at GABA receptors.
- Gabapentin interacts with NMDA receptors, but its analgesic effects are likely unrelated.

Efficacy and Use

- A number of rat studies have investigated the effects of gabapentin on signs of neuropathic pain, such as hyperalgesia and allodynia. Other studies indicate a role for gabapentin in decreasing incisional pain and arthritis.[12]
- Gabapentin appears to be best suited for pain of neuropathic origin.
- Exact indications and efficacy for gabapentin have not yet been determined.
- Most information related to pain and gabapentin has been derived from anecdotal case reports in humans and animals:
  - Neuralgia after herpes zoster infection.
  - Diabetic neuropathy: It is unclear whether veterinary patients develop this problem.
  - Neuropathic cancer pain: When gabapentin is added to an opioid regimen for patients who are only partially opioid responsive, they experience significantly better analgesia. These patients also experience less allodynia.
  - Burning and lancinating pain is more likely to respond to gabapentin compared to dull aching pain.

- Gabapentin does not alter nociceptive/pain thresholds; therefore it does not produce analgesia but assists other drugs in producing analgesia.
- Gabapentin has different effects in normal patients compared with those with inflammatory pain states.
  1. In the absence of any pathological pain, gabapentin may actually facilitate nociceptive responses at the level of the spinal cord dorsal horn neurons.
  2. Gabapentin dose-dependently inhibits dorsal horn responses to inflammatory-induced pain.
- Gabapentin decreases allodynia related to mechanical pressure and cold but does not affect nociceptive thresholds.
- Gabapentin reduces hyperalgesia when given systemically or intrathecally.
- Given prophylactically, gabapentin can inhibit hyperalgesia related to incisional, peripheral nerve, and thermal injury.
- A number of clinical animal studies have been performed to gather more specific information regarding the uses and effects of gabapentin, but controlled data is not yet available.

Dosing
- Although dosing has not been established in dogs or cats, the following recommendations are extrapolations from humans. It is important to remember that no analgesia research exists for dogs and cats using gabapentin. Gabapentin has been investigated as an antiepileptic drug in dogs, with dosing between 800 and 1500 mg daily.
- 1.25 to 4.0 mg/kg PO daily as a start.
- Doses may be able to be escalated up to 50 mg/kg or even higher.

Pharmacology
Gabapentin is highly bioavailable in dogs. It is metabolized by the liver and almost exclusively excreted by the kidneys. Its pharmacokinetics are not changed by multiple dosing. The half-life is about 3 to 4 hours.

Side Effects
In human clinical trials the side effects occur in 25% or less of patients.
- Sleepiness.

- Fatigue.
- Weight gain with chronic administration.

Special Issues

The use of gabapentin for analgesia has been only anecdotally reported in clinical veterinary patients.

MAGNESIUM

Mechanism of Action

Central sensitization is mediated by a cascade of events, including neuronal depolarization and NMDA receptor phosphorylation, resulting in an increase in a cell's excitability. Activation of the NMDA receptor involves removal of a magnesium block. Presumably, administration of magnesium may decrease wind-up. Intrathecal magnesium may also potentiate the effect of morphine and delay the onset of opioid tolerance.[13]

Efficacy and Use

- Little information exists concerning magnesium use for animal pain. It has been used intravenously for treatment of headache, postoperative pain, and neuropathic pain and subarachnoidally for allodynia and as an adjunct to intrathecal morphine.[14-15]
- A dose of 5 to 15 mg/kg IV has been extrapolated from humans. This dose is used for refractory cardiac dysrhythmias in dogs with no apparent side effects.
- In one study, humans received a 50 mg/kg IV bolus followed by 8 mg/kg/hr as an adjuvant to perioperative analgesia management with fentanyl.[16]

Pharmacology

Magnesium is predominantly an intracellular ion. The pharmacology of magnesium is under investigation in animals.

Side Effects and Toxicity

In humans, minor side effects include headache, hypotension, and internal heat sensation.

Special Issues

Measurement of plasma magnesium may be misleading because it may not reflect its intracellular component.

KETOROLAC (TORADOL)

Mechanism of Action

Ketorolac is a nonsteroidal antiinflammatory drug (NSAID) that produces analgesia similar to μ-opioid agonists such as morphine or oxymorphone. It is available in oral and parenteral formulations. It functions in a similar mechanism as other NSAIDs and should be used with caution because there may be a high incidence of side effects.

Efficacy and Use

- Ketorolac is indicated for the management of moderate-to-severe pain that typically would require an opioid.
- While its use is limited to 5 days in humans, dogs and cats should not receive more than two treatments because of the potential for side effects.[17]
  - Dogs
    1. Postsurgical pain: 0.3 to 0.6 mg/kg IV or IM every 8 to 12 hours[17,18,19]
    2. 0.6 mg/kg IM appears to be equipotent to oxymorphone 0.1 mg/kg IM
    3. Nonsurgical orthopedic pain: dogs >30 kg − 10 mg/dog PO once daily for 2 to 3 days.
  - Cats: postsurgical pain: 0.25 mg/kg IM every 12 hours.
  - Misoprostol (2 to 5 μg/kg PO every 8 hours) can be used as prophylaxis against gastrointestinal ulcer prevention in dogs receiving ketorolac.

Pharmacology

Ketorolac, like other NSAIDs, is metabolized by the liver. The pharmacology in dogs is similar to that in humans. It has an elimination half-life of 4.5 hours.[20] The pharmacology in cats is not well described.

Side Effects and Toxicity

- In humans, ketorolac is not used for more than 5 days because of the high likelihood of developing severe side effects such as gastrointestinal bleeding, perforated ulcers, and coagulation disorders. Similar side effects can be expected in dogs.
- Ketorolac should not be used in conjunction with other NSAIDs, corticosteroids, or aspirin.

Special Issues

- Ketorolac should not be used as a preemptive analgesic because of the unpredictability of hypotension under anesthesia and the greater increased risk of renal damage.
- Ketorolac should not be used intraoperatively in patients that may hemorrhage because of the likelihood of inhibiting normal clotting function.
- Ketorolac is contraindicated in patients with renal disease and those at risk for renal impairment caused by hypovolemia and hypotension.

REFERENCES

1. Felsby S, Nielsen J, Arendt-Nielsen L, et al: NMDA receptor blockade in chronic neuropathic pain: a comparison of ketamine and magnesium chloride, *Pain* 64:283-291, 1996.
2. Wilder-Smith OH, Arendt-Nielsen L, Gaumann D, et al: Sensory changes and pain after abdominal hysterectomy: a comparison of anesthetic supplementation with fentanyl versus magnesium or ketamine, *Anesth Analg* 86:95-101, 1998.
3. Mama KR, Golden AE, Monnet E, et al: *Plasma and cerebrospinal fluid concentrations and NMDA receptor binding activity associated with intraoperative administration of low-dose ketamine,* Proceedings of the seventh World Congress of Veterinary Anaesthesia, Bern, Switzerland, 2000, p 78 (abstract).
4. Minto CF, Power I: New opioid analgesics: an update, *Int Anesthesiol Clin* 35:49-65, 1997 (review).
5. Lehmann KA: Tramadol for the management of acute pain, *Drugs* (47 suppl)1:19-32, 1994 (review).
6. Sindrup SH, Anderson G, Madsen C, et al: Tramadol relieves pain and allodynia in polyneuropathy: a randomized, double-blind, controlled trial, *Pain* 83:85-90, 1999.
7. Lintz W, Erlacin S, Frankus F, et al: Biotransformation of tramadol in man and animal, *Arzneimittel-Forschung* 31:1932-1943, 1981.
8. Miranda HF, Pinardi G: Antinociception, tolerance, and physical dependence comparison between morphine and tramadol, *Pharmacol Biochem Behav* 61:357-360, 1998.
9. Pud D, Eisenberg E, Spitzer A, et al: The NMDA receptor antagonist amantadine reduces surgical neuropathic pain in cancer patients: a double blind, randomized, placebo controlled trial, *Pain* 75:349 354, 1998.
10. Eisenberg E, Pud D: Can patients with chronic neuropathic pain be cured by acute administration of the NMDA receptor antagonist amantadine, *Pain* 74:337-339, 1988.

11. Radulovic LL, Turck D, von Hodenberg A, et al: Disposition of gaba-pentin (neurontin) in mice, rats, dogs, and monkeys, *Drug Metab Dispos* 23:441-448, 1995.

12. Mao J, Chen LL: Gabapentin in pain management, *Anesth Analg* 91:680-687, 2000.

13. Ren K, Dubner R: Central nervous system plasticity and persistent pain, *J Orofac Pain* 13:155-163; discussion 164-171, 1999 (review).

14. Crosby V, Wilcock A, Corcoran R: The safety and efficacy of a single dose (500 mg or 1 g) of intravenous magnesium sulfate in neuropathic pain poorly responsive to strong opioid analgesics in patients with cancer, *J Pain Symptom Manage* 19:35-39, 2000.

15. Kroin JS, McCarthy RJ, Von Roenn N, et al: Magnesium sulfate potentiates morphine antinociception at the spinal level, *Anesth Analg* 90:913-917. 2000.

16. Koinig H, Wallner T, Marhofer P, et al: Magnesium sulfate reduces intra- and postoperative analgesic requirements, *Anesth Analg* 87:206-210, 1998.

17. Mathews KA: Nonsteroidal anti-inflammatory analgesics: indications and contraindications for pain management in dogs and cats, *Vet Clin North Am Small Anim Pract* 30:783-804, 2000.

18. Mathews KA, Paley DM, Foster RA, et al: A comparison of ketorolac with flunixin, butorphanol, and oxymorphone in controlling postoperative pain in dogs, *Can Vet J* 37:557-567, 1996.

19. Popilskis S, Jordan D, Laurent L, et al: *Comparison of ketorolac and oxymorphone on postoperative pain relief and neuroendocrine response in dogs,* Proceedings of the sixth International Congress of Veterinary Anesthesia, Thessaloniki, Greece, 1977, p 107.

20. Pasloske K, Renaud R, Burger J, et al: Pharmacokinetics of ketorolac after intravenous and oral single dose administration in dogs, *J Vet Pharmacol Ther* 22:314-319, 1999.

15

Local and Regional Anesthetic Techniques for Alleviation of Perioperative Pain

JAMES S. GAYNOR AND KHURSHEED R. MAMA

- Regional anesthesia: The term implies that a region of the body is affected as opposed to the entire body, as occurs with general anesthesia. The region affected may be very limited or broad in scope.
- Unlike most instances of general anesthesia, during which it is mainly the "perception of pain" that is blocked (by virtue of unconsciousness), local anesthetics block the "transmission of noxious impulses."
- Because the analgesic effects of local anesthetics do not depend on central depression (anesthesia), regional analgesic techniques may be used in a conscious patient.

REGIONAL ANESTHETIC TECHNIQUES

Topical Anesthesia

- Surface, or topical, anesthesia results when the drug is applied to the skin or mucous membrane to cause loss of sensation by paralyzing sensory nerve endings.
- Local anesthetics are widely used on the mucous membranes of the eye, nose, and mouth. Most are ineffectively used on unbroken skin because cornified epidermis limits penetration.
- The recent introduction of a combination of lidocaine and prilocaine in a eutectic mixture has overcome this problem and is now commonly used to provide dermal analgesia for venipuncture and catheterization.

261

- Technique
  1. The fur is clipped over the site to be desensitized.
  2. The lidocaine/prilocaine cream is liberally applied and covered with an occlusive bandage. This is allowed to remain for a minimum of 30 minutes, with 45 to 90 minutes as the ideal.
  3. The cream is wiped off and the procedure is performed.

Anesthesia by Infiltration

- Infiltration anesthesia is perhaps the most common method of regional anesthesia and consists of making numerous subcutaneous (SC) injections of small volumes of local anesthetic solution into the tissues.
- The drug diffuses into surrounding tissue from the site of injection and anesthetizes nerve fibers and endings. Large amounts of relatively dilute solutions are often infiltrated into operative sites.
- Epinephrine (1:200,000) may be used in combination with infiltration of local anesthetic to reduce systemic absorption of the anesthetic agent and prolong the duration of analgesia.
- Acute pain therapy can be continued by infiltration anesthesia for several days by using the PainBuster Soaker (dj Orthopedics, Inc., Vista, California). The local anesthetic is delivered by an elastomeric reservoir (pump), which is filled with local anesthetic (e.g., lidocaine, mepivacaine, ropivacaine). The pump is attached to delivery tubing and a sterile multipore catheter that is placed at the surgical site. The pump delivers local anesthetic at a constant rate (0.5 to 5 ml/hr) for up to 5 days (Fig. 15-1).

Incisional Line Block

- This block is used before surgical incision or after the surgery before complete closure.
- Technique for line block before incision.
  1. Needle: 25 g, 2.5 cm (1 inch) hypodermic.
  2. Insert the needle subcutaneously after a sterile prep.
  3. Aspirate.
  4. Inject enough local anesthetic to produce a noticeable bleb.
  5. Remove the needle and reinsert at the edge of the bleb.
  6. After aspiration, inject more local anesthetic to extend the bleb.
  7. Repeat the process until the length of the incision has been blocked.

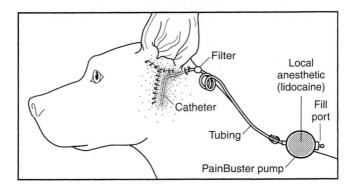

Fig. 15-1 Anesthesia by continuous infiltration of local anesthetic after total ear canal ablation.

BOX 15-1

Caution with Local Anesthetic

Always aspirate for blood before injecting any local anesthetic.

---

8. Bupivacaine (0.5% = 5 mg/ml) with or without epinephrine or lidocaine (2% = 20 mg/ml) with or without epinephrine is often used at a dose of 1 to 2 mg/kg. This solution is then diluted with an equal amount of 0.9% saline to increase the injectate volume.

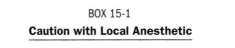

- Technique for incisional block before closing incision (Fig. 15-2).
  1. Needle: 25 g, 2.5 cm (1 inch) hypodermic.
  2. This is done in a sterile manner by the surgeon. Someone must pass the needle and syringe aseptically to the surgeon to prevent contamination.
  3. Insert the needle at one end on the midline of the incision before closing the skin.
  4. After aspiration for blood, inject local anesthetic in a fanlike manner to block subcutaneous and muscular tissues. If this is

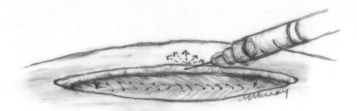

Fig. 15-2 Incisional block.

BOX 15-2

Epinephrine and Local Anesthetic

Epinephrine should be combined with a local anesthetic only for blocks that are not on the distal extremities. This prevents distal ischemia.

---

being performed on the abdominal body wall, inject local anesthetic down to the peritoneum.
5. Remove the needle and reinsert a slight distance away, reinjecting local anesthetic in a fanlike manner.
6. Repeat until the area under the whole incision has been infiltrated.

PERIPHERAL NERVE BLOCK

- This conduction block is produced by injection of local anesthetic in the immediate vicinity of individual peripheral nerves or a nerve plexus.
- Paravertebral nerve blocks in cattle and horses, intercostal nerve blocks, and the brachial plexus block in dogs and cats may be considered examples of peripheral nerve blocks. Intrapleural anesthesia is an alternative to multiple intercostal nerve blocks and may be considered a regional peripheral nerve block.

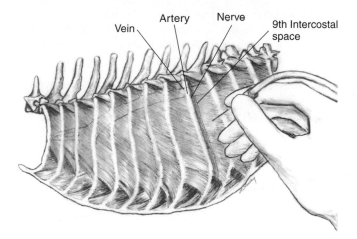

Fig. 15-3 Interpleural block.

Interpleural Block

This block is used to provide analgesia and anesthesia related to thoracic and cranial abdominal pain, especially pain related to pancreatitis.

Needles

- 22 g butterfly catheter
- 20 g, 5 cm (2 inch) through-the-needle catheter
- Preexisting chest tube

Technique (Fig. 15-3)

1. Aseptically prepare the site of catheter insertion.
2. Place the catheter in the ninth intercostal space on the midlateral aspect of the thorax.
3. Aspirate.
4. Inject lidocaine (1.5 mg/kg) first. The patient may momentarily vocalize, since the lidocaine may sting, but the onset of the lidocaine block is rapid.
5. Inject the bupivacaine (1.5 mg/kg) next. If bupivacaine is injected first, the patient will vocalize for 15 to 25 minutes, the amount of time it takes for onset.

6. This procedure can be repeated every 3 to 6 hours.
7. If injecting through a chest tube, a small amount of saline can be used to flush the local anesthetic into the chest.

Positioning
Correct positioning of the patient after injection is unclear. There are several options.

- Roll the patient onto its back so the local anesthetic flows into the paravertebral gutters to block nerves before entering the spinal cord. This is most common in patients under anesthesia because they are easily moved.
- Place the patient in an upright position. This is most common in awake patients.
- Position the patient onto the affected side.
- Position the patient on the unaffected side.
- If interpleural anesthesia does not seem to work, attempt to alter the patient's position to change the distribution of the local anesthetic.

Intercostal Block
- This block is useful for providing analgesia after intercostal thoracotomy and for desensitizing the area around isolated broken ribs.
- Needle: 22 to 25 g hypodermic.

Technique
This technique can be performed intraoperatively before closing the skin from an intercostal thoracotomy or percutaneously in a nonsurgical patient (Fig. 15-4).

1. Perform a sterile prep if performing the intercostal block percutaneously.
2. Blocks are performed two to three spaces cranial and caudal to affected area.
3. The nerves are located on the caudal aspect of the rib behind the vein and artery.
4. Place the needle just caudal to the rib.
5. Aspirate for blood.
6. Inject local anesthetic.
7. Awake patients should be given a combination of lidocaine (1.5 mg/kg) combined with bupivacaine (1.5 mg/kg) to ensure a rapid onset of a block that should last 4 to 6 hours.

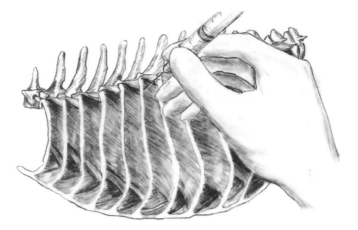

Fig. 15-4 Intercostal block.

8. Patients who are receiving this block intraoperatively can receive only bupivacaine.

Infraorbital Nerve Block

- This block is used to provide anesthesia/analgesia to the upper lip and nose, dorsal aspect of the nasal cavity, and skin ventral to the infraorbital foramen.
- Needle: a 25 g, 2.5 cm (1 inch) hypodermic needle is adequate in virtually all dogs and cats.

Technique (Fig. 15-5)

1. Palpate the infraorbital foramen rostral and distal to the medial canthus of the eye.
2. Insert the needle into the foramen.
3. Aspirate for blood.
4. Deposit a small amount of local anesthetic (usually less than 1 ml).

Mental Nerve Block

- The mental nerve is blocked to provide analgesia to the lower lip.
- Needle: a 25 g, 2.5 cm (1 inch) hypodermic needle is adequate in virtually all dogs and cats.

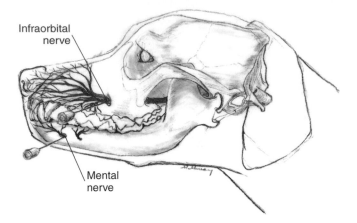

Infraorbital nerve

Mental nerve

Fig. 15-5 Infraorbital and mental nerve blocks.

Technique (See Fig. 15-5)
1. Palpate the mental foramen on the lateral aspect of the mandible just caudal to the canine tooth.
2. Insert the needle into the mental foramen.
3. Aspirate for blood.
4. Inject a small amount of local anesthetic (usually less than 1 ml).

Mandibular Nerve Block
- The mandibular nerve is blocked to provide anesthesia of the ipsilateral incisors, canine tooth, premolars, molars, skin and mucosa of the chin and lower lip.
- Needle: 22 g, 2.5 cm (1 inch) hypodermic needle. Large dogs may require a 3.75-cm needle.

Technique (Fig. 15-6)
1. Aseptically prepare the site medial to the mandible.
2. Place an index finger in the patient's mouth. Palpate the mucosa on the medial aspect of the cheek for the mandibular nerve, which feels like a fibrous band.
3. Insert the needle with the other hand from the ventral-medial aspect of the mandible.

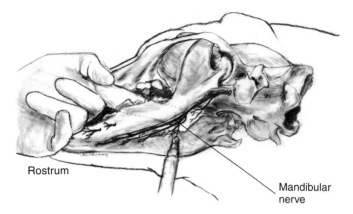

Rostrum

Mandibular nerve

Fig. 15-6 Mandibular nerve block; canine head in right lateral position.

4. The index finger in the mouth guides the needle to placement next to the nerve.
5. Aspirate for blood.
6. Inject a small amount of local anesthetic (usually less than 1 ml).

Forefoot Block

• This block is useful for declaws in cats, toe amputations, or any surgery of the foot distal to the carpus.
• Needle: 25 g hypodermic.
• A combination of lidocaine (1.5 mg/kg) and bupivacaine (1.5 mg/kg) for dogs or cats is used. The total dose should be split between areas to be desensitized. This dose may be diluted if additional volume is necessary

Technique (Fig. 15-7)

1. Insert the needle just distal to the carpus on the proximal-medial aspect of the metacarpus.
2. Always aspirate before injection.
3. Inject a small amount of the combined local anesthetics to produce a small bleb.
4. Insert needle and repeat injections, continuing across the dorsum of the foot to the lateral aspect.

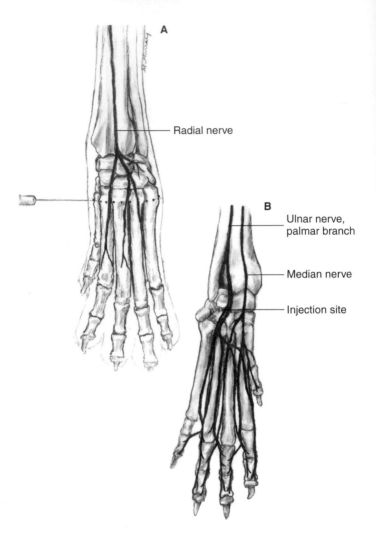

Fig. 15-7 **A,** Forefoot block, dorsal aspect. **B,** Forefoot block, palmar aspect.

5. Complete the block by inserting the needle in the depression just distal to the accessory carpal pad, aspirating, and injecting a small amount of local anesthetic, ensuring a continuous infiltration from the medial aspect to the lateral aspect.

Brachial Plexus Block

A brachial plexus block is used to provide anesthesia distal to the elbow.

Needles

- 22 g, 7.5 cm (3 inch) spinal needle for blind technique.
- 22 g, 7.5 cm (3 inch) insulated needle for guided technique.

Nerve Locator Guided Technique *(Fig. 15-8)*

1. The guided technique is much more accurate and successful in obtaining a good brachial plexus block with a minimal of local anesthetic.
2. Aseptically prepare the area medial to the scapulohumeral joint.
3. Attach one electrode from the nerve locator to the skin; attach the other to the proximal portion of the needle.
4. Insert the needle medial to the scapulohumeral joint, advancing toward the costochondral junction of the first palpable rib, medial to the scapula but outside the thorax.
5. As the needle is inserted, turn on the nerve locator to the highest current setting.
6. As the paw begins to twitch, precisely place the needle to obtain a maximal twitch with as little current as possible.
7. Aspirate for blood.
8. Inject a small amount of local anesthetic until the twitch disappears.
9. Because the brachial plexus is diffuse, perform this technique two more times, fanning the needle dorsal and ventral from the initial placement.
10. Inject a maximum of lidocaine 1.5 mg/kg or bupivacaine 1.5 mg/kg. Typically, considerably less drug is necessary because the local anesthetic is deposited directly on the nerves.

Blind Technique *(Fig. 15-9)*

1. The blind technique only has approximately a 50% success rate using large volumes of local anesthetic.

A

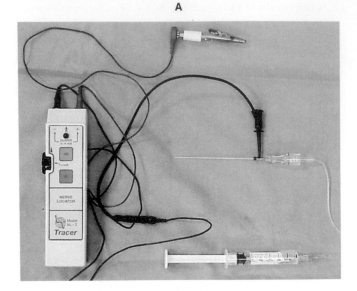

B

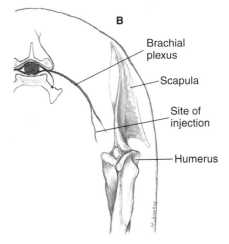

Fig. 15-8 A, Nerve locator. **B,** Brachial plexus.

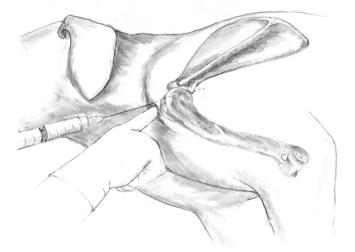

Fig. 15-9 Brachial plexus block.

2. Aseptically prepare the area medial to the scapulohumeral joint.
3. Insert the needle medial to the scapulohumeral joint, advancing toward the costochondral junction of the first palpable rib, medial to the scapula but outside the thorax.
4. Aspirate for blood.
5. Inject local anesthetic while withdrawing the needle 75% of the distance inserted.
6. Reinsert the needle two more times, approximately 30 degrees dorsal and 30 degrees ventral.
7. Aspirate for blood after each insertion, then inject local anesthetic while withdrawing.
8. Local anesthetic dose can be as high as lidocaine 1.5 mg/kg or bupivacaine 1.5 mg/kg.

INTRAARTICULAR ADMINISTRATION

- This route may be used to facilitate diagnosis of lameness as is commonly done in the horse.

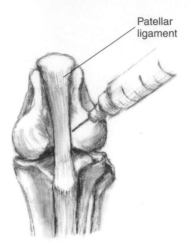

Fig. 15-10 Stifle joint, intramuscular block.

- The technique may also be used to desensitize the affected joint before (preemptive analgesia) and after surgical intervention (e.g., arthroscopy). In small animals, the stifle joint is most commonly injected.
- Needle: 22 g, 2.5 cm (1 inch) hypodermic needle.

Technique *(Fig. 15-10)*
1. Clip and aseptically prepare the joint.
2. Insert the needle lateral to the patellar ligament.
3. Aspirate to ensure that the needle is not in tissue.
4. Inject local anesthetic.
   - Lidocaine 1 to 2 mg/kg
   - Bupivacaine 1 to 2 mg/kg
   - Most medium-to-large dogs stifle hold about 5 ml of fluid.
5. Morphine 0.1 mg/kg can be injected postoperatively to provide analgesia but not anesthesia.

INTRAVENOUS LOCAL OR REGIONAL ANESTHESIA
- This is accomplished by IV injection of large volumes of dilute local anesthetic into an extremity isolated from the rest of the

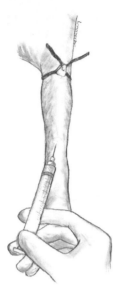

Fig. 15-11 Forelimb Bier block.

circulation by a tourniquet. The tissue distal to the tourniquet is blocked. This technique is also called a *Bier block*.

- The apparent mechanism of action is by diffusion of local anesthetic across blood vessels to local nerves.
- Normal nervous and muscle function returns quickly upon release of the tourniquet, which allows blood flow to dilute the regional local anesthetic concentration.
- Needle: 22 g, 2.5 cm (1 inch) hypodermic needle.

Forelimb Block
Technique *(Fig. 15-11)*
1. Apply an occlusive bandage in a distal to proximal manner to remove blood from the limb.
2. Place a tourniquet proximal or distal to the elbow.
3. Remove the occlusive bandage.
4. Inject lidocaine into the cephalic vein. Onset of block is very fast. Between 1 to 2 ml of 2% lidocaine can be diluted with an

equal amount of 0.9% saline (producing 1% lidocaine). Of the dilute lidocaine, 2 to 4 ml can be injected.

5. Apply a second tourniquet (preferably pneumatic) in the blocked area distal to the first tourniquet. Remove the first tourniquet. This will decrease tourniquet-induced pain.

6. The tourniquet must be removed within 90 minutes to avoid shock, endotoxemia, and potential death on tourniquet release.

Rear Limb Block

Technique

1. This technique is performed similar to that of the IV regional forelimb block.

2. Apply an occlusive bandage in a distal to proximal manner to remove blood from the limb.

3. Apply a tourniquet proximal to the tarsus.

4. Remove the occlusive bandage.

5. Inject lidocaine into the saphenous vein. Onset of block is very fast. Between 1 to 2 ml of 2% lidocaine can be diluted with an equal amount of 0.9% saline (producing 1% lidocaine). Of the dilute lidocaine, 2 to 4 ml can be injected.

6. Apply a second tourniquet (preferably pneumatic) in the blocked area distal to the first tourniquet. Remove the first tourniquet. This will decrease tourniquet-induced pain.

7. The tourniquet must be removed within 90 minutes to avoid shock, endotoxemia, and potential death on tourniquet release.

EPIDURAL ANESTHESIA AND ANALGESIA

- Injecting local anesthetic solution into the epidural space generally at the lumbosacral (LS) space (for dogs, pigs) or the first or second intercoccygeal space (for horses, cows; sometimes referred to as *caudal anesthesia*) produces epidural or extradural anesthesia.

- The anesthetic acts on the posterior spinal nerves before they leave the vertebral column.

- The extent of anesthetic action depends on the spread of the drug and diffusion to neural tissues from the site of injection.

- Long-term administration of drugs is facilitated by placement of an epidural catheter. This technique also facilitates craniad distribution of drug.

- Anesthesia can be produced by using a local anesthetic such as lidocaine or bupivacaine.
- Analgesia can be produced without loss of motor function with the use of an opioid, such as morphine.
- Regardless of the desired effect, the technique of epidural injection is the same.
- Most epidural injections in dogs and cats are performed at the LS space. The spinal cord usually ends at the last lumbar vertebra (L7) in dogs; thus there is less chance of obtaining cerebrospinal fluid (CSF) at this space. The spinal cord usually ends at the first sacral vertebra in cats, making it likely to get CSF if attempting an epidural at the LS space.

Needles
- 8-, 20-, and 22-gauge beveled spinal needles of various lengths are commonly used.
- An alternative is an 18- or 20-gauge blunt-pointed Tuohy epidural needle.

Epidural Injection
Technique
1. Place the patient in lateral or sternal recumbency.
    - Patients with rear limb trauma may not easily be placed in sternal recumbency because of the potential for worsening a fracture. An advantage of the sternal position is the ability to use the hanging drop technique (Fig. 15-12, *A*).
    - Virtually all patients can be placed in lateral recumbency for this procedure (Fig. 15-12, *B*).
2. Clip and aseptically prepare an area of fur just cranial to wings of the ilium, caudal to the second sacral vertebra and as wide as the lateral aspects of the ilium wings.
3. Locate the LS space by placing the thumb and smallest finger on opposite wings of the ilium. Palpating between these fingers, on midline, is the dorsal spinous process of the sixth lumbar vertebra (L6). A significant space can be felt just caudal to L6. Directly caudal to that space is the dorsal spinous process of L7. Further caudal is a large palpable depression, the LS space.
4. Place the needle perpendicular to the skin on midline in the middle of the space. Sometimes angling the needle tip slightly cranially is beneficial.

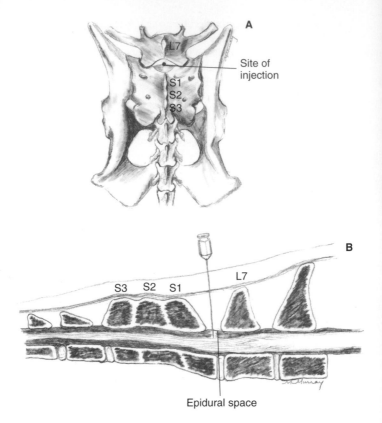

Fig. 15-12 A, Dorsal view of lumbosacral area of a dog. **B,** Lateral view of lumbosacral area of a dog.

5. Insert the needle slowly. Often, resistance can be felt as the needle passes through the ligamentum flavum at the top of the vertebral canal. At this point, the needle is in the epidural space.
    •   Remove the stylet of the needle. If blood comes from the needle, the needle should be removed. If CSF is encountered, use half the dose of local anesthetic. Opioid doses, in general, do not need to be changed.

- Inject 1 ml of air with a glass syringe to verify placement. There is minimal resistance of a glass syringe plunger on a glass barrel. If the air stays in the space without pushing the syringe plunger back, the needle is likely to be in the correct place. If injection of air leads to resistance and pushing back of the plunger, the needle is not in the desired location.

Alternative Hanging Drop Technique
1. Place the patient in sternal recumbency.
2. Remove the stylet before puncturing the ligamentum flavum.
3. Place a drop of sterile saline in the hub of the needle.
4. As the needle passes through the ligamentum flavum into the epidural space, the negative pressure in the space sucks in the saline. This is a definitive sign of proper needle placement.
5. Stabilize the needle and administer the drug slowly over a 1-minute period. Minimal resistance should be encountered on injection.

Placement of an Epidural Catheter
Technique
1. The technique is identical to placement of an epidural described previously except that a Tuohy needle is used.
2. Insert the catheter through the needle a distance that will stay in the epidural space and is equal to the depth of the needle in the skin plus approximately 1 to 3 inches.
3. Remove the needle by securing the catheter and needle together and withdrawing from the skin. This helps prevent shearing off the catheter in the epidural space.
4. The advantage of epidural catheter placement is the ability to provide epidural anesthesia or analgesia for days without the trauma of repeated epidural punctures.

Dilution and Administration of Morphine and Bupivacaine for Continuous Epidural Administration
1. Dilute preservative-free morphine (1 mg/ml) with sterile preservative-free 0.9% saline to a concentration of 0.5 mg/ml by adding equal amounts of saline to the morphine.
2. Add 1 ml of bupivacaine (0.75%) to 5 ml of the dilute preservative-free morphine. This produces a solution of bupivacaine (1.25 mg/ml) and morphine (0.42 mg/ml).

3. The solution is administered at a rate of 0.03 to 0.05 ml/kg/hour. This delivers morphine at a rate of 0.3 to 0.5 mg/kg/24 hours.
4. If rear limb motor paralysis occurs, the bupivacaine should be diluted into 11 ml of dilute morphine solution and administered at the rate described previously to deliver the same morphine dose but a considerably lower bupivacaine dose.

SPINAL ANESTHESIA

- Spinal anesthesia is produced by injecting local anesthetic into the subarachnoid space.
  - This can be accomplished at the LS space in cats.
  - This can be accomplished at L5 to L6 or L6 to L7 vertebrae in dogs.
- Because the vertebral level of termination of the spinal cord varies among animal species, this form of anesthesia is technically more difficult than epidural injection in other veterinary species.
- Local anesthetic doses for subarachnoid injection are usually 50% of doses for epidural injection.
- Opioid doses do not need to change for subarachnoid injection.

SUGGESTED READINGS

Muir WW, Hubbell JAE, Skarda RT, et al: *Handbook of veterinary anesthesia,* ed 3, St Louis, 2000, Mosby.

Thurman JC, Tranquilli WJ, Benson GJ: *Lumb & Jones' veterinary anesthesia,* ed 3, Baltimore, 1996, Williams & Wilkins.

16

Complementary and Alternative (Integrative) Pain Therapy

ROMAN T. SKARDA

Nonpharmacologic neuromodulation therapies such as acupuncture, electroacupuncture (EAP) or percutaneous acupoint electrical stimulation (PAES), transcutaneous electrical nerve stimulation (TENS), percutaneous electrical nerve stimulation (PENS), laser therapy, and pulsed magnetic field therapy (PMFT) are safe techniques for providing pain relief in humans and animals, either as a supplement to conventional pain therapy or alone (Box 16-1). All six modalities produce an analgesic effect. Acupuncture and related techniques are effective therapies for acute and particularly chronic pain in animals (Fig. 16-1). Most of the information provided focuses on the dog and horse because of the paucity of published information on other species. Little information is available for the cat. A more extensive reference list and the addresses of manufacturers of equipment are provided because of the relative lack of familiarity of most veterinarians and their assistants with this topic.

- Electrical stimulation is more intense than manual manipulation of needles.
- PAES-induced analgesia has been used successfully in many patients with chronic pain and in patients whose pain was resistant to conventional TENS.
- Electrical current is essential for producing analgesia with PAES, TENS, PENS, laser, and PMFT techniques.
- Use of both PAES and PENS at acupuncture points and dermatomes produces an even more profound and longer-lasting analgesic effect in patients with acute and chronic pain syndromes than either modality alone.

BOX 16-1
Definitions

Acupuncture is the manual stimulation of acupuncture points based on traditional Chinese medicine (TCM).

Electroacupuncture (EAP) or **percutaneous acupoint electrical stimulation (PAES)** is the electrical stimulation of acupuncture points based on classic Chinese principles.

Transcutaneous electrical nerve stimulation (TENS) is the electrical stimulation of dermatomes, myotomes, and sclerotomes that correspond to the specific sensory nerves originating at the site(s) of the painful stimuli by using surface electrodes.

Percutaneous electrical nerve stimulation (PENS) is similar to TENS except that those areas are stimulated by using needles and electrical stimulation percutaneously.

Laser therapy is the noninvasive form of stimulation by application of polarized light over acupuncture points, injuries, and lesions to stimulate healing within the tissues.

Pulsed magnetic field therapy (PMFT) is a method of applying a magnetic field with an extremely low range of frequencies to the cell to change the electrical potentials of nerves and other cells and normalize the flow of ions and nutrients in the cell for promoting the healing of damaged tissues.

- PAES, TENS, laser therapy, and PMFT are beneficial complementary methods for the control of pain in numerous clinical disorders of small and large animals (Box 16-2).

PERCUTANEOUS ACUPOINT ELECTRICAL STIMULATION

- High-risk surgical patients or patients who have orthopedic or neurologic surgery, gastric-dilatation-volvulus syndrome, dystocia, and toxic pyometra may be good candidates for PAES-induced analgesia.
- Selective cesarean section is the most ideal indication for using PAES analgesia because it does not produce central nervous system (CNS) and respiratory depression of the fetus.
- The PAES or TENS treatment is usually given in addition to standard analgesics such as systemically administered opioid

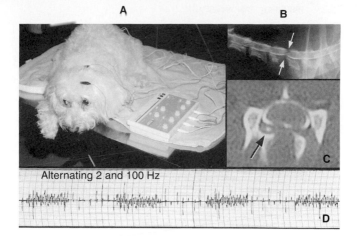

Fig. 16-1 A, Bichon Frise (11 years old) with relief from severe chronic neck pain during PAES. **B,** Myelographic radiograph of the lateral projection of the caudal cervical spine of the dog, indicating extradural spinal cord compression (as indicated by *arrows*) at the cervical vertebrae C5/C6. **C,** Axial computed tomographic image at the level of the C6 vertebra, indicating calcified disk material *(arrow)* displacing the spinal cord dorsally at the right side of the spine. The defect of vertebral body after vertebral decompression is visible. **D,** Biphasic stimulation with alternating 2-Hz and 100-Hz frequencies. Recorded at 25 mm/sec and 5 mV/cm.

BOX 16-2
Types of Pain Treated with PAES

- Localized, sharp pain from inflammation of nerves or nerve roots in small dogs attributable to compression by intervertebral disks, spondylopathy, and cauda equina syndrome (neuritic pain; Fig. 16-1).
- Localized, sharp pain from inflammation of nerves or nerve roots in large dogs and horses ("wobbler" syndrome) attributable to compression of the spinal cord, intervertebral disks, and spondylopathy (neuritic pain).
- Localized, constant, and aching pain originating from musculoskeletal damage (hip dysplasia, osteoarthritis) and bone metastases (inflammatory and somatic pain).
- Pain from metabolic, immunologic, or direct physical effects on segments of the nervous system (neuropathic pain).
- Miscellaneous pain from degenerative myelopathy, trauma, and canine acral lick dermatitis.
- Surgical analgesia.

agonists (e.g., morphine, hydromorphone), transdermal opioid patch (e.g., fentanyl), intravenous infusion of lidocaine, and non-steroidal antiinflammatory drugs (NSAIDs) (e.g., phenylbuta-zone, carprofen, ketoprofen, etodolac, meloxicam). The PAES and TENS supplements helped do the following:

- Increase patient comfort.
- Reduce the dose, dose interval, or both of pain medication.
- Reduce length of time pain therapy was required.
- Shorten time of hospitalization.

Potential Types of Surgery Performed with Analgesia Induced by Percutaneous Acupoint Electrical Stimulation

Dog

- Cesarean section.
- Ovariohysterectomy.
- Abdominal laparotomy.
- Gastric and intestinal surgery.
- Nephrectomy.
- Splenectomy.
- Umbilical hernioplasty.
- Removal of mammary and skin tumors.
- Ear cropping.
- Craniotomy.
- Open reduction and repair of long bone fractures.

Horse, Cattle, Sheep, Pig

- Castration.
- Orchidopexy.
- Dystocia.
- Reposition of prolapsed uterus.
- Surgery of anal and vaginal region.
- Relief of dystocia.
- Surgery on esophagus and rumen.
- Repair of navel and umbilical hernia.
- Surgery on the bladder and urethra.
- Orthopedic surgery (bones, joints).
- Experimental studies.

Other Clinical Use of PAES in Animals

Other indications for using PAES are paresis or paralysis of facial nerves, the radial nerve, or the tibial nerve; trigger point therapy;

BOX 16-3

Contraindications for PAES

- Pregnant animals (except for cesarean section or if uterine tone is poor) because of the risk of spontaneous abortion.
- Extremely debilitated animals.
- Extremely febrile animals.
- Local skin infection.
- Local malignancies.
- Severe blood coagulopathies:
  - Platelet dysfunction.
  - von Willebrand's disease.
- Traumatic disk injury in the first 24 hours.

---

muscle atrophy; postoperative ileus; and postoperative vomiting and nausea.

Risks

The complication rate associated with acupuncture and PAES administration to animals appears to be low. If the techniques are performed properly, complications do not occur. Contraindications for PAES are listed in Box 16-3.
- Contact dermatitis.
- Local hematoma (bleeding from a punctured blood vessel).
- Local infections.
- Pneumothorax (punctured lung).
- Convulsions.
- Nerve damage.

Equipment

Quality products, pricing, and service of various acupuncture needles and equipment for PAES and TENS can be obtained from suppliers listed in Appendix 16-1.

Acupuncture Needles

- Depending on the size of the patient and the location of selected points, filiform stainless steel 1.25- to 10-cm needles are used (Box 16-4).

Fig. 16-2 A, Package with 10 sterile acupuncture needles (Hwato, size 0.3 × 25 mm) for single use. **B,** CEPES-laser Combi-Plus-Soft-Laser. **C,** Pointer-Plus hand-held unit for locating and stimulating acupuncture points transcutaneously (TENS). **D,** Acu-Vet hand-held unit for locating and stimulating acupuncture points transcutaneously (TENS). **E,** Electro-Acupuncture Unit IC-4107 for locating and stimulating acupuncture points percutaneously (PAES). Further description can be found in the text.

> ### BOX 16-4
> ### Variation in Gauge Size of Needles
>
> - Human acupuncture needles, 29- to 34-gauge.
> - Veterinary acupuncture needles:
>   - 22- to 26-gauge for large animals.
>   - 26- to 30-gauge for small animals.

- Good quality acupuncture needles are manufactured in China (Hwa-To needle [Fig. 16-2, *A*], Hua-Xia needle), Japan (Seirin and Addiquipp needles), and Korea (DBC, Han-il, CW, Taki, and Detox needles).
- Acupuncture needles should be sterilized at 120° C for 30 minutes at 15 lb pressure.
- The needles are inserted at acupuncture points to the correct depth; they are taped or sutured firmly in position and are connected in pairs to the output socket of an acupuncture electrostimulator for PAES treatment.

Acupuncture Electrostimulators
Many different types of electrostimulators made in China, Japan, the United States, Canada, Europe, and Australia are on the market. There is little standardization of equipment (Box 16-5).

Hand-Held Units (Point Finders). Point finders can help in determining the proper location of acupuncture points.

- A hand-held unit (Pointer Plus, M.E.D. Servi-Systems Canada, Ltd [Stittsville, Ontario, Canada] or OMS Medical Supplies, Inc.,

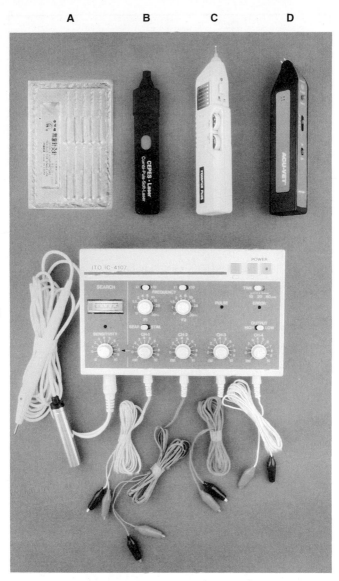

BOX 16-5

Ideal Equipment has the Following Characteristics:

1. Strength and portability.
2. Battery-operated.
3. Outputs for at least six to eight electrodes.
4. Delivers a bipolar waveform $(+)$ and $(-)$ at each electrode to prevent electrolytic injury from prolonged use of monopolar waveform.
5. Delivers a square or spike biphasic waveform.

Braintree, Massachusetts) for locating and stimulating acupuncture and trigger points that uses 10 Hz, 1 to 25 V, and 1 to 50 mA is shown in Fig. 16-2, *C*.

- A second hand-held point locator and therapy unit (ACU-VET, Integra Animal Health, Moraga, California) for noninvasive EAP mode (2.5 Hz) and TENS mode (60 to 80 Hz) is shown in Fig. 16-2, *D*.

Multiple Electronic Acupuncture Device. A multiple electronic acupuncture device is needed to produce PAES at several sites and over longer periods. A compact, attractive, and lightweight model (ITO 4107, OMS Medical Supplies, Inc.) is shown in Fig. 16-2, *E*. The ITO 4107 has the following characteristics:

- It reflects the latest in research and clinical practice in Japan.
- It detects acupuncture and auricular points. Point detection is also displayed by sound and meter.
- It stimulates four pairs of acupuncture needles for analgesia and therapy.
- It generates an equal biphasic pulse form, which has been designed to minimize electrolysis damage to the needles. The polarity of the four channels may be reversed every 30 seconds automatically.
- Two frequencies can be varied between 1 and 300 Hz.
- Automatic safety controls prevent accidental shocking when treatment is initiated or settings are changed.
- It operates on 6 standard 1.5-V size AA batteries.

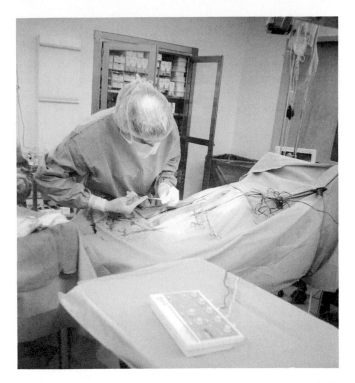

Fig. 16-3 Great Dane, 73 kg; preparation for pyometra surgery. Anesthesia was induced with 2% lidocaine (2.0 mg/kg IV) and propofol (2.0 mg/kg IV), intubation with an endotracheal tube (outer diameter = 14 mm), maintenance of anesthesia with isoflurane (0.5%/2 liters O_2) and PAES at SP 6, ST 36, ST 25 (bilateral) and paraincisional, with 2 Hz/100 Hz alternating frequencies.

Restraint

Technique in Small Animals

- Small animals are generally operated on in lateral, dorsal, or ventral recumbency.
- A sedative or analgesic and small doses of general anesthetics are needed in 50% to 95% of cases to facilitate surgery (Fig. 16-3).

- The animal's elbows and hocks are tied with bandages and secured to the operating table.
- A tape bandage may be tied around a dog's jaws to prevent biting.
- The owner or an attendant should comfort and speak to the nonanesthetized dog from time to time during PAES treatment.

Technique in Large Animals

- EAP for surgical analgesia may be performed in horses and cattle restrained in the standing position or in dorsal, lateral, or ventral recumbency.
- Restraint during nonsurgical PAES treatment may not be necessary if the inserted acupuncture needles are taped or sutured to the skin and are connected to an EAP stimulator that is firmly secured to the horse (Fig. 16-4).
- Usual methods for restraint (e.g., stockade, chute, cattle crate), as applied for surgery performed with local anesthesia, may be used in the standing animal.
- Nervous animals may be given a sedative or analgesic intravenously.

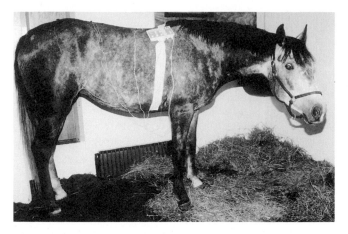

Fig. 16-4 PAES of an unrestrained horse (Warmblood mare, 610 kg, 5 years old, with fracture of transverse process of third cervical vertebra) in its stall. Acupuncture needles are placed at BL 18, BL 23, BL 25, and BL 28 bilaterally and are connected via paired leads to the EAP stimulator (ITO JC 4107), which is secured to the horse with a bandage.

- Recumbency may be induced with a short-acting, intravenous anesthetic.
- Recumbent animals should be securely restrained with ropes.

Selection of Acupuncture Points
General Statements
- Point combinations for induction of hypalgesia sufficient for surgery vary with the operative site and preference of the surgeon.
- Points are generally chosen based on meridian (channel) theory of human acupuncture.
- Acupuncture points in animals have the same names and codes as in humans; they are transposed to animals from human acupuncture anatomy.
- Acupuncture meridians have several courses:
  - Superficial course (from the first to the last point on the meridian).
  - Deep course (going to the organ of the meridian).
  - Collateral course (linking to interior and exterior parts of the body). This may explain why a treatment plan may include a liver point for operation on the eye, a heart point for operation on the tongue, and a kidney point for operations on the ear and bone.
- The area of analgesia is generally related to the site of electrostimulation.
- Segmental or adjacent segmental acupuncture points are selected because the acupuncture stimulus can spread over several segments by ascending and descending collateral branches.

Acupuncture Point Selection in Dogs
- The most commonly used acupuncture points along the two sides of the spine in the dog and surgery sites are summarized in Box 16-6. These points are believed to be similar for the cat but have not been accurately defined or published.
- Most points for surgery in the forelimb, neck, and head are in the forelimb.
- Most points for surgery in the hind limb are in the hind limb.
- Most points for abdominal surgery are on the hind limb, paralumbar region, and ventral abdomen.
- The anatomic locations of various acupuncture points for producing analgesia in the dog are illustrated (Fig. 16-5).

BOX 16-6

**Location of Acupuncture Points
for Producing Analgesia**

For surgery in all areas:
  BL 23 +/or SP 6; LI 11 + Japanese point In Ko Ten; ST 36 +
  Japanese point Bo Ko Ku
For surgery on the head, neck, thorax, and front limb:
  PC 6 + TH 5
For surgery on the abdomen and hind limbs:
  SP 6 + ST 36 and paraincisional for laparotomy
For surgery on high-risk dogs:
  LI 4 + LI 11 + SP 6 + ST 36
For back surgery:
  BL 23 + BL 40 + BL 60 + ST 36 + GB 34

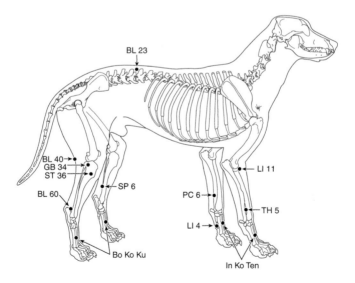

Fig. 16-5 Locations of various acupuncture points to induce analgesia in dogs.

BOX 16-7

Abbreviations and Anatomic Locations of Acupuncture Points in the Dog

1. LI 4 (Large Intestine point 4): between the first and second metacarpal bones, approximately in the middle of the second metacarpal bone on the radial side.
2. LI 11 (Large Intestine point 11): at the end of the lateral cubital crease, halfway between the biceps tendon and the lateral epicondyle of the humerus, with the elbow flexed.
3. PC 6 (Pericardium point 6): at 2 ribs-width above the transverse crease of the carpus between the tendons of the flexor digitorum superficialis and flexor carpi radialis.
4. TH 5 (Triple Heater 5): 2 ribs-width above the carpus, on the cranial aspect of the interosseus space between the radius and ulna.
5. In Ko Ten: between metacarpal bones 2 and 3.
6. BL 23 (Bladder point 23): at one to two ribs-width lateral to the caudal border of spinous process of the second lumbar vertebra.
7. ST 36 (Stomach point 36): one finger-width from the anterior crest of the tibia, in the belly of the musculus tibialis cranialis.
8. GB 34 (Gallbladder point 34): in the depression anterior and distal to the head of the fibula.
9. BL 40 (Bladder point 40): in the center of the popliteal crease.
10. SP 6 (Spleen point 6): three ribs-width directly above the tip of the medial malleolus, on the posterior border of the tibia.
11. BL 60 (Bladder point 60): in the depression, between the lateral malleolus and tendon calcaneus, level with the tip of the lateral malleolus.
12. Bo Ko Ku: between metatarsal bones 2 and 3.

- The abbreviations and locations of these points for producing analgesia by the International Veterinary Acupuncture Society (IVAS) are described in Box 16-7.

Acupuncture Point Selection in Horses (Fig. 16-6)
Abdominal Surgery
- Lung point 1 (LU 1) + Triple Heater point 8 (TH 8) are stimulated using the following technique:
  - One needle is inserted in LU 1 (caudal to the shoulder in the second intercostal space) for a depth of 3 to 5 cm (positive pole).

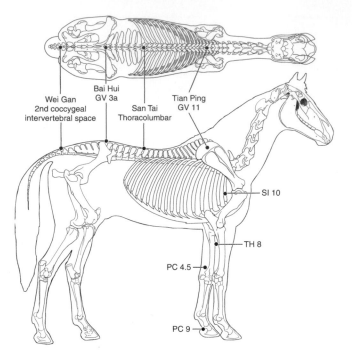

Fig. 16-6 Locations of various acupuncture points to induce analgesia in horses.

- A second needle is placed at TH 8 (approximately one hand-width ventral to the elbow joint, on the lateral side) and is inserted ventromedially caudal to the radius/ulna to reach the pericardium 4.5 point (PC 4.5), subcutaneously dorsal to the "chestnut" (negative pole).
- A third needle is inserted at Small Intestine point 10 (SI 10), which is located on the caudal border of the deltoids and between the long and lateral heads of the triceps brachii.
- A fourth needle is inserted in the center depression between the bulbs of the heel on the forelimb to reach the Pericardium 9 point (PC 9).

Abdominal, Vaginal, and Hind Limb Surgery

- Bai Hui (main point) + Wei Gan (secondary point) + San Tai (tertiary point) + Tian Ping (minor point) + added points on or

near the spinal nerves that supply the surgical area are stimulated with the following technique:
- One needle is inserted in acupuncture point Bai Hui (GV 3a
  point) at the dorsal midline of the lumbosacral space, 3 to
  5 cm deep.
- A second needle is inserted in Wei Gan (at the dorsal midline of
  the second coccygeal intervertebral space), 1 to 1.5 cm deep.
- A third needle is inserted in San Tai (at the dorsal midline of
  the thoracolumbar intervertebral space), 2 to 4 cm deep.
- A fourth needle is inserted at Tian Ping (at the dorsal midline of the fourth or fifth thoracic intervertebral space, GV
  11 point) and advanced cranioventrally 6 to 8 cm.

Acupuncture Point Selection in Cattle
- Most abdominal surgeries in cattle are performed with the animal under local infiltration or regional anesthesia with a local
  anesthetic.
- Electrostimulation at the anterior end of the transverse process of
  the first lumbar vertebra (Yao Pang 1), the posterior end
  of the transverse process of the second lumbar vertebra (Yao
  Pang 2), and the posterior end of transverse process of the fourth
  lumbar vertebra (Yao Pang 4) has been given to nine Korean na-
  tive cattle sedated with 2% xylazine (0.5 ml/kg IM).
  - Currents ranging from 2 to 9 V and a frequency of 30 Hz
    were used.
  - A latency period of 10 to 25 minutes was required to induce
    regional analgesia of the flank.
  - Analgesia for abdominal operations, including four laparot-
    omies, three rumenotomies, and two omentopexies, was con-
    sidered to be good in six heads of nine (68%), fair in one
    (11%), and poor in two (22%).
  - All cattle remained standing.
- Various acupuncture points for producing surgical analgesia in
  cattle have been described.
- The locations of various acupuncture points to induce analgesia
  in cattle are illustrated (Fig. 16-7).

Acupuncture Point Selection in Pigs
- The Akita Veterinary Acupuncture Research Unit in Japan tested
  many point combinations in pigs, including LU 1 and TH 8 penetrating to PC 4.5.

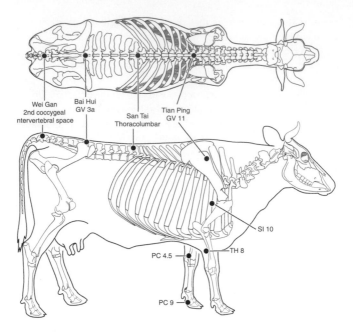

Fig. 16-7 Locations of various acupuncture points to induce analgesia in cattle.

- The most effective points for producing hypalgesia are located in the midline of the thoracolumbar space (point Tian Ping) and lumbosacral spaces (Bai Hui) penetrating almost to the dura mater spinalis.

Precautions for PAES Technique

For precautions, see Box 16-8.

Needle Placement for PAES in Dogs

- Acupuncture points are palpated at precise anatomic landmarks.
- Point finders (see Fig. 16-2, *C* and *D*) are helpful in localizing the points.
- The needles are inserted deeply into the acupuncture points.
  - The needle penetrates completely from TH 5 to PC 6 between the radius and ulna of both limbs. The needle also

---

BOX 16-8
Precautions When Performing PAES Technique

- A conductive surface (metal table) should not be used.
- Animals should not be wet.
- A bath must not be given 24 hours before the acupuncture treatment.
- The pairs of needles should be attached to each circuit of the electrostimulator by using alligator clips.
- The clips of the electrodes should be firmly attached to the needles, avoiding any entrapment of hairs.
- Each pair of electrodes should be on the same side of the spinal cord.
- Any one pair of leads must not cross the spine between the cervical and thoracic vertebrae (e.g., BL 13 to BL 13; SP 21 to SP 21; LIV 14 to LIV 14) to prevent interference with cardiac function and, on rare occasions, cardiac arrest caused by ventricular fibrillation.
- All control knobs of the stimulator must be set at zero at the beginning and before the needles are taken off at the end of the PAES treatment to prevent electrical spikes to the animal.
- Environmental noise and commotion should be kept to a minimum to keep a conscious animal calm.
- Unnecessary blunt dissection and traction on internal organs must be minimized.

---

penetrates completely through the limb at ST 36 and SP 6 of both hind limbs.

- The needles are twirled, then bent and taped or sutured in position to prevent dislodgement.
- For electrostimulation, the needles are connected in pairs to the output socket of a multiple electronic acupuncture device.
- The leads may be alternated between needles, if more needles than can be stimulated simultaneously are used.

PAES Stimulation

- The power switch is turned on, and the electrical stimulation frequencies F1 and F2 are preferentially set at 2 and 100 Hz, respectively (see Fig. 16-1, bottom strip).
- The output voltage is increased slowly until the needles begin to twitch in time with the frequency of the stimulator at 2 Hz.

BOX 16-9

Intensity of Stimulation

The intensity of stimulation is traditionally increased until muscle fas-
ciculation is seen at 1 to 5 Hz. This produces:
• General analgesia with prolonged induction.
• Prolonged analgesia after cessation of stimulation.
• Analgesia that is endorphin-mediated.
• Analgesia that is reversible by naloxone.

At the high frequency (100 Hz), the muscle goes into local
spasm and the needle vibration is not obvious.
• The output voltage from each control is first increased to maximum tolerance of anesthesia mode, dense-disperse waveform. The
output is then reduced to a level that is tolerated without obvious
discomfort or pain, restlessness, struggling, and vocalization.
• The polarity does not need to be considered if bipolar waveforms
are used. Best results with unipolar waveforms are obtained with
placement of the negative terminal peripherally and placement
of the positive terminal at the vertex.

Amplitude of Stimulation (Box 16-9)
• An intensity of 1 to 3 mA is used clinically to produce nonpainful
fasciculation of the muscles in which the needle is embedded.
• The output current may be slightly increased to 3 to 5 mA during periods of strong painful stimuli, which are caused by incis-
ing the skin, peritoneum, pleura, periosteum, or nerves and by
suturing the peritoneum and skin.
• Higher amplitudes (beyond 5 mA) may cause pain and stress.
Stress-induced analgesia depends in part on diffuse noxious inhibitory control and is not a usual part of acupuncture analgesia.

Onset of Hypalgesia
• The onset and duration of hypalgesia are variable. Segmental
acupuncture analgesia usually occurs rapidly. Generalized opiate
effects take 20 to 40 minutes.
• At least 10 to 30 minutes are generally needed to produce and release endogenous opioid-like peptides: endorphins, enkephalins,

and dynorphins. The morphine-like substances are produced in the hypothalamus and are released into the cerebrospinal fluid (CSF) and blood.
- Analgesia produced by the endogenous opioid-like peptides generally occurs within 20 minutes after acupuncture and PAES administration.
- Induction time for hypalgesia can be prolonged from 20 to 40 minutes, depending on site of surgery, frequency (in Hz) of stimulation, and intensity of stimulation.
- The surgery site is tested for analgesia every 5 minutes after onset of electrical stimulation by grasping the skin with tooth forceps or clamps or by pricking the site with needles.

Duration of PAES Stimulation
- PAES stimulation is continued during the entire operation or for at least 30 minutes to relieve neuropathic inflammatory, somatic, and miscellaneous pain.
- The duration of stimulation may change the mechanism of analgesia from opiate to nonopiate.
- Inadequate or excessive PAES stimulus produces little or no analgesia.
- Long periods of PAES (>3 hours) should not be applied to prevent the development of tolerance.

Published Articles for Humans and Small and Large Animals
Humans
Complementary and alternative (integrative) pain therapy in humans with acupuncture, EAP, TENS, and PENS has been reported (Box 16-10). Analgesia depended on the following:
- Stimulation site
- Frequency (in Hz) of electrical stimulation
- Intensity of electrical stimulation
- Duration of electrical stimulation
- Type of surgical procedure
- The patient's psychologic profile

Small Animals
Complementary and alternative (integrative) pain therapy in dogs and cats with acupuncture or EAP, surgical EAP or PAES, and

---

BOX 16-10
Results with the Use of Acupuncture, EAP, TENS, and PENS

Most investigators have reported the following results with the use of acupuncture, EAP, TENS, and PENS:

- Improved pain relief.
- Decreased narcotic requirements (by up to 50%).
- Shortened recovery room stay.
- Increased postoperative mobility and activity level.
- Reduced postoperative side effects (e.g., pulmonary complications).

---

combined use of acupuncture and EAP has been reported. In one study, surgical analgesia of the abdomen in 20 dogs was produced for periods of 30 to 50 minutes by using a combined technique: xylazine (1.5 mg/kg of body weight, diluted in 10 ml of lactated Ringer's solution) was injected into acupuncture points TH 8, TH 17, BL 23, and SP 6 on both sides of the spine and then after acupuncture needles had been inserted into SP 6, ST 36, GB 34, and ST 25 (bilateral) EAP was applied with 6 to 9 V and 3 Hz to the needles during 20 to 30 minutes of induction and 15 to 20 Hz thereafter for maintenance analgesia during abdominal surgery.

Large Animals
- Variable analgesia in horses, cattle, sheep, and pigs after use of acupuncture and EAP/PAES for complementary and alternative (integrative) pain therapy has been reported.
- Controlled and blinded studies on opioid requirements, duration of surgical recovery, and pulmonary complications of animals treated with complementary and alternative pain therapy have not been reported.

Location, Intensity, and Frequency of Electrical Stimulation
Important determinants of analgesic efficacy in humans are the location of stimulation, the intensity of stimulation, and the frequency (in Hz) of stimulation.

Location of Stimulation

- In rats, the analgesic effect induced by three types of stimulation such as acupuncture, EAP, and TENS has been compared. The results of this study indicated that EAP produces greater analgesic effects when compared with acupuncture, whereas EAP and TENS (2 Hz, 15 Hz, 100 Hz) produced similar effects of increased tail flick latencies in rats.
- In human volunteers, EAP was reported to be more effective than manual acupuncture and as effective as TENS for pain relief.
- EAP at Chinese acupoint Hegu (Large Intestine point 4) and Zusanli (Stomach point 36) and TENS stimulation at dermatomal levels corresponding to the site of surgical incision in humans significantly decreased postoperative requirements for opioid narcotics and incidence of opioid-related side effects.

Stimulation Frequency

- The frequency of stimulation affects both the fibers in a typical sensory nerve and the neurotransmitters in the brain and spinal cord, which are involved in pain perception response.
- A mixed pattern (2 Hz/100 Hz) of electrical stimulation has been used and investigated most in controlled and blinded studies in humans.
- The alternating stimulation at 15-Hz and 30-Hz frequency selection in patients with chronic lower lumbar back pain, when compared with either low (4 Hz) or high (100 Hz) frequencies alone, produced, at the end of a 2-week treatment period, the greatest decrease in pain, improvement in physical activity and quality of sleep, and decrease in requirements for oral opioid narcotics.

Effect of Frequency on Nerve Fibers

Different-diameter nerve fibers have different characteristics, and sinusoid waveform stimulation permits neuroselectivity (Box 16-11). The fiber profile of a typical sensory nerve has been described. It is illustrated in Fig. 16-8.

- C fibers and A-delta (Aδ) fibers conduct pain. The pain conducted by C fibers is dull and burning. Aδ fibers, when compared with C fibers, are 5 to 15 times thicker, transmit impulses 10 times faster, have a lower threshold, and are associated with faster and sharper pain sensations than C fibers.

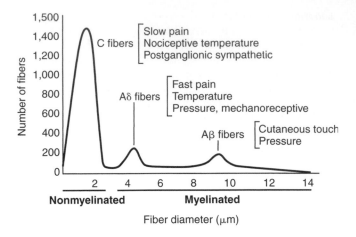

Fig. 16-8 Fiber spectra profile of a sensory C fiber. (From Katims JJ: *Pain Digest* 8:219, 1998.)

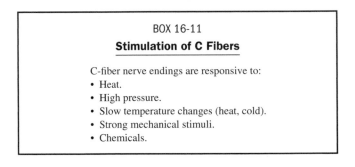

BOX 16-11

Stimulation of C Fibers

C-fiber nerve endings are responsive to:
- Heat.
- High pressure.
- Slow temperature changes (heat, cold).
- Strong mechanical stimuli.
- Chemicals.

- Large-diameter myelinated fibers can respond to the rapid 100-Hz stimulus.
- Small unmyelinated fibers respond to a slow frequency stimulus (2 to 10 Hz) because they require several milliseconds of continuous depolarization to respond.
- PAES and TENS have been demonstrated to excite the classically defined cutaneous A fibers, B fibers, C fibers, and polymodal C fibers (those unmyelinated afferents that are responsive to mechanical and heat stimuli in sympathetic C fibers).

Effect of Frequency on Neurotransmitters

Neurotransmitters involved in acupuncture therapy and pain inhibition include the body's endogenous substances.

- Endorphins: β-endorphin, met-enkephalin, and dynorphin.
- Neurochemical substances: serotonin (5-hydroxytryptamine [5-HT]), norepinephrine, acetylcholine, and dopamine.
- Each of the three families of endorphins, enkephalins, and dynorphins has its specific action and can be precipitated by various techniques of PAES and TENS stimulation.
  - The endorphins act in the brain.
  - The enkephalins act in the brain and spinal cord.
  - Endorphins and enkephalins are powerful modulators of pain arising from the musculoskeletal system.
  - The dynorphins act primarily at the spinal level. Dynorphins are potent blockers of visceral pain.
- Low-frequency stimulation (1 to 2 Hz, 1 to 2 cycles per second) has been reported to increase the release of endorphins and enkephalins over stimulated segments in humans, thereby producing a more generalized analgesia. This was not the case with high-frequency stimulation.
- An increase in the concentration of β-endorphin, but not enkephalin, was detected in human spinal fluid when EAP (2 to 3 Hz during 30 minutes) was given for treatment of recurrent pain.
- High-frequency stimulation (100 Hz) has produced segmental visceral analgesia, attributable to release of dynorphin at the spinal level, and segmental analgesia that was not reversible with naloxone.
- High-frequency/low-intensity stimulation has also resulted in local segmental analgesia, which was not reversed by naloxone.

Effect of Frequency on Analgesia

- Frequencies below 1 Hz and beyond 100 Hz provide no additional benefit.
- Low-frequency stimulation (4 Hz) has been reported to have a greater analgesic effect than high-frequency stimulation (100 Hz) in an experimental study of ischemic pain.
- In contrast, one study indicated that the use of high-frequency stimulation produced greater analgesic effects on cold-induced pain in healthy subjects.

304 PART THREE PAIN MANAGEMENT

- A mild range of frequency (12 to 15 Hz) or alternation of low and high frequencies (2 Hz and 100 Hz) has produced a synergistic analgesic effect by using all three opioid peptides.
- Comparable analgesic effects at both low and high frequencies of stimulation have also been reported in humans.

Mechanism of Acupuncture Analgesia

- The mechanisms of action of acupuncture, EAP (PAES), TENS, and PENS have been extensively reviewed and are still not completely understood.
- The following theories have been described:
  - Specificity.
  - Summation.
  - Pattern.
  - Gate.
  - Two gates.
  - Humeral pain mechanisms.
  - Neurogenic pain mechanisms.
- Analgesia elicited by acupuncture has been described as a result of activation of acupuncture points that are cutaneous areas with high concentrations of nerve endings (particularly Aδ and C fibers), mast cells, capillaries, and venules. These areas have a lower electrical resistance than the surrounding areas.
- After needle stimulation, afferent Aδ and C fibers carry impulses to the spinal cord. The impulses travel through the anterolateral tract of the spinal cord to the hypothalamic-pituitary system, which releases β-endorphin and met-enkephalin into the periaqueductal gray matter (PAG), CSF, and blood. This has two actions:
  - First, β-endorphin and met-enkephalin are released to activate the raphe nuclei and bring into play the descending inhibitory system.
  - Second, a mesolimbic loop of analgesia releasing serotonin and met-enkephalin is activated at the supraspinal level. It is postulated that in patients with chronic pain, the mesolimbic loop is "warmed up."
- The inhibitory pathway affects the dorsal horn cells of the spinal cord (which receives nociceptive impulses) to release the following neurotransmitters to elicit analgesia:
  - Met-enkephalin.
  - Dynorphin.

- Serotonin (5-HT).
- Norepinephrine.
- Acetylcholine.
- After a relatively brief (20 minutes) period of PAES and TENS stimulation, a self-sustained resetting of the pain-modulation pathway is set up, which may well account for the long-term analgesic effects frequently seen in clinical practice.
- Acupuncture needles stimulate nerve endings in the skin and deeper structures such as muscles, tendons, and fascia.
- The large, myelinated group II afferent nerve fibers of type A-beta (Aβ) and A-gamma (Aγ) conduct impulses to the CNS from pressure receptors, stretch receptors, and muscle spindles.

Hypothesis of PAES Analgesic Mechanism

- The acupuncture- and PAES-induced analgesic effects may well result from different sites: peripheral, spinal ("pain inhibition gates"), and central levels of activation of descending brain-based pain inhibition mechanisms, especially the midbrain and hypothalamus.
- Most recent findings indicate that analgesia is produced by electrical stimulation of certain receptor sites in the dorsal horn of the spinal cord, resulting in release of endorphins and enkephalins.
- Alternatively, peripheral electrical stimulation of large sensory afferent nerves modulates nociceptive input in the dorsal horn of the spinal cord, producing analgesia ("gate control theory" of pain).
- One hypothesis is that acupuncture and PAES cause analgesia by stimulation of Aβ and Aγ fibers by releasing endorphin and enkephalin, which attach to serotonin (5-HT) receptors in the substantia gelatinosa (layers II and III of the dorsal horn of the spinal cord) to release serotonin. Serotonin in turn inhibits the release of substance P (NK1), which activates the pain pathway, thereby inhibiting the pain pathway (Fig. 16-9).
- It is also hypothesized that acupuncture and PAES stimulation activate descending inhibitory pathways (Fig. 16-10) through serotonin, norepinephrine, acetylcholine, and nitric oxide.
- Substance P needs to be further investigated in the PAES process.

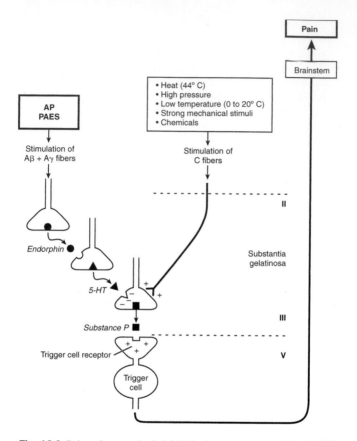

Fig. 16-9 Pain pathway and pain inhibition by acupuncture *(AP)* and PAES. The release and binding of endorphin, serotonin *(5-HT)*, and substance P from and to receptors in the substantia gelatinosa change the pain pattern caused by noxious stimuli into a "nonpain" message.

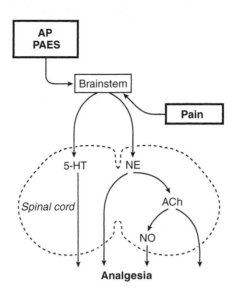

Fig. 16-10 Acupuncture *(AP)* and PAES cause analgesia in large part by activating descending inhibitory pathways, of which descending spinal noradrenergic pathways in the brainstem and spinal cord are among the most important. *5-HT,* Serotonin; *NE,* norepinephrine; *Ach,* acetylcholine; *NO,* nitric oxide.

Advantages of PAES

- PAES can induce hypalgesia sufficient for surgery.
- It can be used in "balanced anesthesia" to greatly reduce the dose of sedatives or analgesics and anesthetic drugs.
- It is advantageous in cesarean section because it has no depressive effects on the fetus.
- It is suitable for animals that are in shock, debilitated, toxic, and have organ disease (heart, lung, liver, kidney) or a low tolerance to general anesthetics.
- When compared with general anesthesia, PAES is a relatively simple and inexpensive technique:
  - Hemorrhage is minimal.
  - Recovery of appetite and gut and bladder function are fast.

- Healing is fast because there is no chemical interference with wound healing.
- Postoperative infection is minimal.
- Postoperative pain is reduced.

Disadvantages of PAES

- An induction period of 10 to 40 minutes (average, 20 minutes) is necessary.
- Sedatives and anesthetics are needed in 50% to 95% of patients to facilitate surgery.
- Physical restraint is necessary.
- Prolonged restraint may be necessary, depending on the skill of the surgeon and tolerance of the patient.
- Muscle relaxation may be inadequate.
- Poor relaxation of abdominal muscles can cause "ballooning" of viscera.
- All sensory inputs except pain are present.
- Manipulation of viscera and organs or traction of mesentery can induce nausea, vomiting, and shock.
- Certain body regions are more sensitive to pain than other regions. Very sensitive tissues are skin, serosa (peritoneum, pleura), periosteum, and nerves.
- There are individual differences with regard to pain threshold and temperament of animals.
- Nervous animals may be good responders but are easily frightened and difficult to restrain despite good analgesia.

Tolerance

- Acupuncture is not for everyone. Tolerance to PAES, which has a time course similar to that seen with repeated doses of morphine, can occur because of fast enzymatic breakdown of enkephalins (met-enkephalin, leu-enkephalin) into nonanalgesic metabolic substances. Tolerance also can occur as a result of stimulation of antiopiate systems by nonopioid endogenous peptides, such as cholecystokinin (CCK) and angiotensin II.
- CCK antagonizes PAES-induced analgesia in rats. CCK may be involved in a constant percentage of animals that are nonresponders to PAES.
- Captopril, the highly specific angiotensin-converting enzyme antagonist, blocks the degeneration of enkephalins. It shows

promise in the reversal of PAES tolerance. It augments analgesia induced by acupuncture-related techniques.

- Antagonism of analgesia by naloxone, an opioid receptor antagonist, provides evidence for the involvement of endogenous opioids in the analgesic effects produced by acupuncture and related techniques—EAP/PAES, TENS, and PENS.

LASER THERAPY

- The term *laser* is an acronym for "Light Amplification by Stimulated Emission of Radiation."
- The light energy is absorbed by the cells within the tissue, resulting in physiologic and metabolic changes involved in the healing process and pain relief.
- Laser therapy is based on photochemical but not thermal effects. The laser energy stimulates the mitochondria for adenosine triphosphate synthesis via the respiratory chain (the so-called oxidative phosphorylation).

Effects of Laser Therapy

- Improved cell respiration.
- Neovascularization.
- Synthesis of collagen/protein.
- Phagocytosis of leukocytes.
- Stimulation of the immune system.

Laser Units Commonly Used in Veterinary Acupuncture

- Helium-neon gas tube (a red light emitter), which produces a wavelength of 632 to 650 nm that can penetrate tissues to a depth of 0.8 to 15 mm.
- Gallium arsenite diode (an infrared light emitter), which produces a wavelength of 904 nm that can penetrate to a depth of 10 mm to 5 cm.

Products of Exact Biofrequencies in Already Programmed or Programmable Lasers

- Optimal energy density.
- Maximum power.
- Exact frequency information.
- Precise application optics (resonance phenomenon).

Conditions Treated by Various Laser Equipment

- Open wounds.
- Burns.
- Ulcers.
- Pressure sores.
- Prevention of proud flesh formation.
- Resolution of swelling from inflammation.
- Musculoskeletal conditions:
  - Back pain and injury.
  - Tendinitis.
  - Suspensory injuries.
  - Ligament injuries.
  - Shin splints.
  - Sprains.
  - Arthritis.
  - Founder.
  - Navicular disease.
  - Quick (5 to 60 seconds) stimulation of acupuncture points.

Failed treatment responses are most likely attributed to delivery of inadequate dosages of energy.

Powerful, Portable, and Rechargeable Battery-Operated Lasers with Interchangeable Attachments to Treat Various-Sized Areas

- Thor DD laser (Electronics Inc., United States).
- Respond 2400 Laser Therapy System (Respond Systems, Inc., United States).
- The Everlase medical laser (M.E.D. Servi-Systems Canada Ltd) is shown in Fig. 16-11. It allows selection of preprogrammed Nogier frequencies for desired therapeutic effects: pain relief, tissue regeneration, and muscle relaxation. The tissue is penetrated by an infrared wavelength of 905 nm and power of pulses of 12,000 mW.
- The CEPES Magnetic laser (M.E.D. Servi-Systems Canada Ltd), which combines both laser and magnetic field therapy in a single, compact instrument (see Fig. 16-2, *B*). It generates a pulsing magnetic field in the electroencephalographic (EEG) (brain wave) range with harmonics up to the MHz level and 0.5 mW red "soft" laser to treat specific ear and body acupuncture points and trigger points.

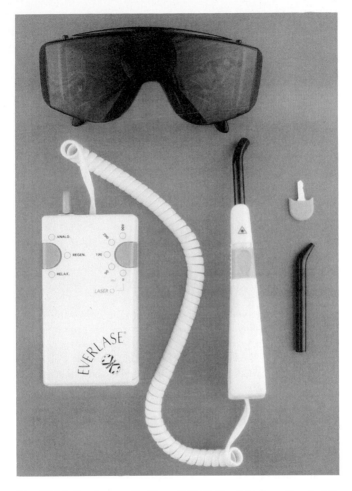

Fig. 16-11 Everlase medical laser (M.E.D. Servi-Systems Canada Ltd, Sittsville, Ontario, Canada) for pain relief, tissue regeneration, and muscle relaxation, with protective eyeglasses.

Advantages of Laser Therapy

- Laser therapy is a safe and painless form of therapy.
- It requires short treatment periods.
- Minimal animal restraint during the treatment is necessary.
- Lasers are especially useful in treating leg acupuncture points in horses and cattle when needle placement is considered challenging and dangerous to the operator.
- Lasers are useful adjuncts to natural healing methods, but they should not be used to replace acupuncture needles.

Disadvantages of Laser Therapy

- The cost for a laser unit is from $2000 to several thousands of dollars, if an option to lease is not available.
- Lasers have a reduced ability to stimulate and balance acupuncture points in comparison with needles.
- Few studies have compared the efficacy of one type of laser with that of another.

PULSED MAGNETIC FIELD THERAPY

- PMFT is a method of applying a magnetic field with an extremely low range of frequencies to the cell for promoting the healing of damaged tissue.
- The concept of using magnets for healing the body goes back thousands of years to ancient Greece, Egypt, and China.
- Recent studies about repair of bone fractures and delayed union fractures have suggested that acupuncture analgesia and healing properties may be mediated by changing electromagnetic fields in the body.
- Pulsating magnetic fields have been used since the 1970s on dogs, small animals, and performance horses, such as show horses and thoroughbred race horses, to alleviate pain originating from acute and chronic sore backs, arthritic joints, inflamed tendons, and inflamed tendon sheaths.
- The size and composition of the magnet determine the strength of the magnetic field, which subsequently determines the depth of tissue penetration.
- During magnetic therapy, the hydrogen and oxygen molecules in the water of blood and iron become magnetically polarized

and align with other components in the blood. The charged molecules aggregate, then travel throughout the body more efficiently, thus allowing the blood's nourishing energy to more effectively support healing and recovery.

Effectiveness of Magnetic Field Therapy

- Magnetic field therapy is effective for pain management and healing at very low power.
- Magnetic field therapy systems use multiform pulses of alternating (oscillating positive and negative) electromagnetic induction fields, which mimic the body's waveforms.
- Frequencies ranging from 0.5 to 5 Hz are beneficial for:
  - Reducing blood loss.
  - Infections.
  - Inflammation.
  - Degenerative joint diseases.
  - Generalized pain.
- Frequencies of 5 to 18 Hz aid in:
  - Muscle toning.
  - Improving circulation.

Accessories That Deliver Pulsating Magnetic Therapy

- Applicator pads.
- Generator.
- Magnetic field tester (e.g., Magna Vet 995 VG System, Integra Animal Health).
- Jackets for dogs and small animals.
- Beds for dogs and small animals.
- Blankets, neck wraps, hocks, and leggings for horses (e.g., Respond Systems, Inc.)
- Legging wraps with or without hoof and knee coils may be used to aid healing of foot injuries (chronic navicular, abscess) and knee injuries.
- Hock boots with two coils are designed for therapy of hocks with trauma, arthritic conditions, spurs, spavin, and poor circulation.
- Neck wraps with four coils relax tight muscles and extend the neck.
- A Bio-Pulse 3000 Magnetic Therapy Blanket System with 10 coils (Respond Systems, Inc.) was produced in 1992 to cover major muscle groups and joints of horses for complete PMFT.

HERBAL REMEDIES

- Herbal medicines rarely produce any complications when given alone; however, they may contribute to the development of interactions and reactions when used in combination with opioids, α_2-agonists, or anesthetics. They are generally discontinued 2 weeks before surgery because of their potential to cause increased bleeding and prolonged recovery from anesthesia.
- Examples are: arnica, angelica, comfrey, bogbean, devil's claw, echinacea, ginkgo, ginseng, garlic, guaiacum, Jamaican dogwood, St. John's wort, thyme, and valerian.
- Herbal remedies may be useful for long-term pain control because of their antiinflammatory and muscle-relaxing effects. They are inadequate for acute traumatic and surgical pain.

LEGAL AND ETHICAL ISSUES

- Legal briefs in the *Journal of the American Veterinary Medical Association* in 1987 indicate that the use of acupuncture needles constitutes a surgical procedure under the state veterinary practice act *(1987 American Veterinary Medical Association [AVMA] Directory)*.
- The *AVMA Directory and Resource Manual 1997* indicated that techniques of using acupuncture needles, moxibustion (heat), injections, low-level lasers, and magnets should be regarded as surgical or medical procedures under state veterinary practice acts. The manual also indicates that veterinarians should complete educational programs before they are considered competent to practice veterinary acupuncture.
- The AVMA guidelines for complementary, alternative, and integrative medicine in 2001 proposed that all veterinary medicine and complementary and alternative veterinary medicine practices, including acupuncture, should be held to the same standards. Claims for safety and effectiveness ultimately should be proven by scientific methods. Practices and philosophies that are ineffective or unsafe should be discarded.
- No regulation, however, exists to ensure the competence of a licensed veterinarian to practice acupuncture and related techniques on animal patients.

TRAINING AND CERTIFICATION

- Training of specialization in veterinary acupuncture can be obtained through the IVAS and Colorado State University.
- IVAS-certified members can also become members of the American Academy of Veterinary Acupuncture (AAVA).
- The addresses, phone numbers, E-mail addresses, and Web sites of the IVAS, Colorado State University, and AAVA are listed in Appendix 16-2.
- The Internet is an excellent source of information on professional acupuncture (see Appendix 16-3).

SUMMARY

- The public interest in complementary and alternative (integrative) pain therapy has opened the door for those in the veterinary medical field to step forward.
- Veterinarians are warming up to acupuncture and acupuncture-related techniques. Some remain unconvinced (see Appendix 16-4).
- Even as the public and professional interest grows, the paucity of research data makes it difficult for the veterinary medical establishment to evaluate its effectiveness.
- Advances in understanding animals' endogenous pain control mechanisms should allow for improvement of therapics aimed at producing analgesia by stimulation, such as acupuncture and PAES.
- Acupuncture and PAES show great promise in the relief of severe, chronic pain.
- Rather than viewing acupuncture- and PAES-induced analgesia as an alternative treatment, veterinarians should regard it as complementary to standard veterinary medical practice.

SUGGESTED READINGS

1987 American Veterinary Medical Association directory, Schaumburg, Ill, 1987, American Veterinary Medical Association.

Akamas JJ: Electroacupuncture anesthesia of dogs, *Jpn J Vet Anesth* 7:70-72, 1976.

Ali J, Yaffe CS, Serrette C: The effect of transcutaneous electric nerve stimulation on postoperative pain and pulmonary function, *Surgery* 89:507-512, 1981.

Almay BG, Johansson F, von Knorring L, et al: Relationships between CSF levels of endorphins and monoamine metabolites in chronic pain patients, *Psychopharmacology* 67:139-142, 1980.

Altman S: Acupuncture therapy in small animal practice, *Compendium Small Animal* 19:1233-1245, 1977.

Bayindir O, Paker T, Akpinar B, et al: Use of transcutaneous electrical nerve stimulation in the control of postoperative chest pain after cardiac surgery, *J Cardiothorac Vasc Anesth* 5:589-591, 1991.

Becker RO, Selden G: The ticklish gene. In Becker RO, editor: *The body electric: electromagnetism and the foundation of life,* New York, 1985, Quill, William Morrow.

Benedetti F, Amanzio M, Casadio C, et al: Control of postoperative pain by transcutaneous electrical nerve stimulation after thoracic operations, *Ann Thorac Surg* 63:773-776, 1997.

Bossut DF, Leshin LS, Stromberg MW, et al: Plasma cortisol and beta-endorphin in horse subject to electro-acupuncture for cutaneous analgesia, *Peptides* 4:501-507, 1983.

Bossut DF, Page EH, Stromberg MW: Production of cutaneous analgesia by electroacupuncture in horses: variations dependent on sex of subject and locus of stimulation, *Am J Vet Res* 45:620-625, 1984.

Bossut DF, Stromberg MW, Malven PV: Electroacupuncture-induced analgesia in sheep: measurement of cutaneous pain threshold and plasma concentrations of prolactin and beta-endorphin immunoreactivity, *Am J Vet Res* 47:669-676, 1986.

Chen L, Tang J, White PF, et al: The effect of location of transcutaneous electrical nerve stimulation on postoperative opioid analgesic requirement: acupoint versus nonacupoint stimulation, *Anesth Analg* 87:1129-1134, 1998.

Cheng RS, Pomeranz B: Electroacupuncture could be mediated by at least 2 pain-relieving mechanisms: endorphin and non-endorphin systems, *Life Sci* 25:1957-1962, 1979.

Cheng RS, Pomeranz B: Electroacupuncture is mediated by stereospecific opiate receptors and is reversed by antagonist of type I receptors, *Life Sci* 26: 631-638, 1979.

Christensen PA, Rotne M, Vedelsdal R, et al: Electroacupuncture in anaesthesia for hysterectomy, *Br J Anaesth* 71:835-838, 1993.

Clement-Jones V, McLoughlin L, Tomlin S, et al: Increased beta-endorphin but not met-enkephalin levels in human cerebrospinal fluid after acupuncture for recurrent pain, *Lancet* 2:946-948, 1980.

Faris PL, Komisaruk BR, Watkins LR, et al: Evidence for the neuropeptide cholecystokinin as an antagonist of opiate analgesia, *Science* 219:310-312, 1983.

Frost EAM, Hsu CY: Neurophysiological pathways in acupuncture, *Am J Acupunct* 3:331-335, 1975.

Ghoname ES, Craig WF, White PF, et al: The effect of stimulus frequency on the analgesic response to percutaneous electrical nerve stimulation in patients with chronic low back pain, *Anesth Analg* 88:841-846, 1999.

Giles LGF, Muller R: Chronic spinal pain syndromes: a clinical pilot trial comparing acupuncture, a nonsteroidal anti-inflammatory drug, and spinal manipulation, *J Manipulative Physiol Ther* 22:376-381, 1999.

Gonzalez MV, Sumano HL, Ocampo LC, et al: Induction of surgical analgesia of the abdomen in dogs by electro-acupuncture, *Brochure Pratique d'Acupuncture Veterinaire* 9:14-15, 1989.

Ha H, Tan EC, Fukunaga H, et al: Naloxone reversal of acupuncture analgesia in the monkey, *Exp Neurol* 73:298-303, 1981.

Hamza MA, White PF, Ahmed HE, et al: Effect of the frequency of transcutaneous electrical nerve stimulation on the postoperative opioid analgesic requirement and recovery profile, *Anesthesiology* 91:1232-1238, 1999.

Han JS, Chen XH, Sun SL, et al: Effect of low- and high-frequency TENS on Met-enkephalin-Arg-Phe and dynorphin A immunoreactivity in human lumbar CSF, *Pain* 47:295-298, 1991.

Han JS, Ding XZ, Fan SG: Is cholecystokinin octapeptide (CCK-8) a candidate for endogenous anti-opioid substrates? *Neuropeptides* 5:399-401, 1985.

Han JS, Terenius L: Neurochemical basis of acupuncture analgesia, *Annu Rev Pharmacol Toxicol* 22:193-220, 1982.

Hansson P, Ekblom A: Afferent stimulation induced pain relief in acute orofacial pain and its failure to induce sufficient pain reduction in dental and oral surgery, *Pain* 15:157-165, 1983.

Harata et al: Acupuncture anesthesia for bovine clinic in the field, *Clin Vet Med* 5:44-48, 1987.

Hargreaves A, Lander J: Use of transcutaneous electrical nerve stimulation for postoperative pain, *Nurs Res* 38:159-161, 1989.

Ho WKK, Wen HL: Opioid-like activity in the cerebrospinal fluid of patients treated with electroacupuncture, *Neuropharmacology* 28:961-966, 1989.

Iamaguti P, Gandolfi W, Nicoletti, et al: Electroacupuncture for abdominal surgery in dogs, *Ver Bras Med Vet* 4:20-22, 1981.

Iseki S et al: Interpretation of analgesia of the abdomen, loin, and rear under electroacupuncture analgesia on the dog, *J Vet Med* 684:39-43, 1978.

Iseki S et al: Interpretation of analgesia of the head and neck under electroacupuncture analgesia on the dog, *J Vet Med* 683:39-43, 1978.

Ishizaki S: Electroacupuncture analgesia in high-risk dogs, *Jpn J Vet Anesth* 8:21-28, 1977.

Jang W, Suh DS, Park NY, et al: Experimental studies on the wound healing under medicament and acupuncture anesthesia in dogs, *Korean J Vet Res* 24:110-119, 1984.

Janssens LA: Acupuncture for thoracolumbar and cervical disc disease. In Schoen AM, editor: *Problems in veterinary medicine: veterinary acupuncture,* Philadelphia, 1992, JB Lippincott.

Janssens LA: Acupuncture for thoracolumbar and cervical disc disease. In Schoen AM, editor: *Veterinary acupuncture: ancient art to modern medicine,* ed 2, St Louis, 2001, Mosby.

Janssens LA, Rogers PA, Schoen AM: Acupuncture analgesia: a review, *Vet Rec* 122:355-358, 1988.

Janssens LAA: Analgesic acupuncture in veterinary small animal practice. In *Acupuncture in animals,* Proceedings 167, Australian Veterinary Acupuncture Association, Sydney, 1991, pp 89-91.

Janssens LAA: Canine disc disease: a survey of acupuncture therapy. In Janssens L, editor: *Some aspects of small animal acupuncture,* Brussels, 1989, Belgian Acupuncture Society.

Janssens LAA, Rogers PAM, Schoen AM: Acupuncture analgesia. In *Acupuncture in animals,* Proceedings 167, Australian Veterinary Acupuncture Association, Sydney, 1991, pp 83-87.

Jessel T, Iversen L: Opiate analgesics inhibit substance P release from rat trigeminal nucleus, *Nature* 268:724-727, 1977.

Jin Y: *Electroacupuncture anesthesia (EAA) in the dog,* International Conference on Veterinary Acupuncture, Beijing, 1987, p 106.

Johnson MI, Ashton CH, Bousfield DR, et al: Analgesic effect of different frequencies of transcutaneous electrical nerve stimulation on cold-induced pain in normal subjects, *Pain* 39:231-236, 1989.

Kaneko et al: *Angiotensin II as a physiological opioid antagonist,* International Narcotic Research Conference, Cape Cod, Massachusetts, June 1985, p 181 (abstract).

Katims JJ: Electrodiagnostic functional sensory evaluation of the patient with pain: a review of the neuroselective current perception threshold and pain tolerance threshold, *Pain Digest* 8:219-230, 1998.

Kazawa et al: Laparotomy using electro-acupuncture anesthesia in cattle, *J Vet Clin* 154:10-14, 1976.

Kho HG, Robertson EN: The mechanisms of acupuncture analgesia: review and update, *Am J Acupunct* 25:261-281, 1997.

Kitazawa K, Ohno K, Kadono H: Studies on electroacupuncture analgesia in the dog: confirmation of the effect, *Jpn J Vet Anesth* 6:7-14, 1975.

Kitazawa K, Ohno K, Kadono H: Studies on electroacupuncture analgesia in the dog, *Jpn J Vet Anesth* 7:70-72, 1976.

Klide AM: Acupuncture for treatment of chronic back pain in the horse, *Acupunct Electrother Res Intl J* 9:57-70, 1984.

Klide AM: Use of acupuncture for the control of chronic pain and for surgical analgesia. In Short CE, Van Pomack A, editors: *Animal pain,* New York, 1992, Churchill Livingstone.

Kothbauer O: Ueber die Analgesierung einer Enterzitze, *Oesterr Aerztezeitung* 28:103-137, 1973.

Kothbauer O: Ein Kaiserschnitt bei einer Kuh unter Akupunkturanalgesie [Cesarean section in a cow under acupuncture analgesia], *Wien Tierarztl Monatsschrift* 62:394-396, 1975.

Lakschmipathi GV, Ramakrishna O: A study of the effects of acupuncture analgesia in buffalo calves, *Am J Acupunct* 16:165-168, 1988.

Lianfang H: Involvement of endogenous opioid peptides in acupuncture analgesia, *Pain* 31:99-121, 1987.

Lopes MD, Luna SPL, Alvarenga FL, et al: *Clinical and neurological signs of newborn dogs after cesarean section using inhalation anesthesia or electroacupuncture,* Proceedings of the twenty-fourth annual International Congress on Veterinary Acupuncture, Chitou, Taiwan, 1998, pp 132-133.

Luna SPL, Taylor PM: *Effect of electroacupuncture on endogenous opioids, AVP, ACTH, cortisol and catecholamine concentrations measured in the cerebrospinal fluid (CSF), peripheral and pituitary effluent plasma of ponies,* Proceedings of the twenty-fourth annual International Congress on Veterinary Acupuncture, Chitou, Taiwan, 1998, pp 172-174.

Martin BB Jr, Klide AM: The use of acupuncture for the treatment of chronic back pain in horses: stimulation of acupuncture points with saline injection solutions, *J Am Vet Med Assoc* 190:1177-1180, 1987.

Martono: *Experimental trials on the use of acupuncture as anesthesia in performing surgery on small animals,* Reports of Scientific Session of the third Congress of the Federation of Asian Veterinary Association, 1982, pp 67-69.

McCallum MI, Glynn CJ, Moore RA, et al: Transcutaneous electrical nerve stimulation in the management of acute postoperative pain, *Br J Anaesth* 61:308-312, 1988.

Melzack R, Wall PD: Pain mechanisms: a new theory, *Science* 150:971-979, 1965.

Nam TC, Seo KM, Chang KH, et al: *Acupuncture anesthesia in animals, I Electro-acupuncture regional analgesia in cattle,* Proceedings of the twenty-fourth annual International Congress on Veterinary Acupuncture, Chitou, Taiwan, 1998, pp 67-72.

Nam TC, Seo KM, Chang KH, et al: *Acupuncture anaesthesia in animals. II. Introduction of local and general analgesia by electroacupuncture in dogs,* Proceedings of the twenty-fourth annual International Congress on Veterinary Acupuncture, Chitou, Taiwan, 1998, pp 72-84.

O'Boyle MA, Vajda GK: Acupuncture analgesia for abdominal surgery, *Mod Vet Pract* 56:705-707, 1975.

Park HS, Suh DS: A study on blood coagulation and bleeding time under electroacupuncture anesthesia and medicament anesthesia in the dog, *Korean J Vet Res* 28:193-198, 1988.

Petermann U: *The role of laser acupuncture in equine back problems,* IVAS 2000 World Congress, Vienna, 2000, pp 144-147.

Pomeranz B, Chiu D: Naloxone blockade of acupuncture analgesia: endorphin implicated, *Life Sci* 19:1757-1762, 1976.

Rogers PAM: Acupuncture analgesia for surgery in animals. In *Acupuncture in animals,* Proceedings 167, Australian Veterinary Acupuncture Association, Sydney, 1991, pp 341-360.

Rogers PAM et al: Stimulation of the acupuncture points in relation to therapy of analgesia and clinical disorders in animals, Wright Scitechnica, Bristol, *Vet Annual* 17:258-279, 1977.

Rupniak NMJ: Use of substance P receptor antagonists as research tools in psychopharmacology, *Neurotransmissions* 15:3-10, 1999.

Salar G, Job I, Mingrino S, et al: Effect of transcutaneous electrotherapy on CSF beta-endorphin content in patients without pain problems, *Pain* 10:169-172, 1981.

Schmidt R, Schmelz M, Ringkamp M, et al: Innervation territories of mechanically activated C nociceptor units in human skin, *J Neurophysiol* 78:2641-2648, 1997.

Sculerati M, editor: *1997 American Veterinary Medical Association directory and resource manual,* Schaumburg, Ill, 1997, American Veterinary Medical Association.

Shafford HL, Hellyer PW, Crump KT, et al: Use of pulsed electromagnetic field for treatment of post-operative pain in dogs: a pilot study, *Vet Anaesth Analg* 29:29-35, 2002.

Sjölund B, Terenius L, Eriksson M: Increased cerebrospinal fluid levels of endorphins after electroacupuncture, *Acta Physiol Scand* 100:382-384, 1977.

Skarda RT: *Introduction to canine acupuncture: hip dysplasia,* Waltham Forum Video Series (50 min), Veterinary Learning Systems, Division of Medimedia, USA Inc, NJ, 1998.

Skarda RT: Acupuncture analgesia. In Muir WW, Hubbell JAE, Skarda RT, et al, editors: *Handbook of veterinary anesthesia,* ed 2, St Louis, 2000, Mosby.

Skarda RT, Tejwani GA, Muir WW, et al: *Cutaneous analgesic, hemodynamic and respiratory effects, and beta-endorphin concentration in lumbar spinal fluid after bilateral percutaneous electrical stimulation of acupoints BL 18, 23, 25, and 28 in healthy mares,* IVAS 2000 World Congress, Vienna, 2000, pp 118-121.

Smith CM, Guralnick MS, Gelfand MM, et al: The effects of transcutaneous electrical nerve stimulation on post-cesarean pain, *Pain* 27:181-193, 1986.

Solomon RA, Viernstein MC, Long DM: Reduction of postoperative pain and narcotic use by transcutaneous electrical nerve stimulation, *Surgery* 87:142-146, 1980.

Still J: Acupuncture for laparotomy in dogs and cats: an experimental study, *Am J Acupunct* 15:155-165, 1987.

Still J: *Acupuncture in anesthesiology,* Proceedings of the twenty-fourth annual International Congress on Veterinary Acupuncture, Chitou, Taiwan, 1998, pp 184-185.

Strauss S: *Acupuncture and the endogenous opioids,* Medical Pain Education's home page, 1999, Available online: http://www.pain-education.com/ HTML/POINTS2-a.htm.

Suh DS, Ha CS, Lee CY: Experimental studies on the acupuncture anesthesia in dogs, *Korean J Vet Res* 23:111-117, 1983.

Suh DS, Han BK: Experimental studies on the acupuncture prescription for electroacupuncture analgesia of cattle, *Korean J Vet Clin Med* 6:53-61, 1989.

Takagi J, Yonehara N: Serotonin receptor subtypes involved in modulation of electrical acupuncture, *Jpn J Pharmacol* 78:511-514, 1998.

Toyota S, Satake T, Amaki Y: Transcutaneous electrical nerve stimulation as an alternative therapy for microlaryngeal endoscopic surgery, *Anesth Analg* 89:1236-1238, 1999.

Tseng CK, Tay AA, Pace NL, et al: Electro-acupuncture modification of halothane anaesthesia in the dog, *Can Anaesth Soc J* 28:125-128, 1981.

Tsunoda Y, Sakahira K, Nakano S, et al: Antagonism of acupuncture analgesia by naloxone in conscious man, *Bull Tokyo Med Dent Univ* 27:89-94, 1980.

Ulett GA, Han S, Han JS: Electroacupuncture: mechanism and clinical application, *Biol Psychiatry* 44:129-138, 1998.

Urano Y et al: Clinical effects of electroacupuncture anesthesia of dogs, *J Vet Med* 679:26-35, 1978.

van Tulder MW, Cherkin DC, Berman B, et al: The effectiveness of acupuncture in the management of acute and chronic low back pain: a systematic review within the framework of the Cochrane Collaboration Back Review Group, *Spine* 24(11):1113-1123, 1999.

Walsh DM, Ligett C, Baxter D, et al: A double-blind investigation of the hypoalgesic effects of transcutaneous electrical nerve stimulation upon experimentally induced ischemic pain, *Pain* 61:39-45, 1995.

Wang B, Tang J, White PF, et al: Effect of the intensity of transcutaneous acupoint electrical stimulation on the postoperative analgesic requirement, *Anesth Analg* 85:406-413, 1997.

Wang J, Mao L, Han JS: Comparison of the antinociceptive effects induced by electroacupuncture and transcutaneous electrical nerve stimulation in the rat, *Int J Neurosci* 65:117-129, 1992.

Warfield CA, Stein JM, Frank HA: The effect of transcutaneous nerve stimulation on pain after thoracotomy, *Ann Thorac Surg* 39:462-465, 1985.

White SS, Bolton JR, Fraser DM: Use of electroacupuncture as an analgesic for laparotomies in two dairy cows, *Am Vet J* 62:52-54, 1985.

Wright M, McGrath C: Physiologic and analgesic effects of acupuncture in the dog, *J Am Vet Med Assoc* 178:502-507, 1981.

Xie H et al: *Influence of electroacupuncture stimulation on pain threshold and neuroendocrine responses in horse,* Proceedings of the twenty-fourth annual International Congress on Veterinary Acupuncture, Chi-tou, Taiwan, 1998, p 167.

Xu J, Liu Z: Acupuncture analgesia. In *Acupuncture teaching materials,* 1999, China Agricultural University.

Young GH: Regional analgesia in dogs with electroacupuncture, *California Vet* Nov:11-13, 1979.

Yung CR, Chan WW, Lin JH: *Electroacupuncture anesthesia for surgery in dogs,* Reports of Scientific Session of the fourth Congress of the Federation of Asian Veterinary Association, 1983, pp 67-69.

APPENDIX 16-1
ACUPUNCTURE SUPPLIES

M.E.D. Servi-Systems Canada Ltd.
8 Sweetnam Drive
Stittsville, Ontario
Canada K2S 1G2
1-613-836-3004
1-800-267-6868 Canada and U.S.
http://www.medserv.ca

OMS Medical Supplies, Inc.
1950 Washington Street
Braintree, MA 02184
Order toll free: 1-800-323-1839
Information: 781-331-3370
Fax: 781-335-5779
http://www.omsmedical.com

LHASA Medical, Inc.
539 Accord Station
Accord, MA 02018-0539
Order toll free: 1-800-722-8775
Information: 781-335-6484
Fax: 781-335-6296
http://www.lhasamedical.com

The Supply Center
6829 Canoga Avenue, Suite 5
Canoga Park, CA 91303
818-710-6868
Fax: 818-710-6855
http://www.the supplycenter.com

Seirin-America, Inc.
Weymouth, MA 02189
1-800-337-9338
Fax: 781-340-1637
http://www.SeirinAmerica.com

APPENDIX 16-2
PROFESSIONAL ORGANIZATIONS

The International Veterinary Acupuncture Society (IVAS)
PO Box 1478
Fort Collins, CO 80527-1395
Phone: 970-266-0666
Fax: 970-266-0777
E-mail: Ivasoffice@aol.com

American Academy of Veterinary Acupuncture (AAVA)
PO Box 419
Hygiene, CO 80533-0419
Phone: 303-722-6726
Fax: 303-772-6726
E-mail: aavaoffice@aol.com

Colorado State University
Dr. Narda Robinson
Veterinary Teaching Hospital
Colorado State University
300 W. Drake Road
Fort Collins, CO 80523
Phone: 970-221-4535
Fax: 970-491-4100

APPENDIX 16-3

PROFESSIONAL VETERINARY ACUPUNCTURE ARCHIVES, TIPS, AND CHAT ROOMS ON THE INTERNET

PVA-L Archives:
http://www.listquest.com/secure/pvalist/lq/search.htm? In=pvalist
username:pva-l
password:vetacupuncture

PVA-L Tips:
http://users.med.auth.gr/~karanik/english/pva-l/pvaltips.html

PVA-L Chat Room:
http://users.med.auth.gr/~karanik/english/vetchatp.html

APPENDIX 16-4

TITLES AND HYPERLINKS OF FURTHER LITERATURE

1. *Acupuncture, The Facts.* By Stephen Basser, MD
   http://www.skeptics.com.au/journal/acufacts.htm
2. *Horsefeathers: Acupuncture from a Veterinary Perspective.* By David W. Ramey and Jack Raso
   http://www.prioritiesforhealth.com/1102/acu.html
3. *Chinese Herbs: Some Things to Remember.* By Bill Burley
   http://www.seanet.com/~vettf/HOChihb.htm
4. *Magnetic and Electromagnetic Therapy.* By David W. Ramey, DVM
   http://www.seanet.com/~vettf/Homags.htm

PART FOUR

Acute and Chronic Pain Management

17

Choosing and Administering the Right Analgesic Therapy

WILLIAM W. MUIR III

CHOICE OF ANALGESIC THERAPY

The choice of analgesic therapy, whether pharmacologic or non-pharmacologic, should be tailored to each individual animal's needs with the following goals:

- Eliminating or suppressing pain.
- Making the animal more comfortable.
- Eliminating or suppressing pain behavior and promoting normal behavior.
- Returning the animal to maximum function despite residual pain.
- Removing stress or distress.

The pain experience is often multifaceted and always multidimensional. It incorporates physiologic (nociception, autonomic, endocrine), sensory (location, intensity, quality), postural (stance, gait), and behavioral (mood, appetite) responses. Pharmacologic approaches to the treatment of pain must therefore be carefully considered, given the diverse effects, metabolism, and toxicity of the drugs that are used to treat pain and the potential for human abuse of opioid analgesics. Determining the cause, severity, and duration of pain are the three most important factors in the design of a therapeutic plan. The choice of analgesic drugs for treatment of pain produced by a simple elective surgical procedure, for example, may be considerably different from that used for the treatment of osteoarthritis from hip dysplasia. Similarly, the treatment of pain caused by acute inflammatory conditions (abscesses) or abrasions is different from therapy designed to obtund or eliminate pain caused by severe trauma with nerve damage. The choice of drug and dosage recommendations must be individualized to the patient's needs, since serum levels are poor guides to analgesic efficacy and do little more than confirm that the drug is present in the animal's body. The patient's physical status, medical history, and behavior pattern, in addition to the pet owner's compliance with and understanding of therapy, are also factors that must be considered when pain therapy is prescribed. Ultimately the treatment of pain is only as good as our understanding of its causes and the use of therapeutic approaches that target these causes. Research in the basic sciences is currently unraveling many of the mechanisms responsible for pain and will continue to be responsible for the design and manufacture of safer more efficacious therapeutic alternatives.

Anamnesis

The dog's or cat's age, weight, sex, breed, and physical status are important determinants of drug selection and dose (Box 17-1).

Age

Young (less than 12 weeks) and older animals generally require lower dosages of drugs. Drug metabolism and elimination pathways may not be fully developed in the very young or may be impaired because of normal aging or concurrent disease in older animals. Similarly, young and older animals generally demonstrate a more

---

BOX 17-1
Factors to Consider Before Prescribing Analgesic Drugs

- Patients: age, weight, sex, breed, physical status, medical behavior, drug history, and environment
- Cause (mechanism) of pain
- Severity of pain
- Duration of pain
- Route of administration
- Drug efficacy/safety
- Potential for drug toxicity
- Potential for drug interactions
- Clinical experiences

pronounced central nervous system (CNS) response to analgesic drugs that also produce calming or sedative effects.

Weight

Weight should be used only as a guide to determining dose. Animals that are obviously overweight or underweight generally require lower dosages than are recommended. Overweight cats are particularly susceptible to drug overdose, since it may be more difficult to estimate their true lean body weight, in comparison with estimation of lean body weight in overweight dogs. Regardless, all animals, particularly the smaller ones, should be weighed as accurately as possible before institution of drug therapy.

Sex

Scientific studies have demonstrated sex-related differences in drug dose-response characteristics. Clinically, however, drug dosages are rarely affected by sex differences other than by the effects of sex hormones on behavior. More aggressive animals usually require a larger dose.

Breed

Breed differences can have a significant impact on drug selection and dose. Veterinary textbooks should be consulted and the package insert for veterinary-approved drugs should be carefully read before any drug is prescribed. Doberman pinschers, for example, are predisposed to the extrapyramidal side effects produced by many opioid drugs. Some Boxers have demonstrated pronounced side effects and have even died after administration of acepromazine as an adjuvant to opioid analgesia. Himalayan cats frequently demonstrate increased locomotor activity and hyperexcitability when administered standard doses of opioids for pain control.

Physical Status

The patient's physical status is a major determinant of drug dosage and the technique selected to produce analgesia. Sick, depressed, or debilitated dogs and cats may derive more benefit and demonstrate fewer side effects from analgesic techniques (preemptive, constant-rate infusion [CRI]) and nonconventional routes (epidural, transcutaneous) for drug administration. Close patient monitoring must be provided to all dogs and cats that are unconscious or demonstrate signs of cardiorespiratory compromise and are administered intra-venous (IV), intramuscular (IM), or subcutaneous (SQ) analgesic drugs.

History

The patient's medical, pharmacologic, and pain history provide valu-able information regarding the choice of analgesic therapies and the development of short- and long-term analgesic plans. Although typ-ically not emphasized, nonpharmacologic approaches should always be considered as an alternative or in addition to the use of drugs for the treatment of both acute and chronic pain (see Chapter 16).

Medical History

The patient's medical history rarely alters drug selection but does significantly affect drug dosage. Dogs or cats with a history of sig-nificant CNS or behavioral disorders (seizures, aggression, separa-tion anxiety) may demonstrate pronounced CNS or behavioral changes when administered drugs that are known to produce CNS effects in addition to analgesia. The administration of relatively low dosages of opioids to older dogs that have become less social, for example, may produce depression, periods of disorientation, or episodes of aggression lasting for several weeks. Similarly, dogs or cats with diseases that affect drug metabolism and elimination (liver, renal) may demonstrate drug-related side effects if administered standard dosages of drugs.

Pharmacologic History

The patient's response to previous drug therapy, particularly the re-sponse to analgesic and sedative drugs, should be determined. Drug dosages are published as guidelines and should be used as a starting point. Many animals experience one or more side effects (e.g., vom-iting, nervousness, constipation) when drugs are administered chronically. Dogs or cats that are being administered nonsteroidal antiinflammatory drugs (NSAIDs) or behavior-modifying drugs, for example, are more likely to demonstrate exaggerated drug-related effects, side effects, and toxicity than animals that are not receiving medications. Ultimately, analgesic therapy must be tailored to meet the animal's needs, and knowledge of the animal's response to pre-vious analgesic therapies can be very helpful in this regard.

Pain History

The choice of analgesic and the development of an analgesic plan will be most influenced by the duration of the pain (transient, acute, chronic), its severity, and the animal's response to pain. The dog's or cat's pain history may be extremely important in the initial design of an analgesic plan. Some dogs and cats, for example, seem to over-react to the mildest of noxious events, demonstrating exaggerated signs or responses to what would otherwise be considered minimal or moderately painful events. Other dogs and cats may demonstrate little or no response to painful stimuli for several days after the event or until they are examined. Insight as to how the dog or cat has responded to previous painful events helps determine whether the patient is hypersensitive or a stoic and suggests the types and dosages of drugs that will be needed to return a feeling of well-being to the animal. Nervous, hyperexcitable, small-breed dogs that have lived the majority of their lives indoors, for example, generally demonstrate exaggerated responses to minor traumatic events, including physical manipulation, compared with larger, more sedentary outside dogs. Although it is a generalization that is not always true, the last statement emphasizes the importance of knowing the animal's response to pain. Hyperexcitable, hypersensitive dogs or cats, for example, may benefit more from drugs that produce not only analgesia but also mild sedation.

Environment

The patient's environment may provide clues to the factors responsible for initiating pain and pain-associated behaviors. It is important to know whether there are children in the house and how they interact with the pets. Older osteoarthritic dogs, for example, that are required to go up or down stairs may refuse to move and become agitated when coerced. Similarly, younger animals (dogs or cats) that are in pain may become aggressive if disturbed or forced to play.

Owner Expectations

The owners' opinions and expectations regarding pain and pain therapies should be determined. Their ability to administer medications or perform nonpharmacologic therapeutic techniques must be determined. The advantages, disadvantages, and cost of the pain therapy chosen should be explained to every owner. Owners who are unfamiliar with or unsure of the drugs and techniques used for the treatment of pain are much less likely to comply with therapeutic recommendations.

Cause, Severity, and Duration of Pain

General guidelines regarding the cause (inflammatory, mechanical, neuropathic), severity (mild, moderate, severe), and duration (transient, acute, chronic) of pain should be developed and serve as major determinants of the therapeutic plan.

Cause

Pain can be caused by tissue trauma and inflammation, nerve damage or irritation, and unknown factors (idiopathic). Knowing or determining the cause of pain provides insight into its severity and duration, thereby suggesting potential therapeutic approaches. The excruciating pain caused by gastric distention (visceral pain) with or without displacement ("bloat"), for example, may require gastric decompression, the administration of potent opioids, and surgical intervention. Similarly, the severe visceral pain and respiratory distress caused by thoracic trauma with pneumothorax cannot be effectively treated by analgesics alone; antiinflammatory medications, chest tubes, and possibly surgical reconstruction are required when there are fractured or displaced ribs. Dogs with cervical disk disease (neuropathic pain) may temporarily and repeatedly benefit from antiinflammatory (glucocorticosteroids, NSAIDs) and analgesic (opioids) drugs but eventually require surgery for long-term relief of pain. Determining the cause of pain therefore helps determine the importance of the mechanical, inflammatory, and neuropathic components and suggests appropriate remedies (surgery, antiinflammatory medications, analgesics).

Severity

No disease attracts more attention than an animal demonstrating signs of severe pain. It can be safely assumed, regardless of individual animal variability, that the more pronounced the signs, the more pronounced is the pain. With this in mind, it is an obvious conclusion that severe pain requires the administration of drugs and the use of techniques that provide immediate, potent, and sustained analgesic effects. In other words, the severity of the pain determines which and to what extent various analgesic drugs and techniques will be used. Toward this end, many pain scoring systems and variations of these systems have been developed to quantitate, categorize, and evaluate pain and the severity of pain in animals (see Chapter 6). Pain scoring systems are an integral part of patient evaluation and serve as the basis for drug selection, dose determination, and choice of route of administration. A dog or cat with severe pain secondary to tissue trauma caused by an automobile accident, for example, generally requires the IV administration of a potent opioid (hydromorphone) and/or NSAID for immediate-onset, short-term analgesia. Oral antiinflammatory drugs (ketoprofen, carprofen, etodolac) are administered for long-term analgesia. In contrast, a dog or cat subjected to intense transient pain associated with the placement of a large-gauge IV needle (jugular catheter) or the placement of a chest tube may benefit more from the administration of an injectable or topical local anesthetic (lidocaine). Less severe forms of pain generally respond to weaker analgesic drugs administered at lower dosages, thereby decreasing the potential for drug-related side effects and toxicity.

Duration
The duration of pain helps to determine drug(s), drug dose, and duration of therapy. The injection of a local anesthetic may suffice as analgesic therapy for an otherwise normal healthy dog or cat subjected to acute, transient pain. Animals that have experienced moderate to severe pain for extended periods, however, usually require potent analgesic drugs administered in larger dosages because of the plasticity and upregulation of the sensory nervous system. Chronic pain, particularly when associated with or caused by nerve damage, can be responsible for the production of "wind-up," central sensitization, and allodynia (see Chapter 2). Patients with chronic pain often derive more benefit from a combination of analgesic drugs that act by different mechanisms of action than from larger doses of a single drug. Drug combinations, although potentially more cumbersome to administer and more expensive, may offer the advantage of drug synergism and a reduction in drug side effects and toxicity (see Chapter 7). The choice of drug, drug dosage, and therapeutic plan (pharmacologic and nonpharmacologic) may need to be periodically modified or changed to maintain adequate analgesia, prevent development of drug tolerance, and minimize the potential for drug toxicity.

DEVELOPING A TREATMENT PLAN

The development and periodic reassessment of a therapeutic plan is essential for producing adequate and effective short- or long-term analgesia in dogs and cats (Box 17-2). A rational approach to the treatment of pain is most logically based on a clinical appreciation of the various mechanisms responsible for producing pain and a knowledge of which mechanisms are important in the production of clinical pain.

Similar to an understanding of the mechanisms responsible for causing pain, there must be a conceptual and working understanding of the various types of pain (e.g., inflammatory, neuropathic) and its severity. The treatment of severe pain with drugs that are capable of producing only mild analgesic effects is not only ineffective but makes pain harder to treat and increases the likelihood for drug failure or toxicity.

Several different therapeutic approaches should be designed for the treatment of mild, moderate, and severe pain. From a practical standpoint, the cost of therapy should be integrated into these plans. Nonpharmacologic therapies should be considered and suggested whenever appropriate. Educational materials describing the harmful consequences of pain, the advantages of pain therapy, and the advantages and disadvantages of different therapeutic approaches should be made available to help educate pet owners.

Drugs

Drug selection and therapeutic technique should be based on the cause, severity, and duration of pain (see Chapters 6 and 8). Drugs

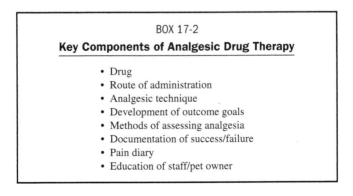

BOX 17-2

Key Components of Analgesic Drug Therapy

- Drug
- Route of administration
- Analgesic technique
- Development of outcome goals
- Methods of assessing analgesia
- Documentation of success/failure
- Pain diary
- Education of staff/pet owner

should be thought of and categorized based on their mechanism of action, analgesic potency, and potential to produce unwanted side effects (Box 17-3). A pain scoring or rating system should be developed or adopted and used for assessing the severity of pain and the success or failure of therapy (see Chapter 6). Clinical experience and familiarity with a select group of drugs is important in achieving a beneficial drug effect.

Opioids

Opioids (e.g., morphine, oxymorphone, butorphanol, codeine) produce mild-to-excellent analgesia with minimal-to-moderate behavior modification or depression. The efficacy of oral opioid administration has not been substantiated in dogs and cats. Transdermal and epidural routes of drug administration offer an alternative to parenteral administration.

α_2-Agonists

α_2-Agonists (e.g., xylazine, medetomidine, romifidine, clonidine) produce good-to-excellent analgesia and moderate-to-profound sedation. Orally administered α_2-agonists are not available. Epidural administration offers an alternative to parenteral routes and is less likely to produce sedation. Clonidine is available for transdermal delivery.

Nonsteroidal Antiinflammatory Drugs

NSAIDs (e.g., aspirin, carprofen, etodolac, ketoprofen) produce mild-to-moderate analgesia and antiinflammatory effects. Oral and

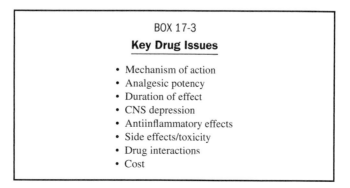

BOX 17-3
Key Drug Issues

- Mechanism of action
- Analgesic potency
- Duration of effect
- CNS depression
- Antiinflammatory effects
- Side effects/toxicity
- Drug interactions
- Cost

parenteral preparations are available. Although NSAIDs are frequently prescribed for chronic use, liver and renal function should be periodically evaluated in animals receiving these drugs.

Local Anesthetics
Local anesthetics produce excellent analgesia but must be administered by injection, and they block both sensory and motor nerve fibers. Some administration techniques (e.g., lidocaine CRI) enhance the anesthetic and analgesic effects of concurrently administered drugs.

Other Drugs
Many drugs, although not noted for their analgesic effects, can produce mild analgesia (e.g., mexiletine, diltiazem) or enhance the analgesic effects of drugs that do (e.g., acepromazine, droperidol). These drugs are often combined with more traditional analgesic therapies to either enhance or prolong (acepromazine-hydromorphone) analgesic drug effects.

Route of Drug Administration
Choosing the appropriate route for drug administration and administration technique can be the deciding factor in producing analgesia while avoiding drug-related side effects or toxicities. The concept of minimal effective concentration, for example, is of limited value in the clinical administration of analgesics, given the wide variation in response to analgesic drugs, despite similar plasma concentrations. Dogs or cats that are sick or that demonstrate signs of CNS depression or cardiovascular or respiratory compromise may not accept or adequately absorb oral medications or may not tolerate the high plasma concentrations produced by IV, IM, or even SQ drug administration compared with alternate routes (e.g., epidural, transcutaneous). The route of drug administration may be more important than the drug administered (Box 17-4).

Oral
The oral route of administration of drugs is preferred for the treatment of most types of chronic and many types of acute pain. Analgesic drugs (NSAIDs) can be administered orally as preemptive analgesia or in conjunction with injectable analgesics to produce additive or synergistic effects. Oral administration of drugs can be

---

BOX 17-4
Routes of Analgesic Drug Administration

- Oral
- Intravenous
- Intramuscular/subcutaneous
- Epidural/subarachnoid
- Transcutaneous/topical
- Sublingual/buccal/transmucosal
- Intranasal/inhalational
- Rectal

---

accomplished in the hospital or at home with minimal to no supervision, drug effects are relatively prolonged, and drug side effects and toxicities are comparatively minimal. Orally administered drugs are subject to first-pass metabolism in the liver, however, which limits their bioavailability, clinical efficacy, and the use of most analgesic drugs, particularly opioids, in dogs and cats (see Chapter 7). Diet, eating behavior, drug formulation, and concurrent diseases can produce prolonged absorption from the gastrointestinal tract and erratic absorption patterns, leading to an inadequate analgesic response. Finally, the owner must comply with dosage schedules for therapy to be effective.

Intravenous
IV administration provides the most rapid and predictable drug effects. Drugs can be administered intravenously as a bolus, slow injection, or CRI. IV drugs must be administered by appropriately trained personnel, and patients must be closely monitored for immediate or delayed adverse drug effects. Drug plasma concentrations are at their highest after IV drug administration, increasing the potential for drug-related side effects and toxicity. Sites of venous access in dogs or cats receiving CRI must be evaluated for signs of extravasation, thrombophlebitis, and generalized inflammation.

Intramuscular and Subcutaneous
Both IM and SQ drug administration are easily performed and provide relatively rapid (5 to 20 minutes) onset of effects. SQ drug

administration is relatively painless if small needles are used. Analgesic drugs can be administered less frequently than required for IV injections, and plasma concentrations are not as elevated, reducing the potential for side effects and drug-related toxicity. The IM administration of drugs can be painful, particularly when larger volumes are administered. Drug absorption is occasionally erratic after IM or SQ drug administration, producing more variable effects than after IV administration. Erratic drug absorption is more likely to occur in dogs and cats with poor peripheral circulation (dehydration, hypovolemia, hypothermia).

Epidural/Subarachnoid (Spinal)

More and more drugs are being investigated for epidural or subarachnoid administration in dogs and cats. Although the epidural route was originally used only for administration of local anesthetics (lidocaine) and opioids (morphine), recent clinical trials have investigated the analgesic effects of epidural administration of NSAIDs (ketoprofen), dissociative anesthetics (ketamine), and α_2-agonists (xylazine, medetomidine). Epidural drug administration produces good-to-excellent analgesia for extended periods (hours) with relatively small drug doses, thereby limiting the potential for side effects and toxicity. The epidural administration of opioids, α_2-agonists, and NSAIDs also avoids the loss of motor control associated with the epidural administration of local anesthetic drugs. The epidural or subarachnoid administration of drugs must be performed by appropriately trained and skilled personnel and requires sterile technique. Epidurally administered drugs should be sterile and preservative-free and should have a relatively poor lipid solubility to limit absorption and prolong effects.

Transdermal and Topical

Few analgesic drugs are available for transdermal (fentanyl, clonidine) or topical (local anesthetics, such as lidocaine and eutectic mixture of local anesthetics [EMLA] cream) administration. Transdermally delivered drugs are easy to administer with minimal training. The drug is absorbed into the blood, bypassing liver metabolism (first-pass elimination), and effects persist for as long as the patch contains drug and remains in contact with the skin, lasting for many hours to days. Transdermal drug delivery is an excellent method for providing preemptive analgesia or "background" analgesia before major surgery and as adjuvant analgesia after a major traumatic event. The potential for drug-related side effects and toxicity is low because of slow drug absorption. Slow drug absorption also prolongs the time to produce analgesia, making it difficult to predict drug effects and titrate drug dosage. Skin irritation develops in some dogs and cats.

Sublingual, Buccal, and Transmucosal

Like transdermal drug delivery, the sublingual, buccal, and transmucosal routes of drug delivery depend on drug absorption from the body surface, in this case the mucous membranes. The absorbed drug is not subjected to first-pass liver metabolism. Although potentially having the same advantages as transdermal drug delivery, the sublingual and buccal routes of drug administration to dogs and cats may not be practical because of the requirement of patient cooperation, the influence of saliva on drug absorption, and the unfamiliar taste produced by many drugs. Regardless, the oral administration of various opioid-containing syrups (e.g., codeine, morphine, buprenorphine) and dextromethorphan results in partial absorption of drug through the mucous membranes, producing mild analgesic effects that last for several hours in dogs and cats.

Intranasal or Inhalational

Intranasal and inhalational drug delivery are similar to sublingual and buccal administration but do not require patient cooperation. Drug absorption is rapid, producing almost immediate drug effects. Few analgesic drugs other than butorphanol have been investigated after intranasal administration.

Rectal

The rectal administration of drugs to dogs and cats is rarely used. Although rectal administration of drugs is easily performed, the bioavailability of rectally administered drugs is poor. Furthermore, rectally administered drugs are generally absorbed slowly, and drug absorption can be interrupted by defecation or straining to defecate.

Techniques for Analgesic Drug Administration

The medical philosophy adopted for drug administration can be as important as the drug selected in determining the therapeutic efficacy of analgesic drug therapy (Box 17-5). The efficacy of butorphanol for all degrees of pain, whether mild or severe, in dogs and cats is not only inappropriate but unsubstantiated. Similarly, the analgesic effects of more potent opioids (e.g., morphine, fentanyl) are generally enhanced by the concurrent administration of NSAIDs and frequently reduce the total amount of opioid required to produce effective analgesia.

Local and Regional Anesthetic Nerve Blocks

Local and regional anesthetic nerve blocks (e.g., infiltration, epidural, intercostal) are valuable adjuncts to the administration of parenteral analgesic medications. Performed properly, these techniques provide excellent analgesia that lasts for several hours with a minimal potential for serious side effects (see Chapter 15).

Preemptive Analgesia

Preemptive (i.e., treatment before pain occurs) analgesic drugs and techniques should be used whenever possible. The earlier pain is treated, the sooner patient well-being and more normal homeostasis can be established. The use of preemptive techniques to treat pain generally reduces drug dosages and the total amount of drug required to maintain analgesia.

Constant-Rate Infusion

A CRI can be used to provide continuous titratable analgesia for extended periods. The use of a CRI to produce a steady-state plasma concentration of drug avoids the peaks (potential side effects or toxicity) and troughs (potential loss of drug effect) associated with re-

---

BOX 17-5

Drug Administration Techniques

- Local/regional anesthesia
- Preemptive analgesia
- Constant-rate infusion
- Compounding
- Drug rotation schedules

peated injectable or oral drug administration. Opioids, local anesthetics, and some anesthetic drugs (e.g., ketamine, tiletamine-
zolazepam [Telazol]) can be administered by CRI to provide excellent analgesia for hours or days. One or two IV bolus drug doses
(bolus + CRI) are usually administered in conjunction with the initiation of CRI to help establish and sustain therapeutic plasma drug
concentrations until steady-state drug concentrations are reached
(see Chapter 7).

Multiple Low Dosing
The administration of multiple low doses of analgesic drugs by IV
or IM injection is similar to CRI because a lower dose of drug is
administered more frequently, thus minimizing peak and trough
drug concentrations and the potential for toxicity and ineffective
drug plasma concentrations, respectively. This technique can be
used when CRI cannot be used or is technically difficult to perform
and is well suited for high-risk patients in which higher-dose bolus
administration is more likely to produce unwanted side effects. This
technique, however, is labor intensive and more disturbing to the
patient than CRI.

Multiple Routes
The same or different analgesic drugs can be administered by multiple routes to produce immediate and sustained drug effects. The IV
administration of a drug in conjunction with its IM or SQ administration produces immediate drug effects, which are sustained for a
longer duration, depending on the rate of absorption and pharmacokinetics of the drug administered. This technique is particularly
useful for drugs that have intermediate (1 to 2 hours) to short (<30
minutes) half-lives. Repeated IM administration of morphine in
conjunction with the placement of a fentanyl patch (transcutaneous
drug delivery), for example, can be used to initiate opioid analgesia
(morphine) until effective plasma concentrations of fentanyl are
reached, which may take 6 to 12 hours (see Chapter 9).

Multiple Drug Administration
The administration of two or more analgesic drugs, either sequen-
tially or together in solution (compounding), is an effective method
of improving and enhancing analgesic drug effects. Generally
speaking, drugs that act by different mechanisms of action are

---

BOX 17-6
How to Respond to Therapeutic Failure

- Reevaluate patient
- Reevaluate treatment plan: drug, dose, technique
- Reevaluate owner compliance
- Reevaluate patient environment
- Reevaluate nonpharmacologic treatments
- Consider adjuvant therapies
- Consider drug tolerance/interactions
- Consider behavioral modification

---

additive and frequently supraadditive (synergistic) when administered at the same time. Synergism allows lower doses of each drug to be administered, decreasing the potential for the development of drug-related side effects or toxicity.

Drug Rotation Schedules

The rotation of drugs that act by the same general mechanism or different mechanisms (e.g., opioids, NSAIDS) may help prevent the development of drug tolerance and drug-related toxicities. Intermittent dosage schedules (3 days on, 2 days off) and alternate administration of carprofen with etodolac or codeine, for example, may help to sustain analgesic drug effects and avoid toxicities unique to single-drug therapy.

WHAT TO DO WHEN THE THERAPEUTIC PLAN DOES NOT WORK

Anyone who has treated dogs or cats in pain is familiar with therapeutic failure. There are many causes for pain and many factors that influence the patient's response to painful sensations and the effects of analgesic therapies (Box 17-6). Behavior modifying drugs or techniques and changes in the home environment may be required to effectively treat pain in some animals. Lack of owner compliance with prescribed recommendations should be considered as one possible cause of therapeutic failure.

SUGGESTED READINGS

Asburn MA, Lipman AG: Management of pain in the cancer patient, *Anesth Analg* 76:402-416, 1993.

Bushnell TG, Justins DM: Choosing the right analgesic, *Drugs* 46(3):394-408, 1993.

Practice guidelines for acute pain management in the perioperative setting: a report by the American Society of Anesthesiologists Task Force on Pain Management, Acute Pain Section, *Anesthesia* 85:1071-1081, 1995.

18

Acute Pain Management
A Case-Based Approach

JAMES S. GAYNOR AND WILLIAM W. MUIR III

The following are specific case examples of animals in pain. The nature of the case and the rationale and specific treatment are described in detail. Each case presents a unique aspect or problem as it relates to management of pain. Various drugs and procedures are mentioned, including drug dosages. More detail on each drug and procedure are provided in other portions of this book. All patients should be considered healthy unless otherwise noted. These case examples are described to provide multiple alternative examples of pain management in dogs and cats.

CANINE OVARIOHYSTERECTOMY (Box 18-1)

This is an example of analgesic management for a dog undergoing ovariohysterectomy (OHE) in a practice that discharges surgery patients on the same day as surgery.

> **SIGNALMENT:** *6-month-old female mixed breed weighing 20 kg.*
> **PROBLEM:** *Most clients do not like to take their pet home sedated. A veterinarian usually will be called if an animal is sedated into the early evening. The challenge is to provide adequate analgesia without sedation overnight.*
> **SOURCE OF PAIN:** *The pain from an OHE is multifold. There is definitely abdominal wall pain from the incision. There is probably also some visceral pain from manipulation of the uterus, ovaries, and associated ligaments.*

BOX 18-1
Canine Ovariohysterectomy

- Somatic and visceral pain
- Mild-to-moderate intensity
- Surgically induced tissue trauma
- Acute onset and short duration

Treatment and Rationale

Although some practitioners may believe that OHEs are not painful, strong evidence suggests that they are. Many dogs that undergo OHE do not outwardly exhibit pain in the presence of humans. Therefore as for any other surgical procedure, it is best to treat pain preemptively, then follow up with the appropriate postoperative drugs.

Preemptive Analgesia

Appropriate preemptive analgesia would be a μ-opioid agonist such as morphine or hydromorphone. This dog received morphine 1 mg/kg SQ combined with acepromazine 0.02 mg/kg and atropine 0.04 mg/kg. The acepromazine was added to the premedication for tranquilization. The atropine was added to offset the vagal-induced bradycardia associated with the morphine.

Immediate Postoperative Analgesia

Morphine has a duration of action of approximately 4 to 6 hours when administered at this dose subcutaneously. Because most OHEs are relatively short (20 to 40 minutes), most dogs will not require additional drugs at extubation. If an OHE is performed in the morning, an additional dose of morphine (0.5 to 1.0 mg/kg SQ) may be required 4 to 6 hours later in order to get the patient through the rest of the day. Morphine will provide maximal analgesia for the immediate postoperative period.

Analgesia at the End of the Day

Dogs are treated with nalbuphine 1.0 mg/kg SQ to ensure several more hours of analgesia with no sedation as the dog leaves the practice with the owner.

24-Hour Analgesia

The pain that ensues from an OHE is usually moderate. Analgesia can be maintained with a nonsteroidal antiinflammatory drug (NSAID), such as ketoprofen or carprofen. The NSAID should be administered after the procedure during recovery to avoid potential hypotension-related problems.

* Ketoprofen 2 mg/kg SQ
* Carprofen 4 mg/kg SQ

3-Day Analgesia

Some practices like to provide approximately 3 days of analgesia for their OHEs. Several options exist.

* Carprofen 1.0 mg/kg PO bid. Carprofen should not be administered orally if another NSAID was originally administered parenterally. This particular dog received this protocol.
* Transdermal fentanyl 2 to 3 μg/kg/hr (Box 18-2).

BOX 18-2

Canine Ovariohysterectomy

* Preemptive analgesia: morphine 1 mg/kg SQ
* Postoperative analgesia: morphine 0.5 to 1.0 mg/kg SQ
* Analgesia at the end of the day: nalbuphine 1.0 mg/kg SQ
* 24-hour analgesia: ketoprofen 2 mg/kg SQ or carprofen 4 mg/kg SQ
* 3-day analgesia: carprofen 1.0 mg/kg PO bid or morphine 0.5 to 0.75 mg/kg PO qid or transdermal fentanyl 2 to 3 μg/kg/hr

---

CANINE OVARIOHYSTERECTOMY 2 (Box 18-3)

This is an example of an analgesic protocol used for dogs who stay one night in the hospital after OHE.

SIGNALMENT: *6-month-old female mixed breed dog weighing 8 kg.*
PROBLEM: *The goal is to provide analgesia for 24 hours. The problem is that the facility is not staffed in the evening to provide redosing of analgesics.*
SOURCE OF PAIN: *The pain from an OHE is multifold. There is definitely abdominal wall pain from the incision. There is probably*

also some visceral pain from manipulation of the uterus, ovaries, and associated ligaments.

BOX 18-3

Canine Ovariohysterectomy

- Somatic and visceral pain
- Mild-to-moderate intensity
- Surgically induced tissue trauma
- Acute onset and short duration

Treatment and Rationale

OHEs, like other surgical procedures, are painful. Patients should receive preemptive and postoperative analgesics.

Preemptive Analgesia

This dog received morphine 7.5 mg SQ (approximately 1 mg/kg) 30 minutes before anesthesia was induced. This dog also received acepromazine 0.02 mg/kg and atropine 0.04 mg/kg combined with the morphine and given subcutaneously. The acepromazine was added to the premedication for tranquilization. The atropine was added to off-set the vagal-induced bradycardia associated with the morphine.

Immediate Postoperative Analgesia

Morphine has a duration of action of approximately 4 to 6 hours when administered at this dose subcutaneously. Because most OHEs are relatively short (20 to 40 minutes), most dogs will not require additional drugs at extubation. This OHE was performed in the morning, so an additional dose of morphine at 1.0 mg/kg SQ was administered to get the patient through the rest of the day. Morphine will provide maximal analgesia for the immediate postoperative period.

Analgesia at the End of the Day

Because no one was available to redose morphine after 6:00 PM, this dog received buprenorphine 0.01 mg/kg SQ. The advantage of buprenorphine is that it has a relatively long duration of action, approximately 2 to 12 hours. The analgesia is not as good as that produced by morphine, but it should be adequate, especially if an NSAID is administered postoperatively.

24-Hour Analgesia

The pain that ensues from an OHE is usually moderate. Analgesia can be maintained with an NSAID such as ketoprofen or carprofen. The NSAID should be administered after the procedure during recovery to avoid potential hypotension-related problems.

- Ketoprofen 2 mg/kg SQ
- Carprofen 4 mg/kg SQ (Box 18-4)

BOX 18-4

Canine Ovariohysterectomy

- Preemptive analgesia: morphine 1 mg/kg SQ
- Postoperative analgesia: morphine 1.0 mg/kg SQ
- Analgesia at the end of the day: buprenorphine 0.01 mg/kg SQ
- 24-hour analgesia: ketoprofen 2 mg/kg SQ or carprofen 4 mg/kg SQ

CANINE CASTRATION (Box 18-5)

SIGNALMENT: *10-month-old male dog weighing 30 kg.*
SOURCE OF PAIN: *Castration results in mild-to-moderate visceral pain postoperatively.*

BOX 18-5

Canine Castration

- Visceral pain
- Mild-to-moderate intensity
- Surgically induced tissue trauma
- Acute onset and short duration

Treatment and Rationale

Preemptive Analgesia

This dog was premedicated with acepromazine 0.04 mg/kg for calming, atropine 0.04 mg/kg to prevent vagal-induced bradycardia, and oxymorphone 0.1 mg/kg for analgesia, all combined and administered subcutaneously.

Immediate Postoperative and 24-Hour Analgesia

Because the pain from castration is believed to be mild to moderate, ketoprofen 2.2 mg/kg SQ can be administered during recovery (Box 18-6).

BOX 18-6

Canine Castration

- Preemptive analgesia: oxymorphone 0.1 mg/kg SQ
- Immediate postoperative and 24-hour analgesia: ketoprofen 2.2 mg/ kg SQ

FELINE OVARIOHYSTERECTOMY (Box 18-7)

This is a case of a cat that will go home the same day as surgery.

SIGNALMENT: *6-month-old female domestic short hair weighing 3 kg.*
PROBLEM: *Providing analgesia that will be sufficient throughout the night when the cat is in the owner's care.*
SOURCE OF PAIN: *The source of pain is a combination of surgical trauma to the abdominal wall and visceral pain from tension on ligaments.*

BOX 18-7

Feline Ovariohysterectomy

- Somatic and visceral pain
- Mild-to-moderate intensity
- Surgically induced tissue trauma
- Acute onset and short duration

Treatment and Rationale

Preemptive Analgesia

This cat was premedicated with morphine 0.25 mg/kg SQ for analgesia combined with xylazine 0.5 mg/kg for additional analgesia and good sedation and atropine to prevent bradycardia induced by the other two drugs. The morphine should last 4 to 6 hours in a cat.

Postoperative Analgesia

This requires a multimodal approach.

- Before the subcutaneous tissues and skin were closed, a local anesthetic incisional block was infused. Bupivacaine (0.5%) with epinephrine (1:200,000) was used. An amount calculated as 1.5 mg/kg was drawn up, then diluted 1:1 with normal saline solution. This block should last 8 to 12 hours.
- Ketoprofen 2.2 mg/kg SQ was administered at the end of the procedure. This should last 24 hours (Box 18-8).

BOX 18-8

Feline Ovariohysterectomy

- Preemptive analgesia: morphine 0.25 mg/kg + xylazine 0.5 mg/ kg SQ
- Postoperative analgesia: bupivacaine incisional block + ketoprofen 2.2 mg/kg SQ

FELINE CASTRATION (Box 18-9)

SIGNALMENT: *8-month-old male Abyssinian cat weighing 3 kg.*

PROBLEM: *Providing analgesia without sedation so the owner can take the cat home the same day as surgery.*

SOURCE OF PAIN: *Visceral pain related to spermatic cord and cremaster muscle tension. This pain is probably mild to moderate.*

BOX 18-9
Feline Castration

- Visceral pain
- Mild-to-moderate intensity
- Surgically induced tissue trauma
- Acute onset and short duration

Treatment and Rationale
Preemptive Analgesia
This cat was premedicated with morphine 0.25 mg/kg SQ for analgesia combined with xylazine 0.5 mg/kg for additional analgesia and good sedation and atropine to prevent bradycardia induced by the other two drugs. The morphine should last 4 to 6 hours in a cat.

Postoperative Analgesia
Ketoprofen 2.2 mg/kg SQ was administered at the end of the procedure. This should last 24 hours (Box 18-10).

BOX 18-10
Feline Castration

- Preemptive analgesia: morphine 0.25 mg/kg + xylazine 0.5 mg/ kg SQ
- Postoperative analgesia: ketoprofen 2.2 mg/kg SQ

DECLAW: FRONT PAW (Box 18-11)

SIGNALMENT: *1.5-year-old castrated male domestic long-hair cat weighing 5.5 kg.*

PROBLEM: *Declaw pain has been one of the most difficult sources of pain to treat in cats. Anecdotally, some owners believe their cats are much meaner after being declawed, presumably from the intense pain experienced.*

SOURCE OF PAIN: *This is severe pain originating from severed ligaments and potentially traumatized bone and periosteum.*

BOX 18-11

Declaw: Front Paws

- Somatic pain
- Severe intensity
- Surgically induced tissue trauma
- Acute onset and short duration

Treatment and Rationale
Preemptive Analgesia

- This cat was premedicated with morphine 0.5 mg/kg SQ for analgesia combined with xylazine 0.5 mg/kg for additional analgesia and good sedation and atropine to prevent bradycardia induced by the other two drugs. The dose of morphine was considerably higher than that used for most other procedures in cats because of the pain intensity. The morphine should last 4 to 6 hours in a cat.

- Before surgery, a declaw local anesthetic block was performed by using bupivacaine (0.75%) 1.5 mg/kg split between the two front paws (see Chapter 15). This block lasts approximately 3 to 6 hours. Bupivacaine without epinephrine should be used in peripheral blocks such as this. The epinephrine component causes vasoconstriction and decreased perfusion to the periphery, potentially resulting in tissue ischemia.

Postoperative Analgesia

A multimodal approach to analgesia is crucial because of the severe nature of this pain.

- Ketoprofen 2.2 mg/kg SQ was administered at the end of the procedure. This should provide centrally mediated analgesia for up to 24 hours.

- Four hours after the initial morphine dose, another dose of morphine at 0.5 mg/kg SQ was administered. This ensured that good analgesia was present as the bupivacaine wore off.
- Buprenorphine 0.005 mg/kg SQ was administered 3.5 hours after the last morphine dose. Although buprenorphine does not provide the same degree of analgesia as morphine, it has a longer duration of action and should help keep the cat comfortable throughout the night, along with the ketoprofen.
- Butorphanol was specifically not used in this case because of its comparatively low analgesic potency. Butorphanol can only provide moderate degrees of analgesia (Box 18-12).

BOX 18-12

Declaw: Front Paws

- Preemptive analgesia: morphine 0.5 mg/kg + xylazine 0.5 mg/kg SQ; bupivacaine declaw block
- Postoperative analgesia: ketoprofen 2.2 mg/kg SQ; morphine 0.5 mg/kg SQ 4 hours after local anesthetic infiltration
- Overnight analgesia: buprenorphine 0.005 mg/kg SQ 3.5 hours after the last morphine administration

---

INCISOR EXTRACTION (Box 18-13)

SIGNALMENT: 12 year-old spayed female miniature poodle, weighing 9 kg, with periodontitis requiring extraction of two left lower incisors. This dog also has mitral regurgitation with a 2/6 systolic murmur. There are no apparent signs of heart failure.

PROBLEM: Providing analgesia for several days after anesthesia and tooth extraction.

SOURCE OF PAIN: *There is mild-to-moderate pain arising from the tooth root and surrounding soft tissue.*

BOX 18-13

Incisor Extraction

- Somatic pain
- Mild-to-moderate intensity
- Inflammatory and surgically induced tissue trauma
- Acute onset and short duration

Treatment and Rationale

Preemptive Analgesia

A multimodal approach was required for this dog.

- This dog was premedicated with hydromorphone 0.1 mg/kg IM for analgesia, along with glycopyrrolate 0.01 mg/kg to prevent hydromorphone-induced bradycardia.
- A left mental nerve block was performed by using bupivacaine 0.5 ml (0.75%). This dose was equivalent to approximately 0.4 mg/kg. A low dose can be used because the nerve being blocked is in a very small area, requiring a small volume of local anesthetic.

Postoperative Analgesia

- The dentistry took only 30 minutes. Therefore the hydromorphone lasted approximately another 4 hours. The dog was then given nalbuphine 1.0 mg/kg SQ to provide several hours of analgesia without sedation so it could be discharged to go home.
- This dog was also prescribed oral liquid morphine (4 mg/ml) 0.5 mg/kg to be administered 3 to 4 times a day. This was to provide analgesia for mild pain for several days (Box 18-14).

BOX 18-14

Incisor Extraction

- Preemptive analgesia: hydromorphone 0.1 mg/kg IM; bupivacaine mental nerve block
- Postoperative analgesia: nalbuphine 1.0 mg/kg SQ
- Multiday analgesia: oral liquid morphine 0.5 mg/kg PO tid-qid

---

MAXILLECTOMY (Box 18-15)

SIGNALMENT: *8-year-old spayed female terrier mix weighing 9 kg.*
PROBLEM: *Mass just behind right upper canine requiring a partial maxillectomy.*
SOURCE OF PAIN: *Bone and soft tissue surgical trauma.*

BOX 18-15
Maxillectomy

- Somatic pain
- Moderate-to-severe intensity
- Inflammatory and surgically induced tissue trauma
- Acute onset and short duration

Treatment and Rationale

Preoperative Analgesia

- This dog was premedicated with hydromorphone 0.2 mg/kg SQ to provide preemptive analgesia and atropine 0.04 mg/kg SQ to prevent vagal-induced bradycardia.
- An infraorbital nerve block was performed by using bupivacaine 2.5 mg (0.5%). This provided regional anesthesia to the nose, which was being partially resected.

Postoperative Analgesia

This dog received a fentanyl bolus 2 μg/kg IV, followed by a fentanyl infusion of 3 to 5 μg/kg/hr IV. Occasionally, the dog appeared dysphoric. As a result, it was administered acepromazine 0.01 mg/kg IV (Box 18-16).

BOX 18-16
Maxillectomy

- Preemptive analgesia: hydromorphone 0.2 mg/kg SQ; bupivacaine infraorbital block
- Postoperative analgesia: fentanyl bolus 2 μg/kg IV, followed by fentanyl infusion 3 to 5 μg/kg/hr IV

MANDIBULECTOMY (Box 18-17)

SIGNALMENT: *8-year-old spayed female golden retriever weighing 25 kg.*

PROBLEM: *This dog had a mass under the left lower canine tooth, diagnosed as osteosarcoma by previous biopsy. This required a complete rostral mandibulectomy, resecting 2.5 cm of mandible. The extensive bone cutting results in significant pain.*

SOURCE OF PAIN: *The pain originates from cut bone and periosteum along with some severed nerves. This usually results in severe pain.*

BOX 18-17

Mandibulectomy

- Somatic pain
- Moderate-to-severe intensity
- Inflammatory and surgically induced tissue trauma
- Acute onset and short duration

Treatment and Rationale

Preemptive Analgesia

Mandibulectomies can be very painful and difficult to treat. This case, like most cases of potential severe pain, warrants a multimodal approach to analgesia.

- Parenteral analgesia: This dog received morphine 1.0 mg/kg SQ as part of her premedication, along with acepromazine and atropine.
- Local anesthesia: Local anesthetic blocks are very useful for helping to prevent wind-up secondary to the surgical insult, resulting in a patient that may be easier to keep comfortable postoperatively.
  - Mental nerve blocks are useful for cranial mandibulectomies. This dog's mandibulectomy was planned to resect bone caudal to the mental nerve. As a result, a mental nerve block was not used.
  - Mandibular nerve blocks are useful for providing local anesthesia to the ramus of the mandible. This dog received bilat-

eral mandibular nerve blocks with bupivacaine 7.5 mg at each site. This low dose of local anesthetic is possible because the local anesthetic is deposited directly over the nerve.

- Ketamine was administered as a bolus 0.5 mg/kg IV, immediately before surgical stimulation, followed by a ketamine infusion, 10 μg/kg/min, to help prevent wind-up and dysphoria postoperatively.
- The PainBuster System (dj Orthopedics, Inc., Vista, California) was used to provide a constant infusion of lidocaine (2 ml/hr) for 3 days (see Chapter 15).

Postoperative Analgesia

- This dog began receiving a fentanyl infusion, 3 μg/kg/hr, after a fentanyl bolus 2 μg/kg IV, immediately after intubation. The infusion was adjusted as necessary throughout the night. It was discontinued 24 hours after surgery.
- The ketamine infusion was lowered to 2 μg/kg/min for the next 24 hours.
- This dog became anxious 12 hours after surgery. Acepromazine 0.01 mg/kg IV was administered, which calmed the dog and presumably also made it care less about its pain.

Multiday Analgesia

This dog was discharged from the hospital approximately 24 hours after surgery. The PainBuster System provided adequate analgesia for 3 days and was replaced with carprofen 50 mg PO bid for another 3 days. The dog exhibited normal behavior at home (Box 18-18).

BOX 18-18

Mandibulectomy

- Preemptive analgesia: morphine 1.0 mg/kg SQ; bupivacaine mandibular nerve block; ketamine microdose infusion
- Immediate postoperative analgesia: fentanyl bolus 2 μg/kg IV, followed by fentanyl infusion 3 μg/kg/hr IV
- Multiday analgesia: PainBuster System; carprofen 2 mg/kg PO bid

NASAL BIOPSY (Box 18-19)

SIGNALMENT: *12-year-old spayed female mixed breed dog weighing 7 kg.*

PROBLEM: *This dog has a 4-month history of epistaxis requiring rhinoscopy and potential biopsy.*

SOURCE OF PAIN: *Stimulation of nasal mucosa.*

BOX 18-19

Nasal Biopsy

- Visceral pain
- Mild-to-moderate intensity
- Surgically induced tissue trauma
- Acute onset and short duration

Treatment and Rationale

Premedication

This dog was very calm and required little premedication for restraint purposes. Nonetheless, she was administered oxymorphone 0.05 mg/kg SQ for some basal analgesia and to achieve an inhalant anesthetic–sparing effect. Atropine 0.02 mg/kg SQ was administered to prevent vagal induced bradycardia from the opioid.

Xylazine

Even with the oxymorphone, it was predicted that adequate analgesia to prevent movement would be difficult to achieve as the rhinoscope approached the back of the nasal passage. When scoping and biopsy became very stimulating, despite oxymorphone and high doses of isoflurane, xylazine 0.1 mg/kg IV was administered. Even though this dose is miniscule compared with that on the label, it provides good analgesia, especially in conjunction with an opioid, with which it is synergistic. Xylazine administration decreased movement and allowed completion of the procedure. Alternatively, medetomidine 10 µg/kg IV could have been administered.

Postoperative Analgesia

Postoperative pain is probably minimal after rhinoscopy and nasal biopsy. As such, no analgesics were administered (Box 18-20).

BOX 18-20

Nasal Biopsy

- Preemptive analgesia: oxymorphone 0.05 mg/kg SQ
- Intraoperative analgesia: xylazine 0.1 mg/kg IV
- Postoperative analgesia: none

SHOULDER SURGERY (Box 18-21)

SIGNALMENT: *2-year-old castrated male Labrador retriever mix weighing 41 kg.*
PROBLEM: *Osteochondritis dissecans (OCD) of the left shoulder.*
SOURCE OF PAIN: *Articular cartilage defect and surgical trauma.*

BOX 18-21

Shoulder Surgery

- Somatic pain
- Moderate intensity
- Inflammatory and surgically induced tissue trauma
- Acute onset; 3 to 5 days' duration

Treatment and Rationale

Preemptive Analgesia

This dog was premedicated with buprenorphine 0.01 mg/kg for analgesia along with acepromazine 0.02 mg/kg for calming and atropine 0.02 mg/kg to offset vagal-induced bradycardia. All drugs were combined in one syringe and administered subcutaneously. Buprenorphine was administered with the intent of providing long-term analgesia.

Postoperative Analgesia

The dog had a very rough recovery from anesthesia and surgery. Because part of the recovery problem was believed to be due to pain, a test dose of IV fentanyl (2 μg/kg) was administered. Because of occupation of the μ receptors by buprenorphine, fentanyl had little effect. The dog was then administered medetomidine 1 μg/kg IV, which calmed the dog considerably. Ketoprofen 2 mg/kg SQ was also administered. Medetomidine administration was repeated approximately every 90 minutes for 4 hours. Four hours after surgery, morphine 1.0 mg/kg SQ was administered, then repeated every 5 hours until the next morning (Box 18-22).

BOX 18-22

Shoulder Surgery

- Preemptive analgesia: buprenorphine 0.01 mg/kg SQ
- Postoperative analgesia: medetomidine 1 μg/kg IV; ketoprofen 2 mg/kg SQ; morphine 1 mg/kg SQ

ELBOW SURGERY (Box 18-23)

SIGNALMENT: *18-month-old female Bernese Mountain dog weighing 34 kg.*
PROBLEM: *This dog had OCD of the right elbow joint.*
SOURCE OF PAIN: *Articular cartilage defect and surgical trauma.*

BOX 18-23

Elbow Surgery

- Somatic pain
- Moderate intensity
- Inflammatory and surgically induced tissue trauma
- Acute onset; 3 to 5 days' duration

Treatment and Rationale
Preemptive Analgesia
This dog was premedicated with oxymorphone 0.1 mg/kg for analgesia along with acepromazine 0.015 mg/kg for calming and glycopyrrolate 0.01 mg/kg to help prevent oxymorphone-induced bradycardia. All drugs were combined in one syringe and administered subcutaneously.

Postoperative Analgesia: Multimodal

- On closing of the joint capsule, a combination of morphine 2.5 mg and bupivacaine 7.5 mg was injected into the joint space.
  - The morphine should bind articular opioid receptors to provide some degree of analgesia.
  - The bupivacaine should block sodium channels and provide good analgesia for 4 to 8 hours.
- This dog woke up feeling very comfortable. It began receiving sustained-release oral morphine, 30 mg twice daily, 6 hours after surgery. Administration of carprofen was also started the morning after surgery.
- The dog remained comfortable for the 4 days it received the morphine (Box 18-24).

BOX 18-24
Elbow Surgery

- Preemptive analgesia: oxymorphone 0.1 mg/kg SQ
- Postoperative analgesia: morphine 2.5 mg + bupivacaine 7.5 mg intraarticular
- Multiday analgesia: sustained-release morphine 1 mg/kg PO bid; carprofen 1.0 mg/kg PO bid

---

RADIUS/ULNAR FRACTURE REPAIR (Box 18-25)

SIGNALMENT: *10-year-old castrated male mixed breed dog weighing 30 kg.*

PROBLEM: *This dog jumped from the back of a truck and fractured its left radius and ulna 3 days before presentation for anesthesia*

and surgery. It had been stabilized hemodynamically before presentation.
SOURCE OF PAIN: *Fractured bones.*

BOX 18-25
Radius/Ulnar Fracture Repair

- Visceral and somatic pain
- Moderate intensity
- Inflammatory and surgically trauma-induced
- Acute onset

Treatment and Rationale
Preemptive Analgesia: Multimodal
- This dog was premedicated with morphine 1.0 mg/kg for analgesia along with atropine, administered subcutaneously, to prevent bradycardia. No sedative or tranquilizer was used because this dog was very calm.
- After induction of anesthesia and clipping of the leg, a brachial plexus block was performed with bupivacaine 5 ml (0.75%), equivalent to approximately 1.3 mg/kg (see Chapter 15).

Postoperative Analgesia
- This dog was given morphine 1.0 mg/kg SQ on extubation. It was not administered earlier because of concerns about sedation and inability to extubate the patient without protective laryngeal reflexes.
- Two hours later, this dog was administered another dose of morphine 1.0 mg/kg SQ.
- The dog still seemed uncomfortable in response to palpation and was unable to rest comfortably. An electroacupuncture treatment was performed.
  - Small Intestine meridian (SI) 3 to SI 9
  - Large Intestine meridian (LI) 4 to LI 15
  - Pericardium meridian (PC) 6 to PC 3
  - 2.5 Hz alternating current (AC) continuous stimulation for 20 minutes

- This dog was comfortable throughout the night and did not require any additional analgesics or sedation (Box 18-26).

BOX 18-26
Radius/Ulnar Fracture Repair

- Preemptive analgesia: morphine 1.0 mg/kg SQ; bupivacaine brachial plexus block
- Postoperative analgesia: morphine 1.0 mg/kg SQ; electroacupuncture

---

FORELIMB AMPUTATION (Box 18-27)

SIGNALMENT: *12-year-old male golden retriever weighing 38 kg.*
PROBLEM: *Osteosarcoma of the right forelimb.*
SOURCE OF PAIN: *Soft tissue surgical trauma secondary to scapulectomy and forelimb removal.*

BOX 18-27
Forelimb Amputation

- Visceral and somatic pain
- Moderate-to-severe intensity
- Inflammatory and surgically induced tissue trauma
- Acute onset

Treatment and Rationale
Preoperative Analgesia

- This dog was premedicated with morphine 1.0 mg/kg SQ to provide preemptive analgesia and atropine 0.04 mg/kg SQ to prevent morphine-induced bradycardia.
- Microdose ketamine was administered as a 0.5 mg/kg bolus, followed by a 10 μg/kg/min infusion. This was administered throughout surgery. Ketamine blocks N-methyl-D-aspartate

(NMDA) receptors and should help decrease postoperative pain and dysphoria.

Postoperative Analgesia

- A morphine infusion of 0.1 mg/kg/hr was started after a morphine bolus of 0.1 mg/kg IV. This provided continuous analgesia.
- The microdose ketamine infusion was decreased to 2 μg/kg/min for the first 24 hours after surgery.
- This dog required no other drugs to maintain good analgesia while in the hospital (Box 18-28).

BOX 18-28

Forelimb Amputation

- Preemptive analgesia: morphine 1.0 mg/kg SQ; microdose ketamine IV
- Postoperative analgesia: morphine bolus 0.1 mg/kg IV, followed by morphine infusion 0.1 mg/kg/hr; microdose ketamine

---

THORACOTOMY-STERNOTOMY (Box 18-29)

SIGNALMENT: *11-year-old spayed female domestic short-hair cat weighing 3.2 kg.*
PROBLEM: *Pulmonary tumor.*
SOURCE OF PAIN: *Surgery and stretching.*

BOX 18-29

Thoracotomy-Sternotomy

- Visceral and somatic pain
- Severe intensity
- Inflammatory and surgically induced tissue trauma
- Acute onset

Treatment and Rationale

Premedication

This cat was fractious. It was believed that high doses of ketamine or some other nonreversible drug would need to be administered to achieve chemical restraint. As a result, this cat was not premedicated, but anesthesia was box-induced with sevoflurane.

Intraoperative

This cat was administered fentanyl 2 μg/kg IV bolus, followed by 5 μg/kg/hr IV infusion before and during surgery to provide analgesia in addition to that provided by the gas anesthetic.

Postoperative

Before the cat awakened, it was administered lidocaine 1.5 mg/kg and bupivacaine 1.5 mg/kg mixed interpleurally through the chest tube. This was administered every 3 to 6 hours. Fentanyl was also administered as an infusion at 2 to 4 μg/kg/hr. The combination produced good analgesia (Box 18-30).

BOX 18-30

Thoracotomy-Sternotomy

- Preemptive and intraoperative analgesia: fentanyl 2 μg/kg IV, followed by fentanyl 5 μg/kg/hr IV
- Postoperative analgesia: lidocaine + bupivacaine interpleural block; fentanyl infusion 2 to 4 μg/kg/hr IV

INTERCOSTAL THORACOTOMY (Box 18-31)

SIGNALMENT: *4-month-old male Labrador retriever weighing 16 kg.*
PROBLEM: *Patent ductus arteriosus (PDA).*

SOURCE OF PAIN: *Soft tissue surgical trauma plus displacement and stretching of soft tissue, cartilage, and bone.*

BOX 18-31

Intercostal Thoracotomy

- Visceral and somatic pain
- Moderate-to-severe intensity
- Inflammatory and surgically induced tissue trauma
- Acute onset

Treatment and Rationale

Premedication
This dog was premedicated with oxymorphone 0.1 mg/kg SQ for preemptive analgesia along with atropine 0.04 mg/kg to counter increases in vagal tone and acepromazine 0.02 mg/kg for calming.

Time of Closure
At the time of closure, bupivacaine 2 mg/kg was injected caudal to the ribs to block the intercostal nerves at the incision site and two intercostal spaces cranial and caudal to the surgical site.

Postoperative
After extubation, this dog was administered morphine 0.05 mg/kg IV, followed by morphine 0.1 mg/kg/hr for continuous analgesia. The combination of local anesthetic and opioid provided good analgesia in this dog (Box 18-32).

BOX 18-32

Intercostal Thoracotomy

- Preemptive analgesia: oxymorphone 0.1 mg/kg SQ
- Postoperative analgesia: bupivacaine intercostal nerve block; morphine bolus 0.05 mg/kg IV, followed by morphine infusion 0.1 mg/kg/hr IV

LAPAROTOMY: INTESTINAL RESECTION AND ANASTOMOSIS (Box 18-33)

SIGNALMENT: *6-year-old castrated male Labrador retriever weighing 47 kg.*

PROBLEM: *Intestinal foreign body requiring resection and anastomosis.*

SOURCE OF PAIN: *Body wall incisional trauma and abdominal ligament stretching.*

BOX 18-33
Intestinal Resection and Anastomosis

- Somatic and visceral pain
- Moderate-to-severe intensity
- Inflammatory and surgically induced tissue trauma
- Acute onset

Treatment and Rationale

Premedication

This dog was premedicated with morphine, approximately 1.0 mg/kg, for preemptive analgesia, along with acepromazine 0.01 mg/kg for calming and atropine 0.04 mg/kg to prevent bradycardia, all combined and administered subcutaneously.

Preincision Medication

Before surgical stimulation, an epidural injection of morphine 0.1 mg/kg combined with bupivacaine 0.1 mg/kg was attempted at the lumbosacral vertebral space. This was unsuccessful. A subarachnoid injection was performed at the lumbar 6-7 vertebral space. Because of the low dose of bupivacaine, there were no alterations in dose, despite injection in the cerebrospinal fluid instead of epidurally.

- Epidural morphine will provide analgesia, but not anesthesia, for 12 to 24 hours. There is typically no change in morphine dose, regardless of epidural or subarachnoid injection. Epidural morphine may also cause urinary retention. Veterinarians should be aware of this effect because patients may require bladder expression or a urinary catheter postoperatively.

- Epidural bupivacaine can have different effects, depending on dose. As the dose gets larger, motor and sensory blockade occur. Doses used in this dog were very small with the intent of blocking sensory nerve transmission without motor blockade and paralysis. If high doses are intended for epidural injection, they should be halved for subarachnoid injection.

Postoperative Analgesia

After the body wall was closed, but before the skin was sutured, an incisional block was performed by using bupivacaine 40 mg (0.5%) in 1:200,000 epinephrine, diluted to half with sterile normal saline solution. The combination of the subarachnoid drugs and the incisional block produced excellent analgesia. This dog did not experience urinary retention (Box 18-34).

BOX 18-34

Intestinal Resection and Anastomosis

- Preemptive analgesia: morphine 1.0 mg/kg SQ; subarachnoid morphine + bupivacaine
- Postoperative analgesia: bupivacaine incisional block

LAPAROTOMY-CYSTOTOMY (Box 18-35)

SIGNALMENT: *4-year-old male cocker spaniel mix weighing 12 kg.*
PROBLEM: *Urinary calculi requiring laparotomy and cystotomy.*
SOURCE OF PAIN: *Body wall incisional trauma and abdominal ligament stretching.*

BOX 18-35

Cystotomy

- Somatic and visceral pain
- Moderate-to-severe intensity
- Inflammatory and surgically induced tissue trauma
- Acute onset

Treatment and Rationale

Premedication

This dog had a history of idiopathic epilepsy and was extremely nervous and active. He was premedicated with morphine 1.0 mg/kg SQ for preemptive analgesia. Acepromazine was contraindicated because of his seizure history. Xylazine 0.4 mg/kg SQ was administered with the morphine. Xylazine has a synergistic effect with opioids to produce better sedation and analgesia. Atropine 0.04 mg/kg was added to the mixture because both drugs increase vagal tone and can cause bradycardia.

Postoperative

* This dog did not receive epidural morphine or local anesthetic, even though this technique would likely produce good postoperative analgesia. On the basis of this dog's behavior, it was believed that it would be extremely difficult to maintain a urinary catheter without it being chewed out. Because epidural morphine can cause urinary retention and this patient was undergoing bladder surgery, it was best to avoid subjecting the cystotomy incision to excess intraluminal pressure.
* Before skin closure, this dog received an incisional block consisting of bupivacaine 15 mg (0.5%) with 1:200,000 epinephrine diluted in half with 0.9% saline solution. This provided good body wall analgesia for approximately 8 hours.
* Fentanyl 2 to 5 μg/kg/hr was administered as an infusion to provide good abdominal analgesia.
* At good analgesic doses, this dog became dysphoric, requiring intermittent administration of xylazine 0.05 mg/kg IV.
* This dog was discharged from the hospital 30 hours after surgery with no other analgesics (Box 18-36).

BOX 18-36

Cystotomy

* Preemptive analgesia: morphine 1.0 mg/kg + xylazine 0.4 mg/kg SQ
* Postoperative analgesia: bupivacaine incisional block; fentanyl bolus 2 μg/kg IV, followed by fentanyl infusion 2 to 5 μg/kg/hr

PANCREATITIS (Box 18-37)

SIGNALMENT: *12-year-old spayed female miniature schnauzer.*
PROBLEM: *History of vomiting and lethargy for 3 days; abdominal pain; no abdominal obstruction; results of blood work consistent with pancreatitis.*
SOURCE OF PAIN: *Visceral pain associated with pancreatitis.*

BOX 18-37

Pancreatitis

- Visceral pain
- Moderate-to-severe intensity
- Inflammatory
- Acute onset

Treatment and Rationale

- This dog was initially unsuccessfully treated with a continuous infusion of fentanyl 3 to 6 μg/kg/hr after a bolus of 2 μg/kg. The dog was still unable to rest without agitation.
- The second approach to this dog's pain included local anesthetics placed in the interpleural space. Interpleural local anesthetics can provide analgesia for thoracic and cranial abdominal pain. The nerves from the cranial abdomen enter the spinal cord in the thorax.
  - Lidocaine 1.5 mg/kg was injected in the sixth intercostal space through a 22-gauge butterfly catheter. This was injected initially to produce an immediate block.
  - Bupivacaine 1.5 mg/kg was injected after administration of the lidocaine. Bupivacaine has a 15- to 20-minute onset and can cause stinging. The lidocaine prevents the bupivacaine-induced stinging.
  - This technique produced comfort, allowing this dog to sleep. The local anesthetic technique was repeated every 4 hours. The fentanyl infusion was continued at 2 μg/kg/hr (Box 18-38).

BOX 18-38

Pancreatitis

- Unsuccessful analgesia: fentanyl infusion
- Successful analgesia: lidocaine + bupivacaine interpleural block

---

LUMBOSACRAL DISK SURGERY (Box 18-39)

SIGNALMENT: *7-year-old spayed female miniature dachshund weighing 8 kg.*
PROBLEM: *Lumbosacral disk protrusion.*
SOURCE OF PAIN: *Spinal cord swelling and disk entrapment of nerve roots.*

BOX 18-39

Lumbosacral Hemilaminectomy

- Somatic and visceral pain
- Moderate-to-severe intensity
- Inflammatory and surgically induced tissue trauma + underlying disease
- Acute onset

Treatment and Rationale
Premedication
This dog was premedicated with morphine 0.75 mg/kg SQ to provide analgesia along with glycopyrrolate 0.01 mg/kg to help prevent bradycardia.

Intraoperative
This dog received fentanyl 2 μg/kg IV, followed by fentanyl 10 μg/kg/hr to provide good intraoperative analgesia and to decrease the inhalant anesthetic concentration to help maintain cardiac output and

blood pressure. The fentanyl infusion was discontinued 30 minutes before the anticipated finish time to facilitate a timely extubation.

Postoperative

This dog had a very smooth recovery. She remained sedated. The fentanyl infusion was restarted at 3 µg/kg/hr. This dog remained comfortable for the next 36 hours before she was discharged from the critical care unit (Box 18-40).

BOX 18-40

Lumbosacral Hemilaminectomy

- Preemptive analgesia: morphine 0.75 mg/kg SQ
- Intraoperative analgesia: fentanyl bolus 2 µg/kg IV, followed by fentanyl infusion 10 µg/kg/hr IV
- Postoperative analgesia: fentanyl infusion 3 µg/kg/hr IV

TAIL AMPUTATION (Box 18-41)

SIGNALMENT: *6-year-old castrated male domestic long-hair cat.*
PROBLEM: *This cat's tail got caught in a portable house fan, causing a degloving injury and a fracture distal to coccygeal space 4.*
SOURCE OF PAIN: *Bone fracture and soft tissue trauma.*

BOX 18-41

Tail Amputation

- Somatic pain
- Moderate intensity
- Inflammatory and surgically induced tissue trauma + underlying disease
- Acute onset

Treatment and Rationale

Preemptive Analgesia

- This cat received medetomidine 20 µg/kg and morphine 0.25 mg/kg administered together subcutaneously for analgesia and sedation. Atropine 0.04 mg/kg was also administered to prevent bradycardia associated with these drugs.

- After induction of anesthesia, bupivacaine 0.75 mg/kg was injected epidurally at coccygeal space 1-2.

Postoperative Analgesia

- Ketoprofen 2.2 mg/kg SQ was injected during recovery to provide analgesia and as an antiinflammatory agent.
- This cat received morphine 0.25 mg/kg SQ 3 hours after the initial morphine injections (Box 18-42).

BOX 18-42

Tail Amputation

- Preemptive analgesia: morphine 0.25 mg/kg SQ + medetomidine 20 μg/kg SQ; bupivacaine epidural
- Postoperative analgesia: ketoprofen 2.2 mg/kg SQ + morphine 0.25 mg/kg SQ

REAR LIMB AMPUTATION (Box 18-43)

SIGNALMENT: *7-year-old spayed female Rottweiler weighing 42 kg.*
PROBLEM: *Osteosarcoma of the left rear limb, requiring amputation.*
SOURCE OF PAIN: *General surgical trauma.*

BOX 18-43

Rear Limb Amputation

- Somatic pain
- Moderate-to-severe intensity
- Inflammatory and surgically induced tissue trauma
- Acute onset

Treatment and Rationale

Preoperative

- This dog received morphine 1.0 mg/kg for preemptive analgesia and atropine 0.05 mg/kg both combined and administered subcutaneously. No other tranquilizer or sedative was administered.

- Epidural morphine 0.1 mg/kg and bupivacaine 0.3 mg/kg were administered to provide supplemental intraoperative analgesia and postoperative analgesia of 12 to 24 hours' duration.

Postoperative

This dog received a fentanyl infusion 3 to 5 μg/kg/hr IV over the next 24 hours to maintain good analgesia. She was released from the critical care unit and received sustained-release oral morphine 30 mg twice daily for the next 4 days (Box 18-44).

BOX 18-44

Rear Limb Amputation

- Preemptive analgesia: morphine 1.0 mg/kg SQ; morphine + bupivacaine epidural
- Postoperative analgesia: fentanyl bolus 2 μg/kg IV, followed by fentanyl infusion 3 to 5 μg/kg/hr IV
- Multiday analgesia: sustained-release morphine 30 mg PO bid

---

BILATERAL FEMORAL FRACTURE REPAIR (Box 18-45)

SIGNALMENT: *6-year-old spayed female (mixed breed) Australian Shepherd.*
PROBLEM: *This dog slipped off an icy deck and fell 25 feet. Radiographs revealed bilateral comminuted femoral fractures.*
SOURCE OF PAIN: *Broken bones and soft tissue trauma.*

Treatment and Rationale

Preemptive Analgesia

Femoral fracture repairs can be very painful. This case, like most cases of potential severe pain, warrants a multimodal approach to analgesia.

BOX 18-45
Bilateral Femoral Fracture Repair

- Somatic pain
- Severe intensity
- Inflammatory and surgically induced tissue trauma
- Acute onset

- Parenteral analgesia: This dog received morphine 1.0 mg/kg SQ as part of her premedication, along with acepromazine and atropine.
- After the dog was anesthetized, an epidural catheter was inserted in the lumbosacral space and advanced 3 disk spaces cranially. Morphine 0.1 mg/kg along with bupivacaine 0.1 mg/kg was injected through the catheter before surgery. This catheter allowed redosing of epidural analgesics for several days. Placing morphine in the epidural space provided good analgesia for 12 to 24 hours with minimal central nervous system side effects such as sedation. The low dose of bupivacaine provided analgesia by blocking sensory nerve transmission with minimal effect on motor nerve transmission. This allowed the dog to feel its legs in recovery, preventing self-trauma and mutilation, which sometimes occurs after epidural regional anesthesia.

Anesthesia and Surgery
This dog underwent normal anesthesia and surgery.

Postoperative
Postoperatively, this dog woke up in pain and agitated.
- Morphine 0.1 mg/kg IV was administered to provide immediate control of the pain. Morphine was then infused at 0.1 mg/kg/hr to provide analgesia in addition to the epidural morphine. The infusion was continued for 16 hours to get the dog past the immediate postsurgical trauma.

- Acepromazine 0.25 mg IV was administered during recovery because of the agitation. It was redosed 3.5 hours later.
- Epidural morphine 0.1 mg/kg was redosed 12 hours after the initial administration, then at 24-hour intervals for another 3 days, at which time the epidural catheter was removed (Box 18-46).

BOX 18-46

Bilateral Femoral Fracture Repair

- Preemptive analgesia: morphine 1.0 mg/kg SQ; morphine and bupivacaine via epidural catheter
- Postoperative analgesia: morphine bolus 0.1 mg/kg IV, followed by morphine infusion 0.1 mg/kg/hr IV; epidural morphine

---

GENERAL TRAUMA (Box 18-47)

SIGNALMENT: *7-year-old castrated male domestic short-hair cat weighing 3 kg.*
PROBLEM: *Recently hit by car with head trauma, a broken left humerus, and general soft tissue trauma.*
SOURCE OF PAIN: *General soft tissue trauma and fractured bone.*

BOX 18-47

General Trauma

- Somatic pain
- Moderate-to-severe intensity
- Inflammatory and trauma-induced tissue trauma
- Acute onset

Treatment and Rationale

- The immediate goal for this cat was to provide hemodynamic stabilization and good analgesia overnight but be able to assess mentation periodically to help determine the status of the head trauma.
- The use of fentanyl was considered but rejected.
- Remifentanil requires no liver metabolism but is cleared via nonspecific esterases throughout the body. In other species it has a duration of action of 8 to 10 minutes, regardless of infusion time. It appears to be the same in cats. For these reasons, remifentanil was administered to this cat at 6 μg/kg/hr, which seemed to keep the cat comfortable. When neurologic assessment was desired, the remifentanil infusion was discontinued. Assessment was performed 10 minutes later. After assessment, analgesia was rapidly provided by administering a bolus of remifentanil 4 μg/kg, then restarting the infusion (Box 18-48).

BOX 18-48

General Trauma

- Continuous analgesia: remifentanil 6 μg/kg/hr

EXERCISE-INDUCED TRAUMA (Box 18-10)

SIGNALMENT: *4-year-old spayed female mixed breed dog weighing 25 kg.*

PROBLEM: *Limping on right rear limb after first long hike of the year in the mountains.*

SOURCE OF PAIN: *After orthopedic examination was done and radiographs were obtained, it was believed that this dog had mild hip dysplasia of the right coxofemoral joint, resulting in osteoarthritic pain. She had some muscle soreness as well.*

BOX 18-49

Exercise-Induced Trauma

- Somatic pain
- Mild-to-moderate intensity
- Inflammatory and exercise-induced tissue trauma
- Acute onset

Treatment and Rationale

This is acute exercise-induced pain of moderate severity. This dog was treated successfully with carprofen 50 mg, given orally twice daily for 7 days (Box 18-50).

BOX 18-50

Exercise-Induced Trauma

- Analgesia: carprofen 2.2 mg/kg PO bid

19

Chronic Pain Management

A Case-Based Approach

JAMES S. GAYNOR AND WILLIAM W. MUIR III

The treatment of chronic pain is an unresolved problem in veterinary medicine. Other than the rampant and routine use of nonsteroidal antiinflammatory drugs (NSAIDs), no medications or therapeutic regimens, including alternative therapies (e.g., acupuncture, physical therapy, nutriceuticals) have emerged as being especially effective for the long-term treatment of chronic pain in dogs and cats. In other words, regardless of the various success stories, the treatment of chronic pain in veterinary medicine is in its infancy. Regardless of the dearth of validated therapies, we offer some examples for the treatment of chronic pain in dogs and cats with the hope that the future will provide experimentally justified and efficacious alternatives to what we believe is largely an unexplored and currently anecdotal practice.

The following are specific examples of dogs and cats with chronic pain. The likely cause and specific treatments of pain are described in detail. Each example presents a unique aspect or problem as it relates to pain management. Because the examples selected were evaluated and the treatment protocols designed by different veterinarians, diverse therapeutic protocols are used. Various drugs, procedures, and treatment philosophies are described. More detail on each drug and procedure can be found in previous chapters of this book. All patients should be considered systemically healthy unless otherwise noted.

HIP DYSPLASIA (Box 19-1)

Pain control for a dog with degenerative joint disease involving both hips.

SIGNALMENT: *12-year-old female spayed German shepherd dog weighing 36 kg with bilateral hip dysplasia: left hip worse than right.*

ISSUE: *The dog has had chronic osteoarthritis and pain for 8 years. The pain has been getting continuously worse with age.*

CAUSE OF PAIN: *Osteoarthritis (inflammatory pain) of the coxofemoral joints.*

BOX 19-1

Case 1: Canine—Hip Dysplasia

Coxofemoral osteoarthritis.
Moderate-to-severe intensity.
Somatic in origin; tissue inflammation.

TREATMENT AND RATIONALE (Box 19-2)

- This dog was initially administered aspirin as needed on "bad days." The frequency of administration increased over several years, and the owner and the veterinarian became concerned about the possibility of gastrointestinal (GI) or renal side effects.
- Carprofen was initiated as an alternative to aspirin: the dog was given carprofen 25 mg PO bid. This dose was considered low, but the dog was more comfortable within 1 day of initiation of therapy.
- Pain gradually increased in intensity, and the dose of carprofen was increased to 50 mg PO bid. This dose was considered to be high, but the dog was more comfortable without signs of toxicity (e.g., ulcers, abnormal findings in liver or renal chemistry or on hemogram) for approximately 6 months.
- After 6 months, the dog was in pain again. Rather than increasing the dose of carprofen and risking toxic side effects, the veterinarian recommended that therapy be changed to etodolac 10 mg/ kg PO sid.

- Although there are only a few relatively low-toxicity NSAIDs, it is reasonable to expect that if one does not work well, another might work better.
- There is a potential risk, when switching from one NSAID to another in a short period, that additive side effects, such as GI ulceration, may occur. Side effects are more likely to occur in patients that are immunosuppressed.
- Ideally, a washout period of approximately 7 to 10 days should occur between ending administration of one NSAID and starting administration of another.
- If a washout period is not possible, administration of a GI protectant, such as misoprostol, for approximately 1 week to 10 days is advisable. For example, end the administration of one NSAID on the evening of one day and start misoprostol 2 to 5 μg/kg PO bid. Start the new NSAID the following day, continuing with the misoprostol for at least 10 days or longer if necessary.
- Oral opioids (morphine 0.5 mg/kg tid) can be administered in the interim to keep the dog comfortable during the washout period.
- Carprofen was discontinued for 10 days, during which time this dog became more and more uncomfortable. The dog was initially administered etodolac 450 mg PO daily, but this did not seem to provide any improvement in the dog's quality of life.
- The veterinarian and owner discussed the potential of acupuncture for relief of pain.
- Electroacupuncture was instituted twice weekly for 3 weeks, alternating hips at each treatment with the following protocol.
  1. Gallbladder (GB) 29 to GB 30
  2. Bladder (BL) 40 to BL 54
  3. GB 34
  4. Bilateral BL—11
  5. Alternating current, 2.5 Hz, continuous for 20 minutes (for 1 and 2 only)
- The dog became much more comfortable. During the fourth week of acupuncture, the dog received only one treatment.

- Acupuncture therapy was subsequently administered every 4 to 6 weeks. After 2 months, the etodolac dose was decreased to 300 mg PO daily. The dog remained comfortable (see Box 19-2).

BOX 19-2

Case 1: Canine—Hip Dysplasia

First therapy: carprofen 25 to 50 mg PO bid.
Second therapy: etodolac 450 mg PO sid.
Final therapy: electroacupuncture.

CHRONIC AURAL DISEASE (Box 19-3)

SIGNALMENT: *10-year-old castrated mixed breed dog weighing 29 kg.*
ISSUE: *The dog had had chronic otitis externa for over a year. Both ears had been unsuccessfully treated with an intermittent regimen of antibiotics (doxycycline, neomycin) and prednisone during this period. The dog was presented with severe otitis externa and semicontinuous head shaking. The tips of both ears had become traumatized and were bleeding from the constant head shaking.*
CAUSE OF PAIN: *Inflammation of both ear canals and the immediate surrounding tissues. Palpation of both ears caused extreme pain.*

BOX 19-3

Case 2: Canine—Chronic Aural Disease

Chronic otitis externa.
Moderate-to-severe intensity.
Somatic in origin; tissue inflammation.

TREATMENT AND RATIONALE: *The dog was in severe pain, and the owners initially refused surgery. A decision was made to begin an aggressive course of antibiotic therapy combined with analgesics and antiinflammatory drugs to bring the infection and inflammatory condition under control (Box 19-4).*

- Initial therapy: A culture was obtained for bacterial/fungal identification and antibiotic/antifungal agent selection. The dog was sedated (medetomidine 20 μg/kg IM), and the ears were cleaned with a salicylic acid cleanser (Epi-otic; Virbac, Fort Worth, Texas).
  - Antibiotic/antifungal therapy consisted of gentamicin, neomycin, polymyxin B, and myconazole.
  - Prednisolone 1 mg/kg PO sid was administered to reduce inflammation and control pain. Prednisolone therapy was reduced to 0.5 mg/kg PO sid after the first week and continued for an additional 2 weeks.
  - Buprenorphine 0.01 mg/kg IM tid was administered for the first 24 hours to control pain.
- Etodolac 10 mg/kg PO sid was administered as continuous analgesic therapy after discontinuation of prednisolone. Renal (blood urea nitrogen [BUN], creatinine) and liver (aspartate aminotransferase [AST] and alanine aminotransferase [ALT]) tests were performed before treatment and at bimonthly intervals to ensure normal organ function (see Box 19-4).
- Medical therapy was continued for an additional 6 months with moderate success, after which time the owners consented to a unilateral (left) total ear canal ablation. The right ear subsequently responded to the therapy within 4 weeks of surgery.
  - A sterile multipore catheter was buried within the surgical incision at the end of the surgical procedure. This catheter was connected to an infusion bulb (PainBuster System; dj Orthopedics, Inc., Vista, California), which delivered 15 mg of ropivacaine for a period of 50 hours after surgery. The dog demonstrated no signs of pain during the time that the local anesthetic, ropivacaine, was being administered (Fig. 19-1).

BOX 19-4

Case 2: Chronic Otitis Externa

First therapy: prednisolone 1 mg/kg PO.
Second therapy: buprenorphine 0.01 mg/kg IM tid.
Third therapy: etodolac 10 mg/kg PO sid.
Final therapy: total ear canal ablation of left ear canal (intralesional ropivacaine; PainBuster for 50 hours postoperatively).

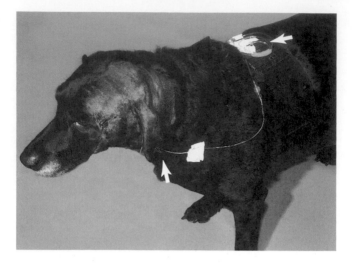

Fig. 19-1 The PainBuster System provides continuous administration of local anesthetic (lidocaine, ropivacaine) into the surgery site for 1 to 5 days.

CHRONIC EPISODIC PANCREATITIS (Box 19-5)

SIGNALMENT: *16-year-old castrated male Persian cat weighing 4.5 kg.*
ISSUE: *The cat had chronic episodic pancreatitis.*
CAUSE OF PAIN: *Chronic, episodic inflammation of the pancreas caused by chronic immune-mediated cholangiohepatitis-pancreatitis.*

BOX 19-5

Case 3: Feline—Chronic Episodic Pancreatitis

Chronic pancreatitis.
Severe intensity.
Somatic in origin; tissue inflammation.

TREATMENT AND RATIONALE: *The cat had severe pain during the pancreatic inflammatory episodes and refused to eat, drink, move, or socially interact. The cat would sit quietly alone for hours, but was noted to periodically stretch and occasionally vocalize (Box 19-6).*

- Initial therapy: The initial therapeutic goal for this cat was to attempt to control pain with intravenous (IV) analgesic drug therapy.
  - Hydromorphone was administered initially as a bolus (0.2 mg/kg IV), followed by an infusion at 0.1 mg/kg/hr. Within 4 hours, the cat was willing and able to drink and eat small amounts. The cat would also stand and move around the cage. The cat was then offered 1 oz of chopped raw bovine pancreatic extract, and cobalamin 150 μg SQ was administered every week for the next 6 weeks.
  - Hydromorphone 0.1 μg/kg/hr was administered for 48 hours and then discontinued. Morphine 0.2 mg/kg SQ was administered during the next 2 days as needed for pain control.

BOX 19-6

Case 3: Chronic Episodic Pancreatitis

First therapy: hydromorphone 0.2 mg/kg IV; 0.1 μg/kg/hr for 48 hours.
Second therapy: morphine 0.2 mg/kg SQ as needed.

RADIATION-INDUCED PAIN (Box 19-7)

SIGNALMENT: *9-year-old spayed female Labrador retriever weighing 31 kg.*
ISSUE: *This dog had a mast cell tumor removed from the lateral aspect of the mid left thigh and had been receiving outpatient radiation therapy in 14 sessions over a 3-week period. The dog continued to experience progressively more severe pain at home. Oral morphine was ineffective, and the dog became recumbent.*
CAUSE OF PAIN: *Radiation-induced soft tissue damage and inflammation.*

BOX 19-7

Case 4: Canine—Radiation-Induced Pain

Radiation therapy.
Severe intensity.
Somatic in origin; tissue inflammation.

TREATMENT AND RATIONALE: *Radiation therapy resulted in tissue inflammation and pain that reduced the dog's quality of life to the extent that she was now recumbent and required continuous care. The owner loved the dog but was extremely concerned that the pain and the dog's deterioration and listless behavior were insurmountable. Pain therapy had to improve the dog's quality of life and attitude for the owner to continue treatment (Box 19-8).*

- Initial therapy: The initial therapeutic goal for this dog was to attempt to control pain with IV drug therapy.
  - A sterile IV catheter was placed in the cephalic vein. Ketamine was diluted and administered as a bolus of 0.5 mg/kg IV, followed by infusion at 1 μg/kg/min. Ketamine was used as an N-methyl-D-aspartate (NMDA) receptor antagonist to help decrease central nervous system (CNS) hypersensitivity and reduce the chronic pain.
  - Fentanyl was administered concurrently, initially as a bolus (2 μg/kg), and followed by an infusion at 5 μg/kg/hr. Within 1 hour, the dog was willing and able to stand and walk.
  - Fentanyl and ketamine were administered for approximately 48 hours, and the dosage of fentanyl was decreased to 2 μg/kg/hr by the end of treatment.
- Long-term therapy: The dog was hospitalized for an additional 48 hours to facilitate the transition to oral drugs.
- Sustained-release morphine 30 mg PO bid was administered for 10 days. It was believed that this dose of morphine would control pain on the basis of the low dose of fentanyl that the dog had received during her initial therapy. This is the same dose of morphine she was receiving before admission to the hospital. The oral dose of morphine was reduced to 30 mg sid for 5 days after the first 10 days. Morphine was then discontinued completely.
- Administration of amantadine (Symmetrel, Endo Laboratories, Chadds Ford, Pennsylvania) was started, 100 mg PO sid, for 5 days with the hope of blocking NMDA receptors and preventing CNS hyperexcitability.
- The dog remained comfortable at home during the rest of her therapy and was last reported to be doing well enough to go outside and serve as a functional pet.

BOX 19-8
Case 4: Canine—Radiation-Induced Pain

First therapy: sustained-release oral morphine 30 mg PO bid.
Second therapy: ketamine 0.5 mg/kg IV, followed by 1 μg/kg/min in
conjunction with fentanyl 2 μg/kg IV, followed by 5 μg/kg/hr,
then 2 μg/kg/hr over 48 hours.
Final therapy: sustained-release oral morphine 30 mg bid for 10 days
and amantadine 100 mg PO sid for 5 days.

FORELIMB AMPUTATION PAIN (Box 19-9)

SIGNALMENT: *7-year-old spayed female husky weighing
25 kg.*
ISSUE: *This dog had osteosarcoma of the right front limb, which
resulted in an uneventful forelimb amputation. Three months later,
the dog was presented with the complaint of intermittently crying
out (episodic pain). The dog was initially administered codeine
30 mg with acetaminophen 300 mg PO bid for 5 days. The pain did
not appear to respond to therapy and became more frequent. On
physical examination, the dog was hyperresponsive to light touch
on the lateral thorax and abdomen but did not have neck or back
pain. The dog was considered to be demonstrating allodynia.*
CAUSE OF PAIN: *The cause of pain was unknown but was
conjectured to be associated with the right forelimb amputation and
therefore possibly related to nerve damage. Pain could be elicited
from the right lateral thorax and abdominal wall.*

BOX 19-9
Case 5: Canine—Forelimb Amputation

Osteosarcoma.
Moderate intensity and allodynia.
Neurogenic and CNS in origin.

TREATMENT AND RATIONALE: *Most traditional analgesic therapies (opioids, NSAIDs) are relatively ineffective for treating injured or diseased nerves (neuropathic pain). The decision was made to treat the dog for pain originating from nerve injury and central sensitization (secondary hyperalgesia) (Box 19-10).*

- Amantadine 100 mg PO sid for 5 days was instituted to block NMDA receptors and decrease central neuronal excitability with the intent of decreasing allodynia.
- Gabapentin 10 mg/kg PO tid was administered for 3 days, followed by 5 mg/kg PO tid for an additional 7 days.
- Sustained-release morphine 30 mg PO bid was administered for 10 days to provide analgesia.
- The owner reported that the dog was comfortable within 2 days. The seventh day after her new analgesic protocol (2 days after discontinuation of the amantadine), allodynia started to develop again. Amantadine 100 mg PO sid was administered for another 10 days, and sustained-release morphine, for another 5 days. The owner did not report a recurrence of pain after the end of the 10-day treatment period. Gabapentin 5 mg/kg PO tid was used, as needed, for 7 to 10 days to control subsequent episodes of pain.

BOX 19-10
Case 5: Canine—Forelimb Amputation

First therapy: amantadine 100 mg PO sid for 5 days concurrent with sustained-release morphine 30 mg PO bid for 10 days.

Second therapy: gabapentin 10 mg/kg PO tid for 3 days, then 5 mg/kg PO tid for 7 more days.

Final therapy: amantadine 100 mg PO sid for 10 days concurrent with sustained-release morphine 30 mg PO bid for 10 days; gabapentin 5 mg/kg PO tid as needed for subsequent episodes.

GENERAL CANCER PAIN (Box 19-11)

SIGNALMENT: *12-year-old female spayed golden retriever weighing 38 kg.*
ISSUE: *The dog was diagnosed and treated for multiple myeloma. There were palpable subcutaneous masses on the right and left thoracic walls and both inguinal regions, and there was a large open sore on the right hock.*
CAUSE OF PAIN: *The dog demonstrated periodic bouts of pain originating from different body locations and hypersensitivity of the subcutaneous masses on palpation. The pain subsided transiently after the initiation of chemotherapy but returned after several weeks, although the dog was in remission.*

BOX 19-11
Case 6: Canine—Multiple Myeloma

Multiple subcutaneous masses.
Mild-to-moderate pain.
Somatic in origin; tissue inflammation.

TREATMENT AND RATIONALE: *The dog was initially treated for cancer with cyclophosphamide 200 mg/m^2 IV, melphalan 20 mg/m^2 PO (10 tablets over 3 weeks), sulfamethoxazole-trimethoprim 30 mg/kg PO bid, and prednisone 1.0 mg/kg PO for 7 days. The origin of the chronic pain was judged to be tumor-associated and inflammatory in origin. A decision was made to begin the dog on an intermittent schedule of NSAID therapy (Box 19-12).*

- Piroxicam 0.5 mg/kg PO every other day was selected as initial therapy because of its synergistic action with anticancer drugs to cause cell death.
- Butorphanol 0.2 mg/kg IM was administered by the owner on an as-needed basis if the pain was judged to be particularly bad.
- Two weeks after initiation of the anticancer therapy, carprofen 2 mg/kg PO bid was selected as an alternative to piroxicam because of its efficacy and comparatively low renal and GI toxicity. Serum liver chemistry values (ALT, AST) were determined at 3-month intervals as a precaution.

BOX 19-12
Case 6: Canine—Multiple Myeloma

First therapy: prednisolone 1.0 mg/kg PO for 7 days.
Second therapy: piroxicam 0.5 mg/kg PO every other day (as needed).
Third therapy: butorphanol 0.2 mg/kg IM as needed.
Fourth therapy: carprofen 2 mg/kg PO bid as an alternative to piroxicam, as needed, for long-term use.

20

Drug Antagonism and Antagonists

WILLIAM W. MUIR III

Drug-related side effects and toxicity are all too common consequences of drug administration, even when recommended drug
dosages and dosing schedules are strictly followed. Some side effects are easily eliminated (e.g., opioid-induced bradycadia and depression), whereas others may be irreversible (e.g., nonsteroidal antiinflammatory drug [NSAID]–induced acute renal failure). Acute
onset of life-threatening side effects or toxicity (e.g., apnea) is particularly problematic because it could result in the animal's death.
Many of the drugs used to produce insensibility and analgesia (anesthetics) or analgesia (opioids, α_2-agonists, local anesthetics) have the
potential to produce a wide variety of side effects and toxicity. Opioids are notorious for their ability to induce bradycadia, depression,
and amplification of the respiratory depressant effects of anesthetic
drugs. α_2-Agonists can induce profound bradycardia, respiratory depression, and sedation in otherwise normal healthy dogs or cats, even
when dosages lower than those recommended by the manufacturer
are administered. The bolus intravenous (IV) administration of benzodiazepines (e.g., diazepam, midazolam), drugs usually considered
to be relatively free of side effects or toxicity, can induce acute collapse, bradycardia, and unconsciousness. The initial response to a
drug-related side effect or toxicity, once identified, should be focused
on its elimination. Fortunately, a variety of pharmacologic drugs and
techniques can be used to diminish or abolish unwanted drug effects.
This chapter focuses on mechanisms of drug antagonism that can be
used to reduce or eliminate the side effects and toxicities produced
by analgesic drugs. Receptor blockade and physiologic drug antagonism are emphasized after a brief discussion of the other methods of
drug antagonism (Box 20-1).

BOX 20-1
Drug Antagonism

- Discontinue drug administration.
- Pharmacokinetic antagonism.
- Competitive antagonism (both drugs bind to the same receptor).
- Physiologic antagonism.

DISCONTINUING DRUG ADMINISTRATION

Stopping the administration of a drug or decreasing its dose or frequency of administration is a simple and effective means of eliminating unwanted drug-related side effects or toxicity. Patients that are receiving drugs chronically (NSAIDs) should be periodically monitored for signs of toxicity (e.g., gastric ulcers, abnormal renal and liver function test results). These procedures, however, are not effective for the immediate termination of acute drug-related side effects or toxicity.

Drug Administration

The dose frequency and route of drug administration can be changed to help decrease the possibility of a drug-related side effect. Decreasing the drug dosage or dividing the dosage for more frequent administration may help minimize peak plasma drug concentrations, thereby decreasing the potential for the development of drug-related side effects.

Route of Administration

Administering drugs by routes that delay drug absorption (e.g., oral, transdermal) prolongs the onset to peak drug effect but decreases peak plasma drug concentrations, thereby decreasing the potential for the development of drug-related side effects.

PHARMACOKINETIC ANTAGONISM

Pharmacokinetic antagonism uses therapies and techniques designed to decrease the plasma concentration of the drug. Toward this end, therapies that decrease or inhibit drug absorption or increase drug elimination should be considered.

Decreasing Drug Absorption

Drug absorption can be decreased or inhibited after oral administration by the coadministration of substances that interfere with drug absorption from the gastrointestinal tract (kaolin, pectin). Alternatively, drugs that induce vomiting (apomorphine) may be administered to limit the amount of drug that is absorbed from the gastrointestinal tract. Local anesthetics are frequently administered with epinephrine to decrease the local blood supply, thereby decreasing their systemic absorption and intensifying their local analgesic actions. Their delayed entry into the blood supply also minimizes their plasma concentrations and the potential for systemic side effects.

Increasing Drug Elimination

Drug elimination can be enhanced by improving or ensuring adequate blood supply to the major organs of elimination (liver, kidneys) for the drug in question. This may require subcutaneous or IV administration of fluids and cardiovascular stimulants (dopamine, dobutamine). The renal excretion of drugs can be increased by administering fluids, optimizing pH, and promoting diuresis (furosemide).

RECEPTOR BLOCKADE (DRUG ANTAGONISTS)

Many analgesic drugs produce their effects by combining with and activating receptors (agonists). Drugs that combine with receptors and produce less than the expected maximal response are referred to as *partial agonists.* For example, two drugs with the same ability to combine (affinity) with a receptor could produce different degrees of analgesia. The drug that produces the maximum effect expected is termed *a full agonist,* whereas the drug that produces less than the expected effect is termed *a partial agonist.* Pure drug antagonists combine with receptors without causing their activation, thereby preventing the effects of full and partial agonists. The affinity of the drug antagonist for the receptor determines how much drug will be necessary to produce an antagonistic effect (high affinity = low amounts of drug). Some drugs combine with and activate receptors, inhibiting receptor occupation of other drugs. These drugs are called *agonists-antagonists.* Drug antagonists and agonist-antagonists compete for the receptor with the agonist or partial agonist, implying that the receptor can only bind to one drug at a time and that the effects of the antagonist or agonist-antagonist are surmountable if enough agonist or partial agonist is administered (see Chapter 7). Butorphanol, for example, is an opioid agonist-antagonist that can be used to antagonize the effects of the pure opioid agonists morphine and hydromorphone while producing opioid agonistic effects. Clinically, most drug antagonists are administered at doses far in excess of what is required to overcome agonist effects. This is an important point, considering that most drug antagonists also reverse the antagonized drug's analgesic effects. Special consideration should be given to the antagonist selected, its dose, and the route of administration; the dose should be titrated to achieve the desired effect whenever possible. Finally, caution is advised whenever a drug antagonist is administered to reverse the sedative effects of a pure or partial agonist, since the return to consciousness may produce overexcitement, agitation, and aggression.

Opioid Antagonists

Naloxone and naltrexone are pure opioid antagonists (i.e., produce no opioid effects) that have high affinity for μ-, κ-, and δ-opioid receptors. Relatively small doses of either drug can be used to rapidly reverse the unwanted or lingering central nervous system (CNS) depression, respiratory depression, and bradycardia produced by opioid agonists or partial agonists. Naloxone is rapidly metabolized and eliminated in dogs and cats, producing relatively short-lived (10 to 20 minutes) effects and predisposing to renarcotization with respiratory depression on occasion. Naltrexone produces effects similar to those of naloxone but has a much longer duration of action, lasting for several hours. Both drugs produce little effect when administered intravenously but can cause hyperalgesia in stressed animals when endogenous opioids (e.g., endorphin, enkephalin) are produced. Similarly, both drugs can reverse the analgesic effects of systemic and parenteral opioid administration and inhibit acupuncture analgesia. The IV administration of large doses of naloxone or naltrexone may produce a state of hyperalgesia in dogs and cats because of the blockade of protective endogenous opioid mechanisms. Intravenous bolus administration of naloxone, although producing rapid reversal of opioid-related side effects, may cause excitement, emergence delirium, and aggression. Unless an emergency situation exists, small doses of either drug should be administered and titrated to produce the desired effect (consciousness) (Table 20-1).

Opioid Partial or Mixed Agonists-Antagonists

Nalorphine, nalbuphine, pentazocine, buprenorphine, and butorphanol are opioids classified as either partial agonists (i.e., produce less than the maximal response) or agonist-antagonists (i.e., activate and block opioid receptors), depending on the opioid receptor in question (see Chapters 8 and 9). They are used clinically to produce analgesia and, on occasion, to reverse the untoward effects (sedation, respiratory depression) of pure opioid agonists (e.g., morphine, hydromorphone, meperidine, fentanyl). Butorphanol, for example, can be administered during recovery from anesthesia and surgery to antagonize prolonged recovery produced by the preanesthetic administration of morphine. Butorphanol administration, if necessary, will increase the level of consciousness, thereby helping prevent respiratory depression in the unstimulated postsurgical patient and produce mild-to-moderate opioid receptor–mediated analgesia. There is also evidence that the administration of small doses of opioid agonist-antagonists (e.g., nalorphine, pentazocine, butorphanol) in conjunction with or after the administration of a pure opioid agonist (e.g., morphine, hydromorphone) may produce additive analgesia. This suggests that analgesia is improved in the

TABLE 20-1
Opioid Antagonists

Drug	Recommended Use*	Emergency Use
Naloxone	5-15 μg/kg IV	50-100 μg/kg IV
Naltrexone	50-100 μg/kg SQ	—
Nalorphine	0.05-0.1 mg/kg IV	—
Butorphanol	0.05-1.0 mg/kg IV	—
Pentazocine	0.1-0.5 mg/kg IV	—
Buprenorphine	5-10 μg/kg IV†	—

SQ, Subcutaneous.
*Repeat as necessary.
†Monitor for respiratory depression.

postoperative patient in which the sedative effects of morphine are partially antagonized. Care must be taken in the selection of partial agonists or agonist-antagonists to antagonize the effects of a pure opioid agonist (morphine, hydromorphone), however, since some partial agonists (buprenorphine) are known to exaggerate the respiratory depressant effects of pure opioid agonists. This effect could become problematic in animals that do not regain consciousness after the administration of buprenorphine.

α_2-Agonists

Yohimbine, tolazoline, and atipamezole are α_2-receptor antagonists, which produce effects by antagonizing both central and peripheral α-receptors (Table 20-2). Both yohimbine ($\alpha_2/\alpha_1 = 40/1$) and tolazoline ($\alpha_2/\alpha_1 = 4/1$) are relatively nonspecific α_2-antagonists compared with atipamezole ($\alpha_2/\alpha_1 = 8500/1$) and occasionally produce hypotension (α_1 blockade) with reflex tachycardia. Tolazoline is also noted for producing histamine release, which can also contribute to hypotension. All three drugs are recommended for the reversal of α_2-agonist–induced (xylazine, medetomidine) side effects, including but not limited to sedation, respiratory depression, bradycardia, and vomiting. The intramuscular (IM) administration of atipamezole produces rapid and complete reversal of α_2-agonist–induced effects, including the elimination of α_2-agonist–induced analgesia. As with the pure opioid antagonists, IV bolus administration of manufacturer-recommended dosages of α_2-agonists should be reserved for emergency or life-threatening situations,

TABLE 20-2
α_2-Antagonists

Drug	Dose
Yohimbine	0.1-0.3 mg/kg IV
	0.3-0.5 mg/kg IM
Tolazoline	0.5-1.0 mg/kg IV
	2-5 mg/kg IM
Atipamezole	0.05-0.2 mg/kg IV
	2-4 × medetomidine dose

since this can also initiate a period of involuntary muscle twitching (jactitations), excitement, delirium, and aggression associated with vomiting, urination, and defecation. Clinically, the IM or subcutaneous administration of atipamezole produces rapid uneventful recovery from α_2-agonist–induced sedation and respiratory depression without significant untoward effects.

Benzodiazepine Antagonists

Diazepam and midazolam are centrally acting muscle relaxants, which are not noted for their analgesic activity but are a frequent component of preanesthetic medications to produce calming and muscle relaxation before surgery. On rare occasions, diazepam and midazolam can induce profound CNS depression and associated respiratory depression. The bolus IV administration of diazepam has also produced bradycardia and hypotension. Flumazenil is a rapidly acting and specific competitive antagonist of diazepam- and midazolam-induced CNS and respiratory depression. Flumazenil is also capable of producing partial reversal of inhalant anesthetic–induced depression. Clinical dosages range from 0.1 mg/kg IV to 0.3 mg/kg IM. Intravenous administration is rarely associated with emergence delirium or signs of excitement. Larger doses (>3 mg/kg IV + infusion) of flumazenil antagonize platelet-activating factor and have been shown to be beneficial in the treatment of hemorrhagic shock.

PHYSIOLOGIC ANTAGONISM

Physiologic antagonism refers to the administration of drugs that do not act as specific receptor antagonists but are administered to produce effects that oppose or cancel the effects of the initial drug (Table 20-3). The administration of fluids or dopamine to oppose the hypotensive effects of inhalant anesthesia is one example of physiologic antagonism. The administration of atropine or glycopyrrolate to treat opioid-induced bradycardia is another example of physiologic antagonism. The wide variety of drugs acting by diverse mechanisms, which are used as analgesics in dogs and cats, have the potential to produce many unwanted side effects. CNS depression or excitement, respiratory depression, bradycardia, hypotension, and muscle twitching are among the most commonly encountered side effects associated with the administration of analgesic

TABLE 20-3

Therapy for Analgesic Drug-Related Side Effects

Problem	Therapy	Dose
Sedation/ depression	Analeptics	
	Doxapram	0.2-0.5 mg/kg IV
	Aminophylline	2-10 mg/kg IV
Excitement/ seizures	Tranquilizers/muscle relaxants	
	Acepromazine	0.05-0.1 mg/kg IV, IM
	Droperidol	0.1-1.0 mg/kg IV, IM
	Haloperidol	0.1-0.5 mg/kg IV, IM
	Diazepam	0.1-0.5 mg/kg IV
	Phenobarbital	1-3 mg/kg IV
	Propofol	1-3 mg/kg IV; 0.1-0.2 mg/kg/min
Vomiting	Antiemetics	
	Ondansetron	0.5 mg/kg IV
	Metoclopramide	0.1-0.3 mg/kg IV
Bradycardia	Anticholinergics	
	Atropine	0.1-0.2 mg/kg IV, IM
	Glycopyrrolate	0.005-0.01 mg/kg IV, IM
Respiratory depression	Respiratory stimulants	
	Doxapram	0.2-0.5 mg/kg IV
	Ventilation	
Hypotension	Catecholamines	
	Dopamine	0.001-0.005 mg/kg/min IV
	Ephedrine	1-5 mg/kg IM

drugs. Behavioral changes are also common side effects of opioids, α_2-agonists, and benzodiazepines and are best treated by changing or discontinuing medication.

Analeptics

Sedation and depression are common side effects of many analgesic drugs. Excessive sedation or depression can produce an unresponsive, listless pet, a reduction in appetite, and the potential for significant respiratory depression, particularly during sleep. This type of response to centrally acting analgesic drugs is best treated by reducing the drug dose or selecting an analgesic that does not produce CNS effects. Clinically, many postoperative patients demonstrate good analgesia but significant CNS depression, requiring semicontinuous monitoring. The decision to be made is whether the patient should be administered a specific drug antagonist (if appropriate) with the risk of reducing or eliminating analgesia. Low doses of the appropriate specific antagonist could be titrated to effect with the hope of producing increased consciousness and little or no loss of analgesia. In some instances, agonist-antagonists (e.g., butorphanol) that counteract unwanted CNS depression and produce analgesia are available. An alternative approach to the administration of a specific antagonist would be to administer a CNS stimulant or analeptic drug. Doxapram is a respiratory stimulant that increases CNS activity in dogs and cats. Although not a specific antagonist, doxapram can counteract the CNS depressant effects of low to moderate doses of α_2-agonists, opioids, and injectable or inhalant anesthetics. Once conscious, most animals remain conscious, but because of doxapram's relatively short half-life, animals administered this drug should be closely monitored to prevent relapse and respiratory depression. Aminophylline, although noted for its bronchodilatory effects, also stimulates the CNS. The IV or IM administration of aminophylline to dogs and cats can shorten recovery from anesthesia, increase alertness, and counteract mild-to-moderate sedation without antagonizing the effects of analgesic drugs. Aminophylline has a much longer duration of action than doxapram.

Tranquilizers/Muscle Relaxants

Nervousness, apprehension, agitation, seizures, and involuntary muscle twitching are all potential side effects associated with the use of traditional centrally acting analgesic medications. These side effects are more frequent when large analgesic drug doses are administered or when these drugs are given to animals with preexisting CNS disorders. Acepromazine is an excellent tranquilizer, which produces adjunctive analgesic and antiemetic effects when combined with opioids. Relatively low IV or IM doses (0.01 mg/kg) can be used to calm nervous or agitated dogs and cats. Although acepromazine is effective, the dose may be difficult to titrate, frequently producing more sedation than needed. Droperidol and haloperidol are butyrophenone tranquilizers noted for their mild calming and antiemetic effects, which can be used as alternatives to acepro-mazine. Droperidol and haloperidol are frequently used as behavior modifiers, and either drug can be used to reduce or eliminate ap-prehension and agitation in dogs and cats. Drug dose should be titrated to the desired effect, and initial dosages of droperidol should not exceed 0.1 mg/kg IV or IM. Diazepam and midazolam are ex-cellent centrally acting neuromuscular blocking drugs that can be used to control involuntary muscle twitching or spasms and seizures. Repeated IV administration (0.1 mg/kg) or infusion (3 to 5 mg/kg hr) may be required to control involuntary muscle spasms or seizures in some animals. Dogs and cats with seizures that do not respond to diazepam or midazolam therapy should be administered phenobarbital (1 to 3 mg/kg IV) or anesthetized with propofol (1 mg/kg IV; 0.05 to 0.1 mg/kg/min). It should be noted that all of the drugs used to produce calming, muscle relaxation, or seizure control are not always effective and occasionally produce aggres-sive behavior (release of suppressed behavior), requiring anesthesia (e.g., propofol: 1 to 3 mg/kg, IV; 0.1 to 0.2 mg/kg/min).

Antiemetics

Nausea and vomiting are common but self-limiting side effects as-sociated with the use of opioid and α_2-agonist drugs. Occasionally, vomiting may persist and result in dyspnea, bradycardia, and the potential for aspiration. Vomiting is particularly problematic when it occurs in association with the induction of, maintenance of, or re-covery from anesthesia. As noted previously, acepromazine, dro-peridol, and haloperidol can be used before or in combination with opioids or α_2-agonists to reduce vomiting. Ondansetron (0.5 mg/kg IV) or metoclopramide (0.2 to 0.5 mg/kg IM) can be used to prevent or eliminate vomiting without producing sedation. Persistent vom-iting in dogs should be treated by infusing metoclopramide (0.01 to 0.02 mg/kg/hr).

Anticholinergics

Sinus bradycardia, first- and second-degree atrioventricular block with ventricular escape beats, and rarely, third-degree atrioventric-ular block may occur after the administration of opioids and partic-ularly α_2-agonists to dogs. Similar cardiac rhythm disturbances, although less common, can occur in cats. Opioid-induced bradyarrhythmias are generally caused by increases in parasympathetic tone and are readily responsive to treatment with either atropine (0.1 to 0.2 mg/kg IV) or glycopyrrolate (0.005 to 0.01 mg/kg IV). α_2-Agonist–induced bradyarrhythmias may be due to increases in parasympathetic tone or decreases in sympathetic tone. Regardless, initial therapy is identical to that for opioids. Anticholinergics should be administered before α_2-agonists (e.g., xylazine, medetomidine) when used as preanesthetic medication.

Respiratory Stimulants

Respiratory depression is an underappreciated and significant side effect associated with IV or long-term drug analgesic administration; it is most common when opioids and α_2-agonists are administered in conjunction with injectable or inhalant anesthetic drugs. Signs of respiratory depression are often subtle, unless marked decreases in respiratory rate or apnea are observed. Respiratory rate and depth should be closely monitored after the IV administration of opioids, α_2-agonists, and benzodiazepines. Doxapram is an excellent CNS and respiratory stimulant but is not a specific drug antagonist and produces only short-term effects. Significant respiratory depression may follow a period of transient respiratory stimulation if consciousness is not produced, since carbon dioxide concentrations (the principle drive to breathing) may have been significantly reduced. Respiratory depression therefore is best treated by careful patient monitoring, appropriate nursing care, and techniques that hasten drug elimination. If necessary, mechanical ventilators should be used to maintain breathing and normal pH and blood gas values.

Catecholamines

Arterial blood pressure should be determined in any patient in whom hypotension is suspected. Hypotension and poor tissue perfusion may occur as a consequence of bradyarrhythmias, vasodilation, and low cardiac output. Clinically, hypotension may result in lethargy, depression, muscle weakness, and marked delays in recovery from anesthesia. Acute hypotension should be treated with appropriate fluids (5 to 10 ml/kg IV, lactated Ringer's solution [LRS]) and the administration of dopamine (1 to 4 μg/kg/min) or ephedrine (1 to 5 mg/kg IV to effect).

SUGGESTED READINGS

Heniff MS, Moore G, Trout A, et al: Comparison of routes of flumazenil administration to reverse midazolam-induced respiratory depression in a canine model, *Acad Emerg Med* 4:1115-1118, 1997.

Muir WW, Hubbell JAE: Drugs used for preanesthetic medication. In Muir WW, Hubbell JAE, editors: *Handbook of veterinary anesthesia,* ed 3, St Louis, 1999, Mosby.

Salonen S, Vuorilehto L, Vainio O, et al: Atipamazole increases medetomidine clearance in the dog: an agonist-antagonist interaction, *J Vet Pharmacol Ther* 18:328-332, 1995.

Schaffer DD, Hsu WH, Hopper DL: Antagonism of xylazine-induced depression of shuttle-avoidance responses in dogs by administration of 4-aminopyridine, doxapram, or yohimbine, *Am J Vet Res* 47(10):2116-2121, 1986.

Thurman JC, Tranquilli WJ, Benson GJ: Preanesthetics and anesthetic adjuncts. In Thurman JC, Tranquilli WJ, Benson GJ, editors: *Lumb & Jones' veterinary anesthesia,* ed 3, Baltimore, 1996, Williams & Wilkins.

21

Cancer Pain Management

JAMES S. GAYNOR

The treatment of cancer has become more commonplace in veterinary practice as knowledge, drugs, and therapeutic techniques evolve. Although some cancers still are not effectively treated, many owners will attempt various measures to prolong their pets' lives.

It is vitally important to attempt to alleviate the pet's pain. It is estimated that cancer pain can be effectively managed in 90% of humans with currently available drugs and techniques (Box 21-1).

OPTIMIZING PAIN MANAGEMENT

There are four main steps to ensure that pain management is optimized in veterinary patients (Box 21-2).

1. Ensure that veterinarians have the appropriate education and training regarding the importance of alleviation of pain, assessment of pain, available drugs and potential complications, and interventional techniques.
2. Educate the client about realistic expectations surrounding pain control and convey the idea that most patients' pain can be managed. This step involves letting the client know that owner involvement in evaluating the pet and providing feedback on therapy is crucial to success. Both the veterinarian and owner should participate in developing effective strategies to alleviate pain. Client involvement also helps decrease the potential feeling of helplessness.
3. Thoroughly assess the pet's pain at the start and throughout the course of therapy, not just when it gets severe.
4. Learn to use opioids and other controlled substances as part of a multimodal approach to pain therapy.

BOX 21-1

Most cancer pain is controllable.

BOX 21-2

Four Steps to Optimize Cancer Pain Control

- Educate yourself on the assessment and alleviation of cancer pain.
- Create real client expectations.
- Assess pet pain regularly.
- Use opioids as part of a *multimodal* approach.

DRUGS AND TECHNIQUES FOR ALLEVIATION OF PAIN

- The general approach to pain management should follow the World Health Organization (WHO) ladder, which is a three-step hierarchy (Fig. 21-1).
- Within the same category of drugs, different side effects for individuals may exist. Therefore, if possible, it may be best to substitute drugs within a category before switching therapies. It is always best to try to keep dosage scheduling as simple as possible. The more complicated the regimen, the more likely that noncompliance will occur.
- Mild-to-moderate pain should be treated with a nonopioid such as a nonsteroidal antiinflammatory drug (NSAID) or acetaminophen.
- As pain increases, some type of opioid should be added to the regimen. As pain becomes more severe, increase the dose of the opioid. Drugs should be dosed on a regular basis, not just as needed, as pain becomes moderate to severe. Continuous analgesia will facilitate maintaining patient comfort. Additional doses of analgesics can then be administered as pain becomes intermittently more severe.
- Adjuvant drugs can be administered to help with specific types of pain and anxiety.

NONOPIOIDS

- Nonopioid analgesics include drugs such as acetaminophen, aspirin, carprofen, ketoprofen, and etodolac.

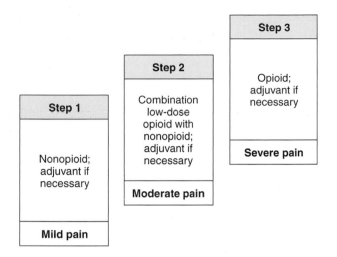

Fig. 21-1 World Health Organization Analgesia Ladder. (From the World Health Organization, Geneva, Switzerland.)

- A complete discussion on NSAIDs can be found in Chapter 10.
- All nonopioids except acetaminophen are considered NSAIDs. Despite the low antiinflammatory activity of acetaminophen, it possesses beneficial analgesic effects, minimal risk of bleeding in thrombocytopenic patients, decreased gastrointestinal effects, and synergism with opioid analgesics such as codeine. Acetaminophen should be avoided in cats because of their inadequate cytochrome P-450–dependent hydroxylation.
- Mild-to-moderate pain, especially that arising from intrathoracic masses, intraabdominal masses, and bone metastases, can be relieved with NSAIDs. NSAIDs have an opioid-sparing effect so that better analgesia can be achieved with lower doses of opioids when pain increases.
- NSAIDs have central analgesic and peripheral antiinflammatory effects mediated through inhibition of cyclooxygenase. The choice of NSAID ultimately depends on available species information, clinical response, and tolerance of side effects.
- Most NSAIDs have been investigated in dogs but not in cats.

Side Effects

- The most common side effect of NSAID administration in dogs is gastric irritation and bleeding caused by loss of gastric acid inhibition and of cytoprotective mucus production normally promoted by prostaglandins and anti–platelet-aggregating activity, respectively.
- Other side effects include renal failure and hepatic dysfunction that may lead to failure.
- NSAIDs, which are more selective for inhibition of cyclooxygenase-2 (COX-2), seem to have fewer gastrointestinal effects and potentially fewer renal effects.
- Selective COX-2 inhibitors, such as carprofen, etodolac, and those soon to be released, should be considered priority NSAIDs in cancer patients. A blood chemistry panel should be performed before initiating NSAID therapy.
- If evidence of liver or renal disease, dehydration, or hypotension exists, another approach to therapy should be considered. Therapy with NSAIDs may also inhibit platelet function, leading to bleeding and oozing. Therapy with NSAIDs should be stopped if this occurs.
- If clinical effectiveness is not achieved with one NSAID, it should be discontinued and another started 7 days later to avoid additive or synergistic cyclooxygenase inhibition effects.
- Aspirin should be avoided in dogs because of the increased possibility of gastrointestinal bleeding, even with buffered formulations.
- Administering misoprostol can help provide gastrointestinal protection during the switchover period. All cancer patients should be closely monitored for gastrointestinal bleeding and thrombocytopenia if receiving NSAID therapy during chemotherapy.

OPIOIDS

- The use of opioids has been discussed in Chapter 9.
- Opioids are the major class of analgesics used in the management of moderate-to-severe cancer pain. They are most effective, predictable, and relatively low risk.
- As a patient's pain increases, the required dose of opioid also increases. Veterinarians may be reluctant to administer high doses of opioids for fear of adverse side effects (Box 21-3).
  1. It is important to remember that veterinarians have an ethical obligation to benefit the patient by alleviating pain.

BOX 21-3

Opioids

- Most effective, predictable analgesics for cancer pain.
- Do not be afraid of high doses as duration and intensity of pain increase.

---

2. Side effects of opioid administration include diarrhea and vomiting initially and constipation with long-term use. Sedation and dysphoria may also occur. The initial gastrointestinal effects occur most frequently with the first injection in the perioperative period and usually do not occur with subsequent dosing. Vomiting and sedation usually do not occur with oral dosing.
3. It is important to discuss with the owner that dosing is very individualized when sending a patient home with oral medications.
   - Adjustment of the dose requires excellent doctor-client interaction.
   - Bradycardia is also possible after opioid administration but is most common if opioids are administered parenterally. If bradycardia occurs, an anticholinergic, such as atropine or glycopyrrolate, should be administered, rather than discontinuing the opioid.
- Full μ agonists, such as morphine, induce the best analgesia in a dose-dependent manner and are not limited by a ceiling effect. As pain increases, larger doses may be administered.
- Morphine is the most commonly used opioid for cancer-related pain. It is available in multiple injectable and oral formulations, including short duration tablets and liquids and sustained-release tablets.
- Oral morphine may be the most effective method for providing longer-term analgesia to dogs and cats with moderate-to-severe pain. Patients receiving analgesics at set dosing intervals should also be provided with some short-duration opioid (fentanyl patch) for breakthrough pain.
- Oxymorphone is available only as an injectable analgesic and may induce panting by changing the temperature set point in the brain.
- Meperidine is very short acting in animals, limiting its use as an analgesic in cancer patients.

- Codeine is available alone or with acetaminophen, allowing some flexibility in choice of oral medications.
- Fentanyl is an injectable drug that is potent and effective. Fentanyl is very appropriate for continuous infusion because it is short acting. This enables the practitioner to alter the dose as necessary from minute to minute to achieve good analgesia and potentially minimal sedation if desired.
- Buprenorphine is an example of a partial μ agonist. It does not produce the same degree of analgesia as does morphine and has a ceiling effect. The advantage of buprenorphine is that it has a long duration of action, 6 to 12 hours. It also has a long time to onset, approximately 40 minutes, even when given intravenously. Because of the inherent lack of maximal analgesia compared to morphine, buprenorphine should only be used for mild-to-moderate cancer pain.
- Another group of opioids are those with κ agonist–μ antagonist effects, of which butorphanol is an example. The analgesia is not as good as that produced by morphine. Even in large parenteral doses, butorphanol produces analgesia of very short duration in dogs, and as such may not be useful for cancer pain.
- Transdermal fentanyl patches can be used as an alternative to oral morphine that provides multiple-day analgesia. Fentanyl patches require 8 to 12 hours to take effect and last 2 to 4 days.
  1. Additional analgesia must be provided during the first 0.5 to 1 day after patch placement.
  2. One problem with transdermal fentanyl is the potential to produce unreliable plasma levels in dogs, probably related to failure of proper patch application or inappropriate dosing.
  3. Fentanyl patches may not provide enough analgesia for severe pain, but they allow lower doses of additional drugs.
  4. Fentanyl patches are expensive and should not be the first approach to chronic therapy.
  5. Transdermal fentanyl is most appropriate in those patients who cannot tolerate oral medication.
- Epidural opioids, especially morphine, have been used as a method for perioperative analgesia. With placement of an epidural catheter, epidural opioids can be administered for days to weeks. See the discussion on epidurals in Chapter 15.

- The appropriate dose of an opioid is a dose that produces analgesia with the fewest side effects.
  1. The need for increased doses often reflects progression of disease.
  2. Long-term use produces opioid tolerance, increasing doses or frequency to achieve equivalent results.
  3. Veterinarians should not be afraid to increase doses when appropriate and should remember the need for analgesia. A distinct advantage of using opioids for pain control is that they are reversible with naloxone or nalmefene if unacceptable side effects occur. Prolonged use may produce constipation, but oral laxatives can help alleviate this problem.

α_2-AGONISTS

- Xylazine and medetomidine are two α_2-agonists approved for use in small animals in the United States. They are uncontrolled parenteral drugs and provide excellent visceral analgesia, but only for 20 minutes to 2 hours.
- Xylazine and medetomidine should not be the first or sole choice for providing analgesia perioperatively to cancer patients because they can greatly reduce cardiac output and tissue oxygenation.
- Xylazine and medetomidine have synergistic effects with opioids. This attribute is useful postoperatively for inducing additional analgesia and alleviating dysphoria.
- Please refer to Chapter 11 for a complete discussion of α_2-agonists.

KETAMINE

- Ketamine has been identified as an N-methyl-D-aspartate (NMDA) receptor antagonist. NMDA receptors are believed to play a role in producing central sensitization and wind-up.
- As an NMDA receptor antagonist, ketamine reduces postoperative pain and cumulative opioid requirements.
- This is accomplished with doses that are much smaller than those for anesthesia.
  1. It is uncommon for patients to develop behavioral or cardiovascular effects.

2. Microdose ketamine may actually decrease the incidence of opioid-induced dysphoria postoperatively.

- Although no clinical animal studies have been completed, intra-operative microdose ketamine appears to provide beneficial effects for a variety of oncology surgical procedures, including limb amputations.
- Ketamine should be administered as a bolus (0.5 mg/kg IV) followed by an infusion (2 to 10 μg/kg/min) before and during surgical stimulation. A lower infusion rate (2 μg/kg/min) may be beneficial for the first 24 hours postoperatively, and an even lower rate (1 μg/kg/min) may be beneficial for the next 24 hours.
- In the absence of an infusion pump, ketamine can be mixed in a bag of crystalloid solutions for administration during anesthesia. Using anesthesia fluid administration rates of 10 ml/kg/hr, ketamine 60 mg (0.6 ml) should be added to a 1-L bag of crystalloid fluids to deliver ketamine at 10 μg/kg/min.

TRANQUILIZERS

- A concern that frequently arises with pain management is concurrent tranquilization and sedation. Most of the drugs used for analgesia usually produce concurrent sedation. As mentioned previously, opioids have mild-to-moderate potential for producing dysphoria.
- Dysphoria becomes more likely when cats are administered dog doses of opioids and when a patient is already experiencing high anxiety in the hospital.
  1. Dysphoric patients can sometimes be treated simply by petting and soothing them or by helping a patient change positions.
  2. Low-dose acepromazine (Table 21-1), both intravenously (IV) and intramuscularly (IM), is reasonable drug therapy for dysphoria. Although acepromazine does not alleviate pain, it calms anxious patients, and they care less about their pain.
  3. For patients in whom acepromazine is contraindicated and for those with bleeding and seizure disorders, the benzodiazepines, diazepam and midazolam, often calm patients.
     - Benzodiazepines should not be used by themselves in most normal alert patients because they frequently cause

TABLE 21-1

Commonly Used Adjuvant Drugs
for Patients with Cancer Pain

Drug	Route	Dose*
Acepromazine	IV	0.005-0.03 mg/kg
Acepromazine	SQ, IM	0.02-0.05 mg/kg
Diazepam/Midazolam (Versed)	IV	0.1-0.2 mg/kg
Xylazine	IV	0.05-0.1 mg/kg
Xylazine	IM	0.2 mg/kg
Medetomidine (Domitor)	IV	0.001 mg/kg
Medetomidine	IM	0.002 mg/kg
Amitriptyline (dog) (Elavil)	PO	1-2 mg/kg q 12-24 hr
Amitriptyline (cat)	PO	2.5-12.5 mg/kg q 24 hr
Imipramine (dog) (Tofranil)	PO	0.5-1.0 mg/kg q 8 hr
Imipramine (cat)	PO	2.5-5 mg/kg q 12 hr

IV, Intravenously; *SQ,* subcutaneously; *IM,* intramuscularly; *PO,* per os (orally); *q,* every.

Other commonly used analgesic drug doses can be found elsewhere in this book (see Chapter 8).

*Doses are the same for dogs and cats unless otherwise described.

excitement. Combined with opioids, sedation usually results.
- A low dose of xylazine, IV or IM, also can decrease dysphoria and increase analgesia in patients who are hemodynamically stable.
4. Patients who develop dysphoria after oral analgesic medications often respond well to oral acepromazine or diazepam. It is important to discern whether the opioid dose is effective before changing the analgesia regimen.

TRICYCLIC ANTIDEPRESSANTS

- Tricyclic antidepressants, such as amitriptyline and imipramine, block the reuptake of serotonin and norepinephrine in the central nervous system. They also have antihistamine effects.

- These drugs have been used in humans for the treatment of chronic and neuropathic pain at doses considerably lower than those used to treat depression. Presumably, they have similar analgesic effects in animals and enhance opioid analgesia as they do in humans.

LOCAL ANESTHETICS

- The use of local and regional anesthetic techniques in small animals was common in the early twentieth century. Recently there has been increased interest in these techniques, probably because of their ability to provide preemptive analgesia and decrease wind-up. Local anesthetic techniques can be used as an alternative or in conjunction with general anesthesia in selected cases.
- Refer to Chapter 12 for a complete discussion of local anesthetics and to Chapter 15 for a description of local anesthetic block techniques.

EPIDURALS

- Refer to Chapter 15 for a discussion of epidural anesthesia, analgesia, and techniques.
- A catheter can be placed in the epidural space to treat severe pain. Maintenance of this catheter requires veterinarian and client vigilance to ensure cleanliness and prevent infection from migrating to the spinal cord. With proper care, an epidural catheter can remain in place for days to weeks.

LOCAL OR WHOLE-BODY RADIATION

- Local or whole-body radiation can enhance analgesic drug effectiveness by reducing metastatic or primary tumor bulk.
- Radiation dose should be balanced between the amount necessary to kill tumor cells and the amount that would affect normal cells.
- Mucositis of the oral cavity and pharynx can develop after radiation to the neck, head, or oral cavities, resulting in impaired ability to eat and drink.
- Mucositis therapies include analgesics, sucralfate, 2% viscous lidocaine, and green tea rinses.

BISPHOSPHONATES

- Bony metastases are one of the most common causes of pain in advanced cancer. Some tumors cause osteoblastic metastases, but most can cause osteolytic lesions.
- Administration of bisphosphonates such as pamidronate reduce pain and pathologic fractures in humans.
- Bisphosphonates accumulate on bone surfaces and inhibit osteoclast-induced resorption, favoring bone formation. This therapy is expensive and has yet to be validated in dogs or cats.

STRONTIUM-89

IV administration of strontium-89 has also been shown to provide analgesia related to bony metastases in approximately 50% of humans, but its use in animals is sparse.

ACUPUNCTURE

- Acupuncture can be used as a pain-relieving modality, often when conventional therapy does not work.
- Acupuncture is also useful in conjunction with other therapies to allow lower doses of drugs that may have significant side effects. Although some practitioners have difficulty accepting acupuncture, it is important to remember that well-documented physiologic theory and evidence for its clinical effects exists.
- Details about acupuncture are discussed in Chapter 16.
- In general, acupuncture analgesia is extremely useful for pelvic pain, radius/ulna and femoral bone pain, and pain caused by cutaneous discomfort secondary to radiation therapy.
- Acupuncture also helps alleviate nausea associated with chemotherapy and some analgesics, and it promotes general well-being.

APPROACH TO PAIN IN THE CANCER PATIENT

- When developing a plan to alleviate pain, it helps to have a paradigm to follow.
- The first principle is to practice a multimodal approach to analgesia. Use drugs in combination that work by different

mechanisms to allow optimal analgesia at the lowest dose possible.

- A simple flow chart (Table 21-2) can help with the sequence of activities related to pain assessment and management. This flow chart emphasizes the use of multiple modalities, beginning therapy with the least invasive methods and advancing treatment to meet the patient's needs.

- Control of cancer pain is within the capabilities of most veterinarians and is achievable in most animal cancer patients with

TABLE 21-2

Flow for the Approach to Management of Surgical Pain

Time	Drugs	Rationale
Preoperative	Morphine	Preemptive, long-lasting analgesia
	± Acepromazine	Tranquilization, calming, anxiolysis
	Atropine/glycopyrrolate	Prevent bradycardia associated with opioid
	Appropriate nerve blocks	Preemptive analgesia, prevent wind-up
	Epidural if applicable	Preemptive analgesia, prevent wind-up
Perioperative	Fentanyl continuous infusion	Decrease cardiovascular effects of inhalant agents; additional analgesia
	Microdose ketamine	Prevent wind-up
Acute postoperative	Appropriate nerve blocks	Analgesia
	Fentanyl continuous infusion	Analgesia adjustable to patient needs
	Microdose ketamine	Prevent wind-up, dysphoria
Postoperative adjuncts	Acepromazine	Anxiolysis, dysphoria
	Diazepam/midazolam	Dysphoria
	Xylazine/medetomidine	Additional analgesia, dysphoria

techniques that are currently available. Pain and its therapy, pain control should be achievable by following these simple ABCs (Box 21-4):

1. Assess the pain. Ask for the owner's perceptions.
2. Believe the owner. The owner sees the pet everyday in its own environment.
3. Choose appropriate therapy, following the WHO ladder.
4. Deliver therapy in a logical, coordinated manner.
5. Empower the clients to actively participate in their pet's well being.

CASE EXAMPLES

The following generic examples, in conjunction with the flow chart, present useful approaches to specific types of pain encountered in oncology practice. The examples recommend specific techniques for the procedure rather than a complete analgesia program.

Lateral Thoracotomy

- Intercostal nerve block
- Interpleural local anesthetic
- Opioid epidural

Sternotomy

- Interpleural local anesthetic
- Opioid epidural

BOX 21-4

ABCs of Cancer Pain Control

A—Assess pain.
B—Believe owner.
C—Choose appropriate therapy and use multimodal therapy.
D—Deliver treatment in a logical manner.
E—Empower clients to participate.

Forelimb Amputation

- Brachial plexus nerve block
- Opioid epidural

Rear Limb Amputation

- Opioid epidural

Cranial Mandibular Surgery

- Mandibular nerve block
- Mental nerve block

Upper Lip and Nose Procedure

- Infraorbital nerve block

Maxillary Surgery

- Maxillary nerve block

Midcaudal Abdominal Surgery

- Opioid epidural (local anesthetic also if caudal abdomen)

Cranial Abdominal Surgery

- Interpleural local anesthetic
- Opioid epidural

  Although not all types of pain can be addressed, pain relief should be considered achievable by following the recommendations and paradigms in this text.

SUMMARY

- Most animals with cancer have pain that can be treated.
- Engage the owners as fully as possible.
- Practice multimodal analgesia.
- If a specific regimen is not working, increase the dose or change protocols.

SUGGESTED READINGS

Cancer pain relief, ed 2, Geneva, 1996, World Health Organization.

Friedland J: Local and systemic radiation for palliation of metastatic disease, *Urol Clin North Am* 26:391-402, 1999.

Fu ES, Miguel R, Scharf JE: Preemptive ketamine decreases postoperative narcotic requirements in patients undergoing abdominal surgery, *Anesth Analg* 84:1086-1090, 1997.

Goisis A, Gorini M, Ratti R, et al: Application of a WHO protocol on medical therapy for oncologic pain in an internal medicine hospital, *Tumori* 75:470-472, 1989.

Golden BD, Abramson SB: Selective cyclooxygenase-2 inhibitors, *Rheum Dis Clin North Am* 25:359-378, 1999.

Jacox A, Carr DB, Payne R, et al: *Management of cancer pain,* Rockville, Md, 1994, Agency for Health Care Policy and Research.

Kasalicky J, Krajska V: The effect of repeated strontium-89 chloride therapy on bone pain palliation in patients with skeletal cancer metastases, *Eur J Nucl Med* 25:1362-1367, 1998.

Merskey H: Pharmacologic approaches other than opioids in chronic noncancer pain management, *Acta Anaesthesiol Scand* 41:187-190, 1997.

Nair N: Relative efficacy of 32P and 89Sr in palliation of skeletal metastases, *J Nucl Med* 40:256-261, 1999.

Sawyer DC, Rech RC, Durham RA, et al: Dose response to butorphanol administered subcutaneously to increase visceral nociceptive threshold in dogs, *Am J Vet Res* 52:1826-1830, 1991.

Shaw N, Burrows CF, King RR: Massive gastric hemorrhage induced by buffered aspirin in a greyhound, *J Am Anim Hosp Assoc* 33:215-219, 1999.

22

Pain Management in the Horse

WILLIAM W. MUIR III AND ROMAN T. SKARDA

Pain is generally one of the first and most dominant signs of injury or disease (e.g., colic) in most horses. Furthermore, the inflammatory responses induced by surgical procedures and anesthesia (e.g., hypotension, ischemia) produces a series of behavioral, neurophysiologic, endocrine, metabolic, and cellular responses (stress response), which can initiate, maintain, and amplify pain.

PAIN PERCEPTION

Nociception (pain perception) can be considered to involve five primary processes: transduction, transmission, modulation, projection, and perception (Fig. 22-1). Pain is normally produced by noxious mechanical, chemical, or thermal activation of small-diameter, high-threshold A-delta (Aδ) and C sensory nerve fibers. Noxious stimuli are transduced into electrical impulses by peripheral pain receptors and subsequently transmitted throughout the sensory nervous system. These electrical impulses are modulated by a variety of endogenous systems (e.g., opioid, serotonergic, noradrenergic) in the dorsal horn of the spinal cord before being transmitted to the brain, where emotional, behavioral, and physiologic responses are initiated.

Physiologic Pain

Pain is considered physiologic when it operates to protect the body by warning of contact with tissue-damaging stimuli. This type of pain is produced by stimulation of nociceptors innervated by high-threshold Aδ (Group III) and unmyelinated C (Group IV) fibers.

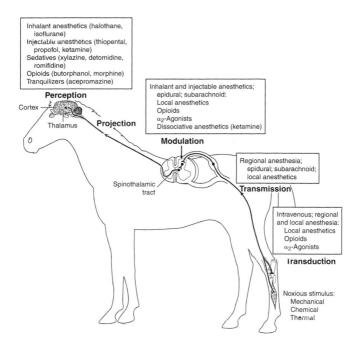

Fig. 22-1 Nociception involves transduction, transmission, modulation, projection, and perception. Various drugs and drug delivery techniques are used to inhibit these processes.

Clinical Pain

"Clinical" pain, by contrast, is produced by peripheral tissue injury or nerve damage. Clinical pain therefore is categorized as inflammatory or neuropathic pain. The term *idiopathic pain* is used to describe pain of unknown origin.

Inflammatory Pain

Inflammatory pain is either somatic (skin, joints, muscles, or periosteum) or visceral (thoracic and abdominal viscera) in origin.

- Somatic pain is easily localized, aching, stabbing, or throbbing, and generally acute. Somatic pain includes cutaneous or incisional pain after operation. Somatic pain is frequently identified as superficial (skin) or deep (joints, muscle, and periosteum).

* Visceral pain is poorly localized, cramping or gnawing, crescendo/decrescendo, and may be referred to cutaneous sites far from the site of injury.

Neuropathic Pain

Neuropathic pain occurs as a direct result of damage to peripheral nerves or the spinal cord, is described as burning, stabbing, and intermittent, and is often unresponsive to treatment.

Both inflammatory and neuropathic pain can produce allodynia, hyperalgesia (primary and secondary), and central nervous system (CNS) and peripheral sensitization to external stimuli (see Chapter 2).

Chemical Mediators of Pain

Chemical mediators of pain and inflammation include histamine, serotonin, bradykinin, leukotrienes, prostaglandins (PGE_2), interleukins (IL-1, IL-6), neutrophil-chemotactic peptides, nerve growth factor (NGF), and neuropeptides, including substance P. These substances enhance the excitability of sensory nerves and postganglionic sympathetic nerve fiber activity, leading to peripheral sensitization, hyperalgesia, and allodynia (see Chapter 2).

Inflammation increases the sensitivity of peripheral terminals of $A\delta$ and C fibers, causes some A-beta ($A\beta$) fibers to express substance P, and stimulates the synthesis and release of NGF, a peptide that increases the synthesis of substance P and calcitonin gene-related peptide (CGRP), stimulates the release of histamine and leukotrienes, and is associated with the development of sensory hyperexcitability and hyperalgesia. The net result of these inflammatory and tissue chemical responses is the development of diverse yet interrelated positive feedback loops, which enhance neural sensitivity and intensify the pain response.

Once transduced, the electrical impulses are transmitted to C-fiber terminals in the dorsal horn, where the excitatory neuropeptides (tachykinins), substance P, neurokinin A (NKA), CGRP, and the amino acid glutamate are released to activate postsynaptic tachykinin (NK1, NK2), CGRP and glutamate (e.g., N-methyl-D-aspartate [NMDA]; amino-hydroxy-methyl-isoxazolepropionate [AMPA], kainate) receptors.

Cumulative increases in the number of electrical impulses produced in dorsal horn cells caused by increased C-fiber stimulus frequency results in increases in excitability of spinal cord neurons and CNS "wind-up." Wind-up contributes to central sensitization, hyperalgesia, and allodynia. A similar phenomenon in the hippocampus has been termed *long-term potentiation (LTP)* and is thought to be the basis for the acquisition of new information and certain forms of short-term memory.

Effects of Pain

Pain is exaggerated by the inflammatory response, which in turn increases the production of pain neurotransmitters (e.g., substance P, CGRP) and increases the excitability of sensory neurons.

- Pain produces a catabolic state, suppresses the immune response, and promotes inflammation, which delays wound healing and predisposes the patient to infection and intensified medical care (see Chapter 3).
- Pain increases patient risk during anesthesia because more drugs are required to maintain a stable plain of anesthesia.
- Pain increases morbidity and the cost of patient care and occupies time better spent on more productive endeavors. These points justify the treatment of pain in all circumstances, which in turn produces a general feeling of mental satisfaction in hospital personnel and owners that patients are not needlessly suffering.

SYSTEMIC DRUG THERAPY

The magnitude of nociceptive input may vary considerably for different injuries or surgical procedures, resulting in a variety of physiologic responses (e.g., heart rate, blood pressure, sympathetic outflow) that require multiple analgesic drugs used in combination (multimodal therapy) and additional adjunctive pain therapy. A wide variety of drug therapies are available for the treatment of pain (Table 22-1 and Box 22-1). Importantly, sedatives, tranquilizers, and opioids modulate CNS processing and the development of hyperalgesia and allodynia. The deliberate administration of analgesic drugs 24 to 48 hours before extensive soft tissue or orthopedic surgery to preempt (minimize) the response to pain, particularly the

TABLE 22-1

Drugs Used to Produce Analgesia in Horses

Drugs	IV Dose (mg/kg)	Effects	Concerns/Comments
Corticosteroids			
Hydrocortisone Sodium succinate	1.0-4.0	Antiinflammatory, analgesic	Laminitis, immune suppression
Dexamethasone Isonicotinate	0.015-0.050	Antiinflammatory, analgesic	Laminitis, immune suppression
Methylprednisolone	0.1-0.5	Antiinflammatory, analgesic	Laminitis, immune suppression
Prednisolone	0.25-1.0	Antiinflammatory, analgesic	Laminitis, immune suppression Tablets: 0.25-1.0 mg/kg PO
Nonsteroidal Antiinflammatory Drugs			
Dipyrone	5-22	Antiinflammatory, analgesic	Potential for GI ulceration and renal toxicity
Phenylbutazone	2-4	Antiinflammatory, analgesic	Potential for GI ulceration and renal toxicity
Flunixin meglumine	0.2-1.1	Antiinflammatory, analgesic	Potential for GI ulceration and renal toxicity
Ketoprofen	1.1-2.2	Antiinflammatory, analgesic	Potential for GI ulceration and renal toxicity
Carprofen	0.5-1.1	Antiinflammatory, analgesic	Potential for GI ulceration and renal toxicity

Opioids

Butorphanol	0.01-0.04	Analgesia (0.5)	Potential for ataxia and disorientation
Pentazocine	0.5-1.0	Analgesia (0.5)	Potential for excitement and increased locomotor activity
Buprenorphine	0.01-0.04	Analgesia (3)	Potential for ataxia and disorientation
Morphine	0.05-0.1	Analgesia (1)	Potential for excitement and increased locomotor activity
Meperidine	0.2-1.0	Analgesia (0.5)	Potential for excitement and increased locomotor activity
Oxymorphone	0.001-0.02	Analgesia (10)	Potential for excitement and increased locomotor activity
Fentanyl	0.01-0.02; 2-100 µg/hr patches/450 kg	Analgesia (100)	Potential for excitement and increased locomotor activity

α_2-Agonists

Xylazine	0.5-1.0	Sedation, analgesia, and muscle relaxation	Potential for bradycardia, hypoventilation, and ataxia
Detomidine	0.01-0.02	Sedation, analgesia, and muscle relaxation	Potential for bradycardia, hypoventilation, and ataxia
Medetomidine	0.01-0.02	Sedation, analgesia, and muscle relaxation	Potential for bradycardia, hypoventilation, and ataxia
Romifidine	0.04-0.08	Sedation, analgesia, and muscle relaxation	Potential for bradycardia and hypoventilation

Numbers in parentheses indicate the analgesic potency of the drug. Higher numbers indicate greater potency.

BOX 22-1

Drugs Used to Produce Analgesia in Horses

Local and Regional Anesthesia
Local anesthetics (lidocaine)
Opioids, α_2-agonists, dissociatives (ketamine)*

Systemic Drugs
Nonsteroidal antiinflammatory drugs (NSAIDs) (phenylbutazone, flunixin meglumine, ketoprofen)
Opioids (morphine, butorphanol)
α_2-Agonists (xylazine, detomidine, romifidine)
Dissociatives (ketamine)
Local anesthetics (lidocaine, mexiletine, -infusion)

Analgesic Adjuncts†
Phenothiazines (acepromazine)
Benzodiazepines (diazepam, midazolam)
Electrolytes (Mg26 salts)
Calcium blockers (diltiazem)

---

*Administered in the epidural or subarachnoid space.
†Drugs that produce little or no analgesia when administered alone.

development of CNS hypersensitivity and resultant hyperalgesia and allodynia, is termed *preemptive analgesia.*

Multimodal Therapy

The combination or sequential administration of analgesics that act by different mechanisms (multimodal therapy) is often advocated to maximize analgesic drug effects (Table 22-2). The administration of two major analgesics (nonsteroidal antiinflammatory drug [NSAID]-opioid, opioid–α_2-agonist) frequently produces supraadditive or synergistic analgesic effects that permit the reduction of individual drug doses and a subsequent reduction in drug-related adverse side effects.

Drug Synergism

Many analgesic drugs are additive or synergistic (supraadditive) when administered together. Synergism or supraadditivity implies

TABLE 22-2

Analgesic Drug Combinations in the Horse

Drug Combination	IV Dose (mg/kg)	Concerns
Acepromazine	0.02-0.05	Hypotension
Butorphanol	0.02-0.05	
Acepromazine	0.02-0.05	Hypotension
Buprenorphine	0.005-0.01	
Acepromazine	0.02-0.05	Bradycardia, hypotension
Xylazine	0.2-0.5	
Xylazine*	0.3-0.5	Bradycardia, ataxia
Butorphanol	0.01-0.05	
Xylazine*	0.3-0.5	Bradycardia
Meperidine	0.5-1.0	
Xylazine*	0.5-1.0	Bradycardia, ataxia
Morphine	0.1-0.5	
Xylazine*	0.5-1.0	Bradycardia
Fentanyl	0.01-0.02	

*Detomidine or medetomidine (0.01-0.02 mg/kg) or romifidine (0.04-0.08 mg/kg) can be substituted for xylazine.

that the combination of two or more products produces more than additive effects. In more qualitative terms, the combination of two drugs produces a better effect (analgesia) than expected. This advantage allows the dose of most drugs to be markedly reduced, thereby reducing the potential for side effects. Drug combinations, which are likely to be synergistic, are produced when drugs that act by separate and distinct mechanisms of action are combined.

- Synergism or supraadditivity has been demonstrated when local anesthetics are combined with opioids or dissociative anesthetics and when NSAIDs are combined with opioids.
- The combination of α_2-agonists with opioids produces excellent clinical analgesia in horses (see Table 22-2). The transdermal delivery of opioids (fentanyl patch; 2 to 100 μg/hr patches/ 450 kg) with low doses of α_2-agonists (e.g., xylazine, detomidine) as needed, provides excellent analgesia for extended periods.

- The administration of adjunctive drugs (tranquilizers) in conjunction with major analgesic drugs may potentiate analgesic effects and produces additional calming effects. Examples include the simultaneous or sequential administration of acepromazine and meperidine (neuroleptanalgesia) or acepromazine and xylazine. Several of the major analgesics (e.g., opioids, α_2-agonists) have the added benefit of being reversible (see Table 22-2).

Preemptive Analgesia

Preemptive analgesia reduces the number and amount of anesthetic drugs required to produce and maintain surgical anesthesia, helps to stabilize the maintenance phase of anesthesia, reduces the total amount of analgesic drugs required to control pain both intraoperatively and postoperatively, and decreases overall patient morbidity associated with surgery and anesthesia. Local anesthetics or NSAIDs combined with low doses of opioids or α_2-agonists are the most routinely administered systemic major analgesic drugs used to provide analgesia for short-term pain therapy (see Table 22-1).

Combination of Opioid Agonists with Agonist-Antagonists

Reversing or antagonizing adverse effects may antagonize the drug's analgesic activity. Interestingly and surprisingly, however, the combination of opioid agonists with agonist-antagonists or "pure" antagonists has shown unexpected analgesic effects. The μ-opioid agonist morphine and κ agonist butorphanol, the μ agonist oxymorphone and κ agonist butorphanol, and the μ agonist morphine and the pure μ-receptor antagonist naloxone produced additive and synergistic antinociceptive effects in humans and cats for reasons that remain poorly defined (Table 22-3).

Other Potentially Effective Methods

Other potentially effective methods for providing long-term analgesia include acupuncture therapy, the judicious administration of NSAIDs, glucocorticosteroids, and regional nerve blocks. Most NSAIDs are cyclooxygenase-1 (COX-1) inhibitors and have the potential for producing gastrointestinal (GI) or renal toxicity, particularly when administered chronically. The preclinical investigation of cyclooxygenase-2 (COX-2) NSAIDs (inhibit COX-2 or inducible COX) will ideally result in the availability of potent analgesic drugs that can be administered chronically without the unwanted GI or renal side effects of COX-1 NSAIDs.

TABLE 22-3
Drug Antagonists

Drug	IV Dose (mg/kg)
Opioids	
Naloxone	0.01-0.02
Nalmefene	0.001-0.005
α_2-Agonists	
Atipamezole	0.1-0.2
Tolazoline	2.0
Yohimbine	0.075
Benzodiazepines	
Flumazenil	0.01
Analeptics (Stimulants)	
Doxapram	0.5-1.0

REGIONAL ANALGESIA

Regional analgesia can be used as an alternative or adjunct to more specific analgesic therapy for the long-term treatment of pain, to provide analgesia for a variety of surgical procedures, and to provide a means to reduce pain while producing minimal side effects (Box 22-2). Many diagnostic and surgical procedures can be performed safely and humanely in the standing horse using sedation, physical restraint, and some form of regional desensitization. The ability to produce effective anesthesia of the spinal nerves requires a working knowledge of the local anatomy, an understanding of the pharmacology of the analgesic drugs used, and the technical proficiency to complete the appropriate injection technique. To achieve spinal analgesia, anesthetic drugs must be deposited in either the epidural or subarachnoid spaces.

Epidural Analgesia

Epidural analgesia is generally easier to perform than subarachnoid anesthesia and has a reduced potential for nerve damage, especially when the injection site is caudal (coccygeal-sacral) to the termination of the conus medullaris. Drugs administered epidurally have a

---

BOX 22-2

**Procedures Amenable to Regional
Anesthetic Techniques**

Standing surgery of the rectum, anus, perineum, tail, vulva, vagina,
   penis, and inguinal region:
   Rectal prolapses
   Perirectal abscesses
   Rectal tears
   Rectovaginal lacerations
   Ovarioectomy
   Removal of urinary calculi
Flank approach to the abdomen:
   Abdominal exploratory
   Uterine torsion
   Loop colostomy
   Surgical embryo transfer
Aid in the relief of postoperative straining
Obstetric manipulations during dystocia
Relief of inflammatory, traumatic, intraoperative and postoperative,
   or chronic pain

---

longer duration of action but produce incomplete, inconsistent, or
asymmetric analgesia because of the presence of a septum within
the epidural space or the influence of fat accumulations.

Subarachnoid Analgesia

Subarachnoid analgesia by contrast produces a more consistent response because the roots of the spinal nerves within the subarachnoid space are not protected by the dura. Lower total drug doses
and more predictable analgesic responses are characteristic of subarachnoid anesthesia. The technique, however, is more difficult to
perform and requires more sophisticated and expensive equipment.

REGIONAL ANALGESIC DRUGS

Historically, local anesthetic drugs (e.g., lidocaine, mepivacaine)
were the only drugs used to produce caudal regional anesthesia
(Table 22-4).

TABLE 22-4

Drugs Used to Produce Regional Analgesia in Horses

Drug	Dosage (mg/kg)	Route	Duration of Analgesia
Local Anesthetics			
Mepivacaine HCl	0.20	S3-S4, S4-S5 (CE)	1-1.5 hr
	0.14-0.25	S2-S3, S3-S4, S4-S5 (CE)	1.5-2 hr
Mepivacaine HCl	0.06	S2-S3 (CSA)	20-80 min
	0.05-0.08	S2-S3 (CSA)	1-1.5 hr
Lidocaine HCl	0.16-0.22	Co1-Co2 (CE)	30-60 min
	0.22-0.44		1-2.5 hr
	0.45		2-3 hr
Lidocaine HCl	0.28-0.37	S3-S4, S4-S5 (CE)	1.5-3 hr
α_2-Agonists			
Xylazine	0.03-0.35	Co1-Co2 (CE)	3-5 hr
Detomidine HCl	0.06	S4-S5 (CE)	2-3 hr
Opioids			
Morphine	0.05-0.10	Co1-Co2 (CE)	8-16 hr
Combinations			
Lidocaine	0.22	Co1-Co2 (CE)	5.5 hr
Xylazine	0.17		
Lidocaine	0.25	Co1-Co2 (CE)	2.5 hr
Butorphanol	0.04		
Morphine	0.20	S1-L6 (CE)	>6 hr
Detomidine	0.03		

CE, Caudal epidural; *CSA,* caudal subarachnoid.

Local Anesthetics

Local anesthetic drugs provide profound relief from pain by preventing the transmembrane flux of sodium ions, thereby inhibiting depolarization of the nerve membrane and the conduction of nerve impulses. Unmyelinated A-alpha (Aα) and C (pain) fibers are preferentially blocked by local anesthetics because of their small size compared with the myelinated Aα and Aβ fibers, which are responsible for proprioception, touch and pressure sensation, and motor activity.

- Local anesthetic desensitization is dose-dependent, nonspecific, and not always predictable. Full analgesic effect occurs within 10 to 20 minutes of drug administration for epidurally administered local anesthetics.
- Additional local anesthetic drug should not be administered during this period to prevent overdosing, which can result in hypotension, and occasionally bradycardia, from sympathetic blockade.
- Complete sensory and inadvertent motor blockade results in marked ataxia and potentially recumbency.

α_2-Agonists

Although local anesthetics are effective analgesics for regional anesthesia, they can produce profound ataxia or recumbency as a result of their nonselective blockade of motor and sensory neurons. α_2-Agonists (e.g., xylazine) produce effective, long-term analgesia with a reduced incidence of intensity of ataxia. Additionally, the notable sedative and cardiopulmonary effects of epidurally administered xylazine are diminished compared with the response after their intravenous or intramuscular administration. α_2-Adrenergic receptors are located throughout the CNS and are found in great numbers in the superficial laminae of the dorsal horn sensory fibers of the spinal cord and brainstem nuclei.

- Epidural administration of xylazine (0.17 to 0.22 mg/kg of body weight [bw]; 1% solution) at the first coccygeal interspace produces surgical analgesia 30 to 45 minutes after administration, which lasts 3.5 hours.
- Epidural administration of 0.06 mg/kg bw detomidine hydrogen chloride (HCl) (1% solution) via an epidural catheter advanced to the caudal sacral (S5 to S4) space produces variable analgesia extending from the coccyx to spinal cord segment S1 and from the coccyx to T16, respectively. Analgesia is achieved within 10 to 25 minutes after drug administration and lasted for over 2 hours.
- Sedation after subarachnoid administration of xylazine or detomidine hydrochloride solution can be prominent.

Opioids

Opioids have been successfully used in humans, dogs, and horses to produce effective caudal regional analgesia with a low incidence of systemic side effects. Their use in horses, however, is relatively limited and for the most part has not provided clinically relevant analgesia. Epidural opioids produce analgesia without motor or sympathetic blockade by reducing the local release of presynaptic neurotransmitters and hyperpolarizing postsynaptic dorsal horn neuronal membranes.

- The onset of opioid drug effects is more rapid with the highly lipid-soluble opiates (e.g., fentanyl). Conversely, less lipid-soluble opiates like morphine are retained within the cerebrospinal fluid (CSF) for long durations after single-dose administration, thereby producing prolonged analgesia (see Table 22-4).
- Epidural opioid administration in horses has been limited primarily to the use of morphine and butorphanol administered alone or in combination with lidocaine.

"Balanced" Epidural Anesthesia

The selective combination of drugs that produce analgesia by different mechanisms (e.g., α_2-agonists and opioids) with subanesthetic concentrations of local anesthetics has the advantage of: (1) reducing the drug dose, (2) enhancing the degree of pain relief, and (3) reducing the adverse effects produced by larger doses of an individual drug. Functional interactions may result from simultaneous action at different sites. For example, activation of both presynaptic and postsynaptic mechanisms simultaneously, by a combination of drugs, may magnify the effects of one drug acting independently at one site.

- The combination of lidocaine with the α_2-adrenergic agonist xylazine, produced a faster onset of analgesia than with xylazine alone and a longer duration than with lidocaine alone (see Table 22-4).
- Butorphanol added to lidocaine increased the duration of both visceral and cutaneous analgesia and extended the area of cutaneous analgesia.
- Morphine sulfate (0.2 mg/kg) in combination with the α_2-adrenergic agonist, detomidine hydrochloride (30 μg/kg), produced profound hind-limb analgesia in horses with experimentally induced tarsocrural joint synovitis. Long-term (14 days) administration of this combination was without apparent adverse systemic effects.
- Ketamine, a noncompetitive NMDA antagonist, may also be an effective regional analgesic when administered epidurally in

combination with drugs that produce their effects by differing mechanisms. Epidural ketamine significantly decreased the amount of halothane required to maintain anesthesia during pelvic limb stimulation in ponies.

REGIONAL ANESTHETIC TECHNIQUES

Various regional nerve blocks have been developed to produce caudal analgesia in standing horses, including caudal epidural analgesia, continuous caudal epidural analgesia, continuous caudal subarachnoid analgesia, segmental thoracolumbar subarachnoid analgesia, and segmental dorsolumbar epidural analgesia. These techniques can be used to perform standing surgery of the rectum, anus, perineum, tail, vulva, vagina, penis, inguinal region, and flank approach to the abdomen; to aid in the relief of postoperative straining; to facilitate obstetric manipulations during dystocia; or the relief of inflammatory, traumatic, postoperative, or chronic pain.

General Considerations

Different injection sites and equipment are required for the various caudal regional anesthetic techniques (Table 22-5). The needle puncture site should be clipped and a surgical, aseptic preparation performed. The skin should be desensitized (superficial block) using a small-gauge needle (25 gauge, 1 in) and 1 to 2 ml of local anesthetic injected subcutaneously to reduce any local discomfort associated with the insertion of larger needles (18 to 16 gauge).

Caudal Epidural Anesthesia (Table 22-6)

Correctly performed, anesthetic deposited epidurally will produce regional anesthesia of the anus, rectum, vulva, vagina, perineum, urethra, and bladder (Fig. 22-2). Caudal epidural anesthesia is produced by inserting a needle between the first and second coccygeal vertebrae (Co1 to Co2). The first coccygeal interspace is readily located in most horses by palpating the first movable coccygeal articulation with the finger while raising and lowering the tail. In obese or well-muscled horses, the site may be difficult to palpate but can be located at the point where the angle of the tail is the steepest, about 5 cm cranial to the origin of the first tail hairs. After desensitizing the skin, an 18-gauge spinal needle with fitted stylet (5 to 7.5 cm) is inserted through the skin perpendicular to the contour of the

---

TABLE 22-5

Equipment for Regional Analgesic Techniques in Horses

Technique	Location of Needle Placement	Equipment Required
Caudal epidural	Co1-Co2	18-gauge, 5-7.5-cm spinal needle
Continuous caudal epidural	Co1-Co2 S1-L6	18-gauge, 10.2-cm Tuohy needle 20-gauge, 91.8-cm epidural catheter or 17-gauge, 19.5-cm Huber point Tuohy needle 30-cm Formocath polyethylene catheter (0.095-cm OD) with spring guide (0.052-cm OD)
Continuous caudal subarachnoid	S1-L6	17-gauge, 19.5-cm Huber point Tuohy needle 30-cm Formocath polyethylene catheter (0.095-cm OD) with spring guide (0.052-cm OD)
Segmental thoracolumbar subarachnoid	S1-L6	17-gauge, 17.5-cm Huber point Tuohy needle 100-cm Formocath polyethylene catheter (0.095-cm OD) with spring guide (0.052-cm OD)
Segmental thoracolumbar epidural*	S1-L6	17-gauge, 17.5 cm Huber point Tuohy needle 100 cm Formocath polyethylene catheter (0.095-cm OD) with spring guide (0.052-cm OD)

*Not recommended for clinical patient.

croup (Fig 22-2, *A*). Alternatively, the 18 gauge needle may be advanced at a 45-degree angle to the skin (Fig 22-2, *B*). A distinct "pop" is generally noted as the needle passes through the dorsal interarcuate ligament, which indicates that the needle is properly placed. Proper needle placement is verified by applying: (1) a drop or two of local anesthetic to the hub of the needle, which should be drawn into the epidural space by the negative pressure ("hanging

TABLE 22-6

Regional Analgesic Techniques in Horses

Technique	Area Blocked	Site of Drug Deposition	Spinal Cord Segments Affected	Indications
Caudal epidural	Caudal region*	Co1-Co2	S2-coccyx	Standing surgery to the anal and perianal regions; obstetric manipulations
Continuous caudal epidural	Caudal region*	S3-S5 S2-S3	S2-coccyx	Extend surgery time for standing procedures, relief of tenesmus, management of chronic pain
Continuous caudal subarachnoid	Caudal region*	S2-S3	S2-coccyx	Extend surgery time for standing procedures of anal and perianal regions
Segmental thoracolumbar subarachnoid	Flank	T18-L1	T12-L3	Standing surgery for flank approach
Segmental thoracolumbar epidural	Flank	T18-L1	T12-L3	Standing surgery for flank approach Not recommended for clinical patients

*Caudal region includes the anus, rectum, vulva, vagina, perineum, urethra, and bladder.

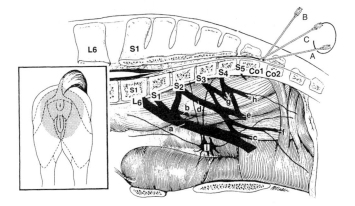

Fig. 22-2 Neuroanatomy and needle placement for caudal epidural anesthesia (*A* and *B*); and needle and catheter placement at Co1-Co2 for continuous caudal epidural anesthesia *(C)*. Ventral nerve branches give rise to the following: *a,* sciatic nerve; *b,* caudal cutaneous femoral nerve; *c,* deep perineal nerve; *d,* pudendal nerve; *e,* distal cutaneous pudendal nerve; *f,* caudal rectal nerve; *g,* pelvic nerve; *h,* caudal rectal nerve; *i,* pelvic plexus. *Inset,* Stippled area delineates extent of subcutaneous desensitization after caudal blockade.

drop technique"); or (2) by aspiration followed by resistance-free injection of 3 to 5 ml of air or local anesthetic. Aspiration of blood or CSF suggests needle placement in the subarachnoid space. If this occurs, the needle should be withdrawn slightly and reaspirated.

- Caudal epidural anesthesia has the advantages of being relatively simple to perform and requires no special equipment, thus limiting cost primarily to that of the drug itself.
- The potential for nerve damage in horses is minimized, since the spinal cord and its meninges end in the midsacral region, cranial to the injection site (see Fig 22-2).
- Disadvantages of the technique include inconsistent results, the limited duration of analgesic action, and the possibility for the development of rear limb ataxia or even lateral recumbency when increased drug doses are administered.

Continuous Caudal Epidural Anesthesia (see Table 22-6)

The limited duration of caudal epidural anesthesia can be overcome by placement of a catheter to provide continuous caudal epidural anesthesia. The establishment of a route for repeated administration of small doses of anesthetic drug extends surgery time, reduces the risk of rear limb ataxia, and avoids the development of fibrosis of the epidural space that results from repeated needle trauma. The disadvantages of catheter placement include greater cost of equipment, complications associated from kinking and curling of the catheter, and lack of documentation for the optimal times and doses required for repeated spinal administration of anesthetic drugs in horses. A 10.2-cm, 18-gauge thin-walled Tuohy needle with stylet is inserted at the first coccygeal interspace, and a 20-gauge Teflon epidural catheter is advanced cranially toward the lumbosacral junction to the desired level (Fig. 22-2, *C*). Alternatively, a 17.5-cm, 17-gauge Huber-point Tuohy directional needle can be used to place and pass a catheter to the caudal portion of the sacral (S3 to S5) epidural space from the lumbosacral intervertebral junction (Fig. 22-3).

• Introduction of morphine and detomidine into an epidural catheter advanced to the lumbosacral region produced effective hind-limb analgesia to the tarsocrural joint, lasting more than 6 hours.

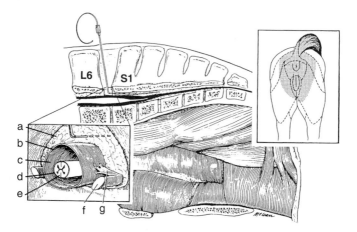

Fig. 22-3 Catheter introduction at the lumbosacral (L6-S1) intervertebral junction for continuous caudal epidural anesthesia. *Left inset,* Proper placement of needle and catheter within the epidural space; *a,* epidural space with fat and connective tissue; *b,* Dura mater; *c,* subarachnoid space; *d,* Pia mater; *e,* spinal chord. *Right inset,* Stippled area delineates extent of subcutaneous desensitization after caudal blockade.

- The caudal epidural injection of 60 to 100 mg of mepivacaine HCl in aqueous solution into a catheter placed at the caudal portion of the sacral (S3 to S5) epidural space produced unilateral or bilateral analgesia extending from spinal cord segment S1 to the coccyx.

Continuous Caudal Subarachnoid Anesthesia
(see Table 22-6)

Continuous caudal subarachnoid anesthesia produces analgesia for prolonged periods in standing horses. The technique is similar to that used to produce continuous caudal epidural anesthesia but provides the added advantage of producing a faster onset of action and shorter duration of effect with reduced drug doses. A 17.5-cm, 17-gauge Huber-point Tuohy needle with stylet is inserted into the subarachnoid space at the lumbosacral (L6 to S1) intervertebral space. Proper placement of the needle in the subarachnoid space is verified by the free flow of spinal fluid from the needle hub. The stylet is removed, and a 20-gauge Teflon catheter (0.036 cm outside diameter) or polyethylene tubing (0.095 cm outside diameter) reinforced with a stainless steel spring guide (0.052 cm outside diameter) is advanced to the midsacral (S2 to S3) subarachnoid space (Fig. 22-4).

- Continuous caudal subarachnoid anesthesia requires approximately one third the amount of drug used to produce the same effect as epidural anesthesia.
- The onset of drug action is faster, and the duration of effect is approximately half as long, conferring the advantage of increased control over the intensity of analgesia and associated side effects.
- The technique, however, carries the risk of trauma to the conus medullaris and associated nerve fibers and is much more difficult to perform than epidural anesthesia.

Segmental Thoracolumbar Subarachnoid Anesthesia
(see Table 22-6)

Segmental thoracolumbar subarachnoid anesthesia is used to produce anesthesia for standing flank surgery in the horse. Segmental thoracolumbar subarachnoid anesthesia requires adherence to strict aseptic technique. A 17.5-cm, 17-gauge Huber-point Tuohy needle with stylet is inserted into the subarachnoid space at the lumbosacral

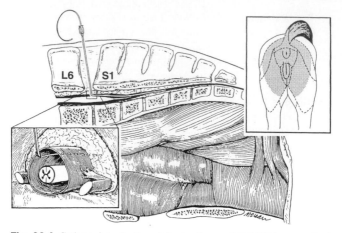

Fig. 22-4 Catheter introduction at the lumbosacral (L6-S1) intervertebral junction for continuous caudal subarachnoid anesthesia. *Left inset,* Proper placement within the subarachnoid space. *Right inset,* Stippled area delineates extent of subcutaneous desensitization after caudal blockade.

(L6 to S1) intervertebral space (Fig. 22-5). The L6 to S1 interspace is located 1 to 2 cm caudal to the cranial edges of the tuber sacral on the dorsal midline. A 100-cm-long catheter with a 0.095 cm outside diameter is passed through the needle and advanced approximately 60 cm to the midthoracic area (see Fig. 22-5). Desensitization of dorsal nerve roots T14 to L3 is produced within 5 to 10 minutes by injecting 1.5 to 2 ml of 2% mepivacaine hydrochloride and lasts for 30 to 60 minutes.

- Anesthesia can be prolonged by fractional bolus administration of half the initial drug dose at approximately 30-minute intervals.
- The advantages of this technique include a rapid onset, minimal drug dosage, and a selective analgesic effect.
- Disadvantages include the potential for traumatizing the conus medullaris, kinking and curling of the catheter, loss of motor control to the pelvic limbs, and meningitis if strict asepsis is not observed.

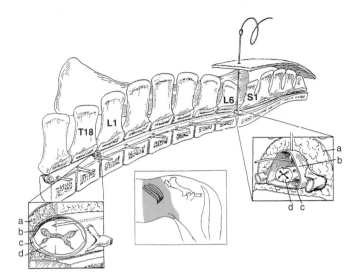

Fig. 22-5 Catheter introduction at the lumbosacral (L6-S1) intervertebral site and advancement to the thoracolumbar junction T18-L1 for segmental thoracolumbar subarachnoid anesthesia. *Left inset,* Proper placement of Tuohy needle and catheter within the subarachnoid space. *Middle inset,* Correctly positioned catheter and spring guide at T18-L1 intervertebral space. *Right inset,* Stippled area delineates extent of subcutaneous desensitization after blockade in the standing horse. *a,* Epidural space with fat and connective tissue; *b,* dura mater; *c,* subarachnoid space; *d,* spinal cord.

Segmental Thoracolumbar Epidural Anesthesia
(see Table 22-6)

Segmental thoracolumbar epidural anesthesia is not commonly used in the horse compared with cattle because it is difficult to perform, provides variable results, and requires special equipment. Furthermore, the T18 to L1 epidural space can be catheterized from the lumbosacral epidural space to desensitize spinal nerves T12 to L2. Segmental (T12 to L2) analgesia involving the flank and extending caudally to the area of the stifle is achieved in 10 to 20 minutes after the injection of 80 mg (4 ml at 2% solution) mepivacaine HCl, with a duration of analgesia lasting approximately 1 to 1.5 hours.

- Segmental thoracolumbar epidural anesthesia should not be routinely used in horses because, as stated previously, it is difficult to perform and requires a specially designed catheter and wire guide.
- Catheter placement carries the risk of catheter kinking or curling at the lumbosacral intervertebral space, causing the injectant to be deposited in the region of the femoral and ischial nerves and predisposing the horse to a loss of pelvic limb function and panic.

Side Effects

Caudal regional anesthesia does carry the risks of nerve or spinal cord trauma, infection and ataxia, and recumbency resulting from motor blockade. Judicious use and application of regional anesthetic techniques, however, provides a low-cost, safe, efficacious means of producing analgesia for many standing surgical procedures and can be used as an adjunct to general anesthesia to reduce the amount of injectable inhalant drug required to maintain surgical anesthesia.

NOTE: The majority of information in this chapter was reprinted from Grosenbaugh DA, Skarda RT, Muir WW: *Equine Vet Ed* 11:98-105, 1999; Muir WW: *Equine Vet Ed* 10:335-340, 1998.

SUGGESTED READINGS

de Leon-Casasola OA, Lema MJ: Postoperative epidural opioid analgesia: what are the choices? *Anesth Analg* 83:867-875, 1966.

Dickenson AH: Mechanisms of the analgesic actions of opiates and opioids, *Br Med Bull* 47:690-702, 1991.

Doherty TJ, Geiser DR, Rohrbach BW: Effect of high-volume epidural morphine, ketamine, and butorphanol on halothane minimum alveolar concentration in ponies, *Equine Vet J* 29:370-373, 1997.

Eisenach JC, Kock MD, Klimscha W: α_2-Adrenergic agonists for regional anesthesia, *Anesthesiology* 85:655-674, 1996.

Fikes LW, Lin HC, Thurman JC: A preliminary comparison of lidocaine and xylazine as epidural analgesics in ponies, *Vet Surg* 18:85-86, 1989.

Gan TJ, Ginsgerg B, Glass PSA, et al: Opioid-sparing effects of a low-dose infusion of naloxone in patient-administered morphine sulphate, *Anesthesiology* 87:1075-1081, 1997.

Gaynor JS, Hubbell JAE: Perineural and spinal anesthesia, *Vet Clin North Am Equine Pract* 7:501-519, 1991.

Green EM, Cooper RC: Continuous caudal epidural anesthesia in the horse, *J Am Vet Med Assoc* 184:971-974, 1984.

Grosenbaugh DA, Skarda RT, Muir WW: Caudal regional anesthesia in horses, *Equine Vet Ed* 11:98-105, 1999.

Grubb TL, Riebold TW, Huber MJ: Comparison of lidocaine, xylazine for perineal analgesia in horses, *J Am Vet Med Assoc* 210:1187-1190, 1992.

Kehlet H, Dahl JB: The value of "multimodal" or "balanced analgesia" in postoperative pain treatment, *Anesth Analg* 77:1048-1056, 1993.

LeBlanc PH: Regional anesthesia, *Vet Clin North Am Equine Pract* 6:693-704, 1990.

LeBlanc PH, Caron JP: Clinical use of epidural xylazine in the horse, *Equine Vet J* 22:180-181, 1990.

LeBlanc PH, Caron SP, Patterson JS, et al: Epidural injection of xylazine for perineal analgesia in horses, *J Am Vet Med Assoc* 193:1405-1408, 1988.

LeBlanc PH, Eberhart SW: Cardiopulmonary effects of epidurally administered xylazine in the horse, *Equine Vet J* 22:189-191, 1990.

Muir WW, Skarda RT, Sheehan WC: Hemodynamic and respiratory effects of a xylazine-morphine sulfate in horses, *Am J Vet Res* 40:1417-1420, 1979.

Muir WW, Skarda RT, Sheehan WC: Hemodynamic and respiratory effects of a xylazine-acetylpromazine drug combination in horses, *Am J Vet Res* 40:1518-1522, 1979.

Muir WW: Anesthesia and pain management in horses, *Equine Vet Ed* 10:335-340, 1998.

Schelling CG, Klein LV: Comparison of carbonated lidocaine and lidocaine hydrochloride for caudal epidural anesthesia in horses, *Am J Vet Res* 46:1375-1377, 1985.

Skarda RT: Local and regional analgesic techniques: horses. In Thurman JC, Tranquilli WJ, Benson GJ, editors: *Lumb & Jones' veterinary anesthesia,* ed 3, Philadelphia, 1996, Williams & Wilkins.

Skarda RT, Muir WW: Segmental thoracolumbar spinal (subarachnoid) analgesia in conscious horses, *Am J Vet Res* 43:2121-2128, 1982.

Skarda RT, Muir WW: Segmental epidural and subarachnoid analgesia in conscious horses: a comparative study, *Am J Vet Res* 44:1870-1876, 1983.

Skarda RT, Muir WW: Continuous caudal epidural and subarachnoid anesthesia in mares: a comparative study, *Am J Vet Res* 44:2290-2298, 1993.

Skarda RT, Muir WW: Caudal analgesia induced by epidural or subarachnoid administration of detomidine hydrochloride solution in mares, *Am J Vet Res* 55:670-680, 1994.

Skarda RT, Muir WW: Analgesic, hemodynamic, and respiratory effects of caudal epidurally administered xylazine hydrochloride solution in mares, *Am J Vet Res* 57:193-200, 1996.

Skarda RT, Muir WW: Comparison of antinociceptive, cardiovascular, and respiratory effects, head ptosis and position of pelvic limbs in mares after caudal epidural administration of xylazine and detomidine hydrochloride solution, *Am J Vet Res* 57:1338-1345, 1996.

Skarda RT, Muir WW, Ibrahim AL: Plasma mepivacaine concentrations after caudal epidural and subarachnoid injection in the horse: a comparative study, *Am J Vet Res* 45:1967-1971, 1984.

Solomon RE, Gebhart GF: Synergistic antinociceptive interactions among drugs administered to the spinal cord, *Anesth Analg* 78:1164-1172, 1994.

Sysel AM, Pleasant RS, Jacobson SD, et al: Efficacy of an epidural combination of morphine and detomidine in alleviating experimentally induced hindlimb lameness in horses, *Vet Surg* 25:511-518, 1996.

Sysel AM, Pleasant RS, Jacobson JD, et al: Systemic and local effects associated with long-term epidural catheterization and morphine-detomidine administration in horses, *Vet Surg* 26:141-149, 1997.

Valverde A, Little CB, Dyson DH: Use of epidural morphine to relieve pain in a horse, *Can Vet J* 31:211-212, 1990.

Drugs Used for the Treatment of Pain and Pain-Related Anxiety in Dogs and Cats

Drug	Trade Name	Dog Dose (mg/kg)	Cat Dose (mg/kg)
Acepromazine	Acepromazine	0.02-0.05 SQ, IM q3-6h 0.005-0.03 IV q1-4h	0.02-0.1 SQ, IM q3-6h 0.005-0.03 IV q1-4h
Amantadine	Symmetrel	3 PO q24h	3 PO q24h
Amitriptyline	Elavil	1-2 PO q12-24h	2.5-12.5 mg/cat PO q24h
Aspirin	Aspirin	10-25 PO q24h	10-25 PO q24-48h
Bupivacaine	Marcaine	1-2 SQ, interpleural	1-2 SQ, interpleural
Buprenorphine	Buprenex	0.01-0.03 SQ, IM, IV q6-12h	0.005-0.03 SQ, IM q6-12h 0.01-0.02 PO tid-qid
Butorphanol	Torbugesic	0.1-0.4 SQ IM q0.75h 0.1-0.2 IV q0.5h	0.2-0.4 SQ, IM q4-5h 0.1 IV q1-2h
Carprofen	Rimadyl Zenecarp	4 SQ single dose 2.2 PO bid-4.4 PO bid	1-4 SQ single dose Not recommended for oral use
Diazepam	Valium	0.1-0.2 IV prn	0.1-0.2 IV prn
Fentanyl	Sublimaze	0.010 SQ, IM 0.002-0.005 IV 2-20 µg/kg/hr IV	0.005-0.010 SQ, IM 0.002-0.005 IV 2-20 µg/kg/hr
Fentanyl: trans-dermal patch	Duragesic	0.002-0.005 mg/kg/hr	0.002-0.005 mg/kg/hr
Flunixin meglumine	Banamine	1.0 PO single dose	1.0 PO single dose

Continued

445

Drugs Used for the Treatment of Pain and Pain-Related Anxiety in Dogs and Cats—cont'd

Drug	Trade Name	Dog Dose (mg/kg)	Cat Dose (mg/kg)
Gabapentin	Neurontin	1.25-4.0 PO q24h	1.25-4.0 PO q24h
Hydromorphone	Dilaudid	0.1-0.2 SQ, IM 0.05-0.1 IV 0.05-0.1 mg/kg/hr	0.05 SQ, IM 0.03-0.05 IV q1h 0.01 mg/kg/hr
Imipramine	Tofranil	0.5-1.0 PO q8h	2.5-5.0 PO q12h
Ketamine (as NMDA receptor antagonist, not anesthetic)	Numerous: Ketalar, Vetalar, Ketset, Ketaflo	0.5 IV, followed by 10 μg/kg/min during surgery, followed by 2 μg/kg/min for next 24 hr	0.5 IV, followed by 10 μg/kg/min during surgery, followed by 2 μg/kg/min for next 24 hr
Ketoprofen	Ketofen, Anafen	1-2 SQ q24h 1 PO q24h	1-2 SQ q24h max 3 days 1 PO q24h max 5 days
Ketorolac	Toradol	0.3-0.6 IV, IM q8-12h	0.25 IM q12h
Lidocaine	Lidocaine	1-2 SQ, interpleural	1-2 SQ, interpleural
Medetomidine	Domitor	0.01-0.02 SQ, IM q1-4h 0.0005-0.001 IV q1h	0.02-0.03 SQ, IM q1-4h 0.0005-0.001 IV q1h
Meloxicam	Metacam	0.2-0.3 IM q24h 0.2-0.3 PO, then 0.1 PO q24h long term	Not recommended 0.3 PO on day 1, followed by 0.1 PO q24h for 4 days, then 0.1 mg/cat PO q24h

446

Midazolam	Versed	0.1-0.4 SQ, IM 0.1-0.2 IV prn	0.1-0.4 SQ, IM 0.1-0.2 IV prn
Misoprostol	Cytotec	0.002-0.005 PO q8h	0.002-0.005 PO q8h
Morphine	Morphine	0.25-1.0 SQ, IM q4-6h 0.05-0.1 IV q1-2h 0.05-0.1 mg/kg/hr 0.1 epidurally q12-24h	0.1-0.5 SQ, IM q4-6h 0.05 IV q1-2h 0.05-0.1 mg/kg/hr IV 0.1 epidurally q12-24h
Morphine sulfate: sustained release	MS Contin	1.0 PO q8-12h	N/A
Morphine sulfate tablets and oral liquid	Morphine sulfate	1.0 PO q4-6h	0.5 PO q4-6h
Naloxone	Narcan	0.002-0.010 IV, SQ, IM	0.002-0.010 IV, SQ, IM
Oxymorphone	Numorphan	0.05-0.1 SQ, IM 0.03-0.05 IV	0.03-0.05 SQ, IM 0.01-0.03 IV
Piroxicam	Feldene	0.3 PO q24h for 3 days then every other day	1 mg/cat PO q24h max 7 days
Tramadol	Ultram	2.5-10 mg/kg PO SID-BID 2-4 IV	Oral dose is unknown 2-4 IV
Xylazine	Rompun, Tranquived	0.05-0.1 IV prn 0.2-0.4 SQ, IM q1-2h	0.05-0.1 IV prn 0.2-0.4 SQ, IM q1-2h

Index

Page numbers followed by *f* indicate figures; by *t*, tables; by *b*, boxes.